THE ULTIMATE
ECHO GUIDE

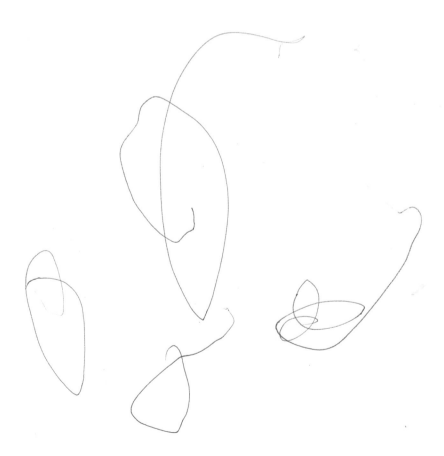

THE ULTIMATE ECHO GUIDE

Editor

Carlos A. Roldan, M.D., F.A.C.C., F.A.S.E.
Professor of Medicine
Department of Internal Medicine
Division of Cardiology
University of New Mexico School of Medicine
Director, Echocardiography Laboratory
New Mexico Veterans Affairs Health Care System
Albuquerque, New Mexico

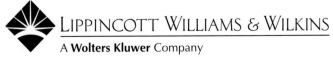

LIPPINCOTT WILLIAMS & WILKINS
A **Wolters Kluwer** Company
Philadelphia · Baltimore · New York · London
Buenos Aires · Hong Kong · Sydney · Tokyo

Acquisitions Editor: Ruth Weinberg
Developmental Editor: Nicole T. Dernoski
Production Editor: Erica Broennle Nelson, Silverchair Science + Communications
Senior Manufacturing Manager: Benjamin Rivera
Compositor: Silverchair Science + Communications
Printer: Quebecor World-Kingsport

© 2005 by LIPPINCOTT WILLIAMS & WILKINS
530 Walnut Street
Philadelphia, PA 19106 USA
LWW.com

Printed in the USA

Library of Congress Cataloging-in-Publication Data

The ultimate echo guide / editor, Carlos A. Roldan.
  p. ; cm.
 Includes bibliographical references and index.
 ISBN 0-7817-4749-X
 1. Echocardiography--Handbooks, manuals, etc. I. Roldan, Carlos A.
 [DNLM: 1. Echocardiography--methods--Handbooks. 2. Heart Diseases--
ultrasonography--Handbooks. WG 39 U47 2004]
 RC683.5.U5U425 2004
 616.1'207543--dc22

                2004006102

10 9 8 7 6 5 4 3 2 1

To my wife, Patricia,
and my children,
Carlos Jr., Paola, and Pablo,
for their love, support, and inspiration

Contents

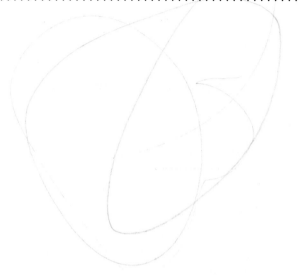

Contributing Authors

Phoebe A. Ashley, M.D.
Staff Cardiologist
Director, Women's Cardiovascular Center
Sacred Heart Medical Center
Director, Intensive Care Unit
McKenzie-Willamette Hospital
Eugene, Oregon

Gerald A. Charlton, M.D., F.A.C.C.
Director, Cardiology Fellowship Program
Assistant Professor of Medicine
Department of Internal Medicine
University of New Mexico School of Medicine
Director, Cardiology Clinical Service
New Mexico Veterans Affairs Health Care System
Albuquerque, New Mexico

Michael H. Crawford, M.D., F.A.C.C., F.A.H.A.
Professor
Department of Medicine
University of California, San Francisco, School of Medicine
Chief of Clinical Cardiology
University of California, San Francisco, Medical Center
San Francisco, California

Anita Kedia, M.D.
Staff Cardiologist
Cardiology Fellowship Programs Co-Director
Lovelace Sandia Health System
Albuquerque, New Mexico

Dara K. Lee, M.D., F.A.C.C.
Staff Cardiologist
Cardiology Division
New Mexico Veterans Affairs Health Care System
Staff Cardiologist
Presbyterian Heart Group
Presbyterian Hospital
Albuquerque, New Mexico

Takashi Miyamoto, M.D.
Cardiology Research Fellow
Division of Cardiology
Cedars-Sinai Medical Center
Los Angeles, California

Juan Carlos Plana, M.D.
Senior Fellow
Section of Cardiology
Baylor College of Medicine
Houston, Texas

Carlos A. Roldan, M.D., F.A.C.C., F.A.S.E.
Professor of Medicine
Department of Internal Medicine
Division of Cardiology
University of New Mexico School of Medicine
Director, Echocardiography Laboratory
New Mexico Veterans Affairs Health Care System
Albuquerque, New Mexico

Robert J. Siegel, M.D., F.A.C.C., F.A.H.A.
Professor of Medicine
University of California, Los Angeles, UCLA School of Medicine
Director, Cardiac Noninvasive Laboratory
Division of Cardiology
Cedars-Sinai Medical Center
Los Angeles, California

Robert A. Taylor, M.D., F.A.C.C.
Assistant Professor Department of Internal Medicine
Division of Cardiology
University of New Mexico School of Medicine
Director, Echocardiography Laboratory
University of New Mexico Health Sciences Center
Albuquerque, New Mexico

Kirsten Tolstrup, M.D., F.A.C.C.
Assistant Professor
Department of Medicine
University of California, Los Angeles, UCLA School of Medicine
Assistant Director, Cardiac Noninvasive Laboratory
Division of Cardiology
Cedars-Sinai Medical Center
Los Angeles, California

William A. Zoghbi, M.D., F.A.C.C., F.A.S.E., F.A.H.A.
John S. Dunn, Sr. Professor of Medicine
Section of Cardiology
Baylor College of Medicine
Director, Echocardiography Laboratory
The Methodist DeBakey Heart Center
The Methodist Hospital
Houston, Texas

Preface

Echocardiography has evolved into a diverse and highly accurate technology. Because of its safety and ease of application, it has become routinely used in the diagnosis, management, and follow-up of patients with any suspected or known heart disease. Consequently, the number of echocardiograms performed continues to increase in most cardiology practices, but the time spent in the interpretation of the studies is likely decreasing. Also, experts do not interpret most echocardiograms. Most currently available echocardiography textbooks are of excellent content and great educational value; they elaborate extensively on theoretical, technical, and clinical concepts of a specific heart disease and include well-established and experimental semi-quantitative and quantitative methods and parameters for assessment of the heart structure and function. Therefore, consultation of these textbooks during daily, routine, high-volume, and fast-paced interpretation or performance of echocardiograms is time-consuming, impractical, and generally not performed. This may result in incomplete and potentially inaccurate interpretation of studies.

The Ultimate Echo Guide should fulfill the need of an easy and fast but complete echocardiography consultation for busy practicing cardiologists, cardiology fellows, echocardiography technicians, and, to some extent, for radiology residents, anesthesiologists, and emergency medicine physicians. The book includes the most currently used and accepted technology and methods but also incorporates the newest data that authors believe are currently of clinical value.

The Ultimate Echo Guide addresses M-mode, two-dimensional (2-D), and Doppler transthoracic (TTE) or transesophageal echocardiography (TEE) of a specific heart disease with a well-organized, succinct approach, with most relevant concepts in echocardiography presented in short bulleted statements and complemented by multiple summary tables and high-resolution digital images.

The Ultimate Echo Guide is multiauthored and includes 16 chapters on the most common heart diseases in which echocardiography plays an important role in diagnosis, management, and follow-up. The first chapter, The Normal Color Doppler Echocardiogram, is followed by chapters on coronary artery disease, ventricular systolic dysfunction, ventricular diastolic dysfunction, pulmonary hypertension and cor pulmonale, mitral regurgitation, mitral stenosis, aortic regurgitation, aortic valve sclerosis and stenosis, tricuspid and pulmonic valve disease, prosthetic valve dysfunction, common adult congenital heart diseases, infective endocarditis, intracardiac masses and systemic embolism, and diseases of the aorta; the book concludes with a chapter on pericardial diseases. For completeness and ease of consultation, most chapters are organized as follows:

Brief introduction
Definition
Common etiologies
Incidence or prevalence, or both
Class I indications for TTE or TEE according to American College of Cardiology/American Heart Association/American Society of Echocardiography guidelines
Discussion of echocardiography techniques (M-mode and 2D; pulsed, continuous, or color Doppler TTE or TEE), including:
    Best imaging planes
    Diagnostic methods
    Diagnostic formulas (when applicable)
    Key diagnostic features
    Pitfalls
Echocardiography parameters that stratify a disease as mild, moderate, or severe
Echocardiography diagnostic accuracy (sensi-

tivity, specificity, predictive values, correlation coefficients)
Echocardiography in the pregnant patient
Echocardiography parameters of poor prognostic value
Echocardiography parameters that indicate need for percutaneous or surgical interventions
Intraoperative or periprocedural echocardiography
Echocardiography follow-up

The chapters purposely have been kept short. Each presents text in bulleted short statements; includes six to eight tables summarizing indications for echocardiography, diagnostic methods, diagnostic accuracy, disease stratification, prognostic indicators, parameters that indicate the need for invasive therapeutic interventions, and follow-up time intervals; includes six to eight multicomponent, high-resolution, digi-

tally acquired echocardiographic images emphasizing a concept, method, formula, or pitfall; and, finally, includes less than 30 highly specific recent references.

For those interested in simplifying the consultative and learning process, we have developed a separate PDA. This contains summaries of relevant concepts, diagnostic methods and formulas, key diagnostic features, tables, and selected illustrations.

The contributing authors and I believe *The Ultimate Echo Guide* fulfills the need for an easy, practical, and complete consultation; enhances understanding and knowledge in echocardiography; leads to a complete and accurate interpretation of echocardiograms; and, most important, may lead to better patient care.

C.A.R.

Acknowledgments

My sincere appreciation to all contributing authors for their outstanding work in the preparation of chapters that make this book and complementary personal digital assistant version valuable educational tools.

Special thanks to Frank Gurule and Aggie Schaeffer, cardiac sonographers of the echocardiography laboratory of the Albuquerque Veterans Affairs Health Care System, for their expert technical assistance in obtaining excellent echocardiographic illustrations.

Thanks to Jim Janis of Medical Media of the Albuquerque Veterans Affairs Health Care System for his expert technical assistance in the preparation of the illustrations for this book.

Finally, special appreciation and thanks to Patricia Roldan for her editorial assistance in the preparation of the content of the book.

C.A.R.

THE ULTIMATE ECHO GUIDE

1

The Normal Color Doppler Echocardiogram

Carlos A. Roldan

■ A complete transthoracic echocardiography (TTE) or transesophageal echocardiography (TEE) (echo) study includes M-mode and two-dimensional (2D) images; pulsed, continuous, and color Doppler images; and tissue Doppler, color M-mode, or contrast echo, if available.

■ These techniques allow an assessment of the size of cardiac chambers; left ventricular and right ventricular wall thickness and wall motion; left ventricular and right ventricular systolic and diastolic function; estimation of left atrial, right atrial, and pulmonary artery (PA) pressures; structure and function of the heart valves; presence of intracardiac shunts; and assessment of the aorta and pericardium (1).

■ Normal echo values of heart chambers and great vessels vary according to age, conditioning, and heredity, but changes according to gender and body surface area are probably not clinically relevant. Thus, in clinical practice, ranges of normal values are probably more clinically useful than mean or indexed values (Tables 1-1 through 1-6) (2–5).

LEFT VENTRICLE

Size and Volume

Best Imaging Planes

■ TTE parasternal long-axis and short-axis views and apical four-chamber and two-chamber views at the level of the papillary muscles' tip to measure left ventricular anteroposterior and mediolateral diameters and volumes.

■ TEE transgastric short-axis and long-axis views at the papillary muscles' level and mid-esophageal four-chamber and two-chamber views with neutral or slight retroflexed position to prevent left ventricular foreshortening.

Diagnostic Methods

■ The most commonly used anteroposterior left ventricular diameters are measured from leading edge of the interventricular septum to leading edge of the posterior wall (Fig. 1-1).

■ Simpson's rule by planimetry of left ventricular end-diastolic and end-systolic volumes

TABLE 1-1. *Normal Values of Left Heart Chambers*

Measurement	Transthoracic echocardiography	Transesophageal echocardiography
Left ventricular anteroposterior – diastole (cm)	3.5–5.7	3.3–5.5
Left ventricular anteroposterior – systole (cm)	2.5–4.3	1.8–4.0
Left ventricular mediolateral – diastole (cm)	3.7–5.6	2.3–5.4
Left ventricular mediolateral – systole (cm)	2.5–4.8	1.8–4.2
Left ventricular volume – end-diastole (mL)	59–157	—
Left ventricular volume – end-systole (mL)	18–68	—
Left ventricular area – end-diastole (cm^2)	18–47	—
Left ventricular area – end-systole (cm^2)	8–32	—
Left ventricular fractional shortening (%)	30–35	30–35
Left ventricular ejection fraction (%)	≥50	≥50
Left ventricular IVS thickness – diastole (cm)	0.6–1.1	0.6–1.1
Left ventricular PW thickness – diastole (cm)	0.6–1.0	0.6–1.0
Left ventricular mass (g)	<294 in men, <198 in women	—
LVOT – mid-systole (cm)	1.8–3.4	—
Left atrial anteroposterior – systole (cm)	2.2–4.5	2.0–5.2
Left atrial mediolateral – systole (cm)	2.5–4.5	2.4–5.2
Left atrial volume (mL)	20–77 men, 15–59 women	—
Left atrial area (cm^2)	9–23	—
Left atrial appendage anteroposterior length (cm)	—	1.5–4.3
Left atrial appendage mediolateral diameter (cm)	—	1.0–2.8

IVS, interventricular septum; LVOT, left ventricular outflow tract; PW, posterior wall.

from 2D TTE or TEE orthogonal four-chamber and two-chamber views is the most commonly used automated method to assess left ventricular volumes.

- Left ventricular end-diastolic volume can be calculated using a simplified method as

$$\left[\begin{array}{c} \text{Maximal long} \\ \text{axis diameter} \end{array} \times \begin{array}{c} \text{maximal short} \\ \text{axis diameter} \end{array} \times 3.44 \right] - 6$$

Normal Values

- By TTE, left ventricular end-diastolic and end-systolic anteroposterior diameters range from 3.4 to 5.7 cm and 2.5 to 4.3 cm, respectively (2–4).
- By TEE, left ventricular diameters range from 3.3 to 5.5 cm and 2.0 to 4.0 cm, respectively (4).
- Normal left ventricular end-diastolic volume ranges from 59 to 157 mL, and the upper limit of normal for left ventricular volume index is 65 mL/m^2. In women, left ventricular volumes are lower than in men.

Pitfalls

- Measurement of left ventricular diameters is subject to error due to variation in cardiac position and shape.

- From TEE mid-esophageal four-chamber view, foreshortening of left ventricle (LV) leads to underestimation of left ventricular volumes and overestimation of ejection fraction (EF).

Wall Thickness and Mass

Best Imaging Planes

TTE parasternal or TEE transgastric long-axis and short-axis views.

Diagnostic Method and Formula

- By M-mode, septal and posterior wall thickness is measured from leading edge to leading edge of the respective wall.
- The left ventricular mass is calculated by M-mode images using the following formula:

0.80 × 1.05 [(septal thickness + posterior wall thickness + left ventricular internal diameter)^3 – (left ventricular internal diameter)^3]

Normal Values

- By M-mode, normal left ventricular end-diastolic wall thickness of the septum and posterior walls is up to 1.1 cm. Posterior wall

TABLE 1-2. *Normal Values of Right Heart Chambers*

Measurement	Transthoracic echocardiography
Right ventricular anteroposterior – end-diastole (cm)	2.5–3.8
Right ventricular anteroposterior – end-systole (cm)	2.0–3.4
Right ventricular mediolateral – end-diastole (cm)	2.1–4.2
Right ventricular mediolateral – end-systole (cm)	1.9–3.1
Right ventricular area – end-diastole (cm²)	11–36
Right ventricular area – end-systole (cm²)	5–20
Right ventricular ejection fraction (%)	≥40
Right ventricular free wall thickness (mm)	2–5
RVOT – mid-systole (cm)[a]	1.8–3.4
Right atrial anteroposterior – systole (cm)[b]	—
Right atrial mediolateral – systole (cm)[c]	2.9–4.6
Right atrial volume (mL)	15–58 men, 14–44 women
Right atrial area (cm²)	8–20

RVOT, right ventricular outflow tract.
[a]By transesophageal echocardiography (TEE), 1.6–3.6 cm.
[b]By TEE, 2.8–5.2 cm.
[c]By TEE, 2.9–5.3 cm.

thickness increases with age from 0.9 cm in 20-year-old subjects to 1.1 cm in those >50 years of age (Fig. 1-1).

■ Normal left ventricular mass and index for men are <294 g and <143 g/m², respectively; for women, normal left ventricular mass and index are <198 g and <102 g/m², respectively (5).

Wall Motion

Best Imaging Planes

■ TTE parasternal long-axis and short-axis and apical views.
■ TEE transgastric short-axis and long-axis as well as mid-esophageal four-chamber and two-chamber views.

Normal Wall Motion

■ Normal resting left ventricular wall motion is best defined by a 30% to 70% increase in systolic endocardial thickening (better defined by M-mode) and less specifically by ≥0.5 cm inward wall motion (Fig. 1-1).
■ A normal wall motion response to exercise or dobutamine demonstrates a hyperdynamic and symmetric systolic endocardial thickening of ≥30%.
■ Each left ventricular wall segment is scored as 1 = normal, 2 = hypokinetic, 3 = akinetic, and 4 = dyskinetic. Thus, a normal global wall motion score is 16, and a normal wall motion score index is 1 (6).

Coronary Artery Supply

■ Basal, mid-, and apical anterior; basal, mid-, and apical anterior septum; and apical lateral walls are supplied by the left anterior descending artery (LAD) (Fig. 1-2).

TABLE 1-3. *Normal Values of Left Heart Valves and Great Vessels*

Measurement	Transthoracic echocardiography	Transesophageal echocardiography
Mitral valve area (cm²)	4–6	4–6
Mitral annulus – diastole (cm)	2.0–3.4	2.0–3.8
Mitral leaflets' thickness (mm)	≤4	0.7–3.0
Mitral regurgitation (%)	38–45	70–80
Pulmonary veins (mm)	8–15	7–16
Aortic valve area (cm²)	3–5	3–5
Aortic annulus – systole (cm)	1.4–2.6	1.8–2.7
Aortic regurgitation (%)	0–2	3–4
Aortic root sinuses – diastole (cm)	2.1–3.5	2.1–3.4
Aortic root – tubule – diastole (cm)	1.7–3.4	—
Aortic arch (cm)	2.0–3.6	—
Descending aorta (cm)	—	1.4–3.0

TABLE 1-4. *Normal Values of Right Heart Valves and Great Vessels*

Measurement	Transthoracic echocardiography	Transesophageal echocardiography
Tricuspid valve area (cm^2)	4–6	4–6
Tricuspid annulus – early diastole (cm)	1.3–2.8	2.0–4.0
Tricuspid leaflets' thickness (mm)	≤4	0.7–3.0
Tricuspid regurgitation (%)	15–78	20–50
Superior vena cava (cm)	—	0.8–2.0
Proximal inferior vena cava (cm)	1.2–2.3	—
Hepatic vein (cm)	0.5–1.1	—
Coronary sinus (cm)	—	0.4–1.0
Pulmonic valve area (cm^2)	3–5	—
Pulmonic valve annulus (cm)	1.0–2.2	—
Pulmonic regurgitation (%)	28–88	20–50
RVOT – mid-systole	1.8–3.4	1.6–3.6
Main pulmonary artery	1.0–2.9	—
Right or left pulmonary artery	0.7–1.7	1.2–2.2

RVOT, right ventricular outflow tract.

- Basal and mid-anterolateral walls are supplied by the LAD or left circumflex (LCX) arteries.
- Basal and mid-inferior walls and basal and mid-inferior septum are supplied by the right coronary artery (RCA). The apical inferior wall is supplied by the RCA or LAD.
- Basal and mid-inferolateral walls are supplied by the LCX artery.

Systolic Function

Ejection Fraction

A normal left ventricular ejection fraction (LVEF) assessed by the Simpson's rule as *end-diastolic volume – end-systolic volume ÷ end-diastolic volume* is ≥50%. However, visual estimation of EF is more commonly used and is a practical, accurate, and reproducible method.

Fractional Shortening

- Defined as *left ventricular end-diastolic – end-systolic diameter ÷ end diastolic diameter* by TTE or TEE. It normally is ≥35%.
- LVEF is estimated as the fractional shortening × the constant 1.7.

E Point Septal Separation

The distance between the most posterior septal endocardium (in systole) and the most anterior

TABLE 1-5. *Normal Left and Right Ventricle Doppler Filling Parameters*

Parameter	Left ventricle		Right ventricle	
	<50 yr	>50 yr	<50 yr	>50 yr
Peak E (cm/sec)	72 ± 14	62 ± 14	51 ± 7	41 ± 8
Peak A (cm/sec)	40 ± 10	59 ± 14	27 ± 8	33 ± 8
E/A ratio	1.9 ± 0.6	1.1 ± 0.3	2.0 ± 0.5	1.34 ± 0.4
Deceleration time (msec)	179 ± 20	210 ± 36	188 ± 22	198 ± 23
IVRT (msec)	76 ± 11	90 ± 17	76 ± 11	90 ± 17
PV/SVC peak systolic (cm/sec)	48 ± 9	71 ± 9	41 ± 9	42 ± 12
PV/SVC peak diastolic (cm/sec)	50 ± 10	38 ± 9	22 ± 5	22 ± 5
PV/SVC atrial reversal (cm/sec)	19 ± 4	23 ± 14	13 ± 3	16 ± 3
Left atrial filling fraction (%)	0.25 ± 0.05	0.35 ± 0.06	—	—

A, late filling; E, early filling; IVRT, isovolumic relaxation time; PV, pulmonary veins; SVC, superior vena cava.

TABLE 1-6. *Normal Aortic and Pulmonic Valve Velocities in Adults <50 Years Old*

Parameter	Aortic valve	Pulmonic valve
Peak velocity (cm/sec)	72–120	44–78
Ejection time (msec)	265–325	280–380
Acceleration time (msec)	83–118	130–185

motion of the anterior mitral leaflet during early (E) left ventricular filling is normally ≤5 mm, but even <7 mm predicts normal left ventricular systolic function (Fig. 1-1) (7).

Mitral Annular Systolic Descent

A systolic descent of the mitral annulus toward the left ventricular apex of >1 cm accurately predicts normal left ventricular systolic function.

Aortic Root Motion

In subjects with normal left ventricular stroke volume (generally but not always associated with normal systolic function), the anterior aortic root motion is >1 cm or 30 to 45 degrees from end-diastole to its maximal anterior systolic excursion (Fig. 1-1).

Stroke Volume and Cardiac Output

- *Stroke volume* is calculated as 0.785 [left ventricular outflow tract diameter (LVOT)]^2 or $\Pi(r)^2 \times$ LVOT velocity time integral (VTI) and is normally >65 mL.

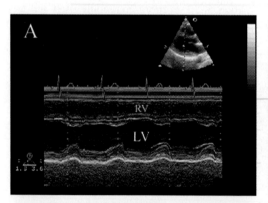
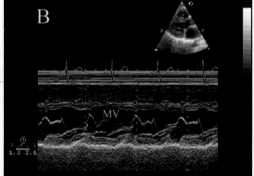
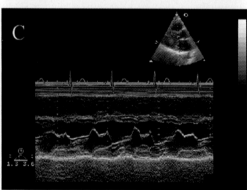
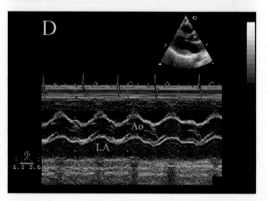

FIG. 1-1. Normal M-mode echocardiogram. This M-mode echocardiogram sweep demonstrates normal heart chambers **(A,D)**, normal left ventricular wall thickness and endocardial thickening **(A)**, normal mitral and aortic valve mobility and thickness **(B–D)**, normal aortic root motion **(D)**, and normal pericardial thickness and echoreflectance **(A–C)**. Ao, aorta; LA, left atrium; LV, left ventricle; MV, mitral valve; RV, right ventricle.

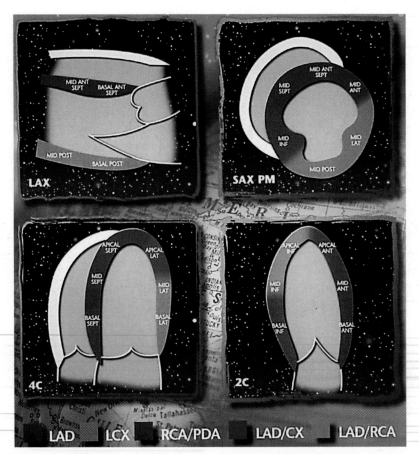

FIG. 1-2. Normal 16 left ventricular wall segments and corresponding coronary artery supply. ANT, anterior; INF, inferior; LAD, left anterior descending artery; LAT, lateral; LCX, left circumflex artery; PDA, posterior descending artery; POST, posterior; RCA, right coronary artery; SEPT, septal. (Courtesy of Biosound, Indianapolis, IN.)

♦ LVOT is measured from TTE long parasternal 2D images.
♦ LVOT VTI by pulsed Doppler is obtained from TTE apical five-chamber view.
■ Cardiac output = stroke volume × heart rate. Normal cardiac output and index are ≥4.5 L/min and ≥3.0 L/min/m², respectively.

Ejection Intervals

■ The isovolumic contraction or preejection period measured by M-mode or pulsed Doppler (from onset of QRS to aortic valve opening or onset of LVOT VTI) is normally short (<60 msec).
■ Ejection period (measured from opening to closing of the aortic valve or from onset to end of LVOT VTI by pulsed or continuous wave Doppler) is normally <160 msec. The initial period of ejection (time from onset to peak velocity of the aortic VTI) is also short (<60 msec).

Rate of Rise of Left Ventricular Systolic Pressure

■ The rate of rise of left ventricular systolic pressure (dP/dt) is an index of systolic function. The rate of rise of mitral regurgitation (MR) peak velocity is an indicator of dP/dt.
■ Thus, dP/dt can be calculated using the Bernoulli equation ($\Delta P = 4V^2$) as the difference in pressure gradients at 3 m/sec and 1 m/sec from onset of MR divided by the time interval

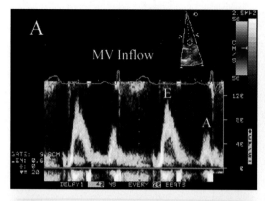

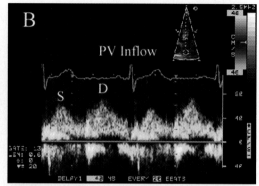

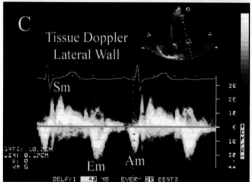

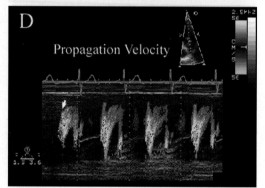

FIG. 1-3. Normal parameters of left ventricular diastolic function in a healthy 26-year-old. **A:** Mitral valve (MV) inflow pattern demonstrates predominant E wave velocity, a short deceleration time, and E/A ratio >1.5. **B:** Pulmonary vein (PV) inflow demonstrates a systolic velocity (S) of smaller amplitude than the diastolic (D) velocity. Atrial reversal velocity was not obtained. **C:** Tissue Doppler of the basal lateral wall demonstrates isovolumetric contraction and biphasic ejection systolic velocities (Sm), early diastolic (Em), and late diastolic (Am) velocities of 20 cm/sec, 20 cm/sec, and 15 cm/sec, respectively. Note on the systolic velocity profile the initial higher and shorter lasting velocities of isovolumic contraction followed by lower but longer-lasting velocities during ejection. **D:** Color M-mode flow propagation velocity measured at the first aliasing isovelocity (*arrow*) was >60 cm/sec.

between these velocities or 32 mm Hg/time interval in seconds.

■ A normal dP/dt is >1,200 mm Hg/sec.

Tei or Myocardial Performance Index

Assess both left ventricular systolic and diastolic function as isovolumic contraction time + isovolumic relaxation time (IVRT)/ejection time. A normal index is >40.

Tissue Doppler

■ Pulsed wave myocardial systolic and diastolic velocities of the ventricular basal segments (lateral, septal, anterior, and posterior/inferior

walls) are indicators of left ventricular and right ventricular systolic and diastolic function (8–10).

■ Spectral gain settings are reduced to record the low velocity and high intensity signals from the myocardial walls, blood flow high velocity signals are filtered out, a 2.5-MHz to 4.0-MHz transducer is used, a sample volume of 2 to 3 mm axial length is used, and the velocity scale is set at 20 cm/sec.

■ The myocardial velocities recorded include the systolic (Sm), early diastolic (Em) and late diastolic (Am).

■ The Sm velocities show an initial higher velocity corresponding to isovolumic contraction and then a biphasic velocity corre-

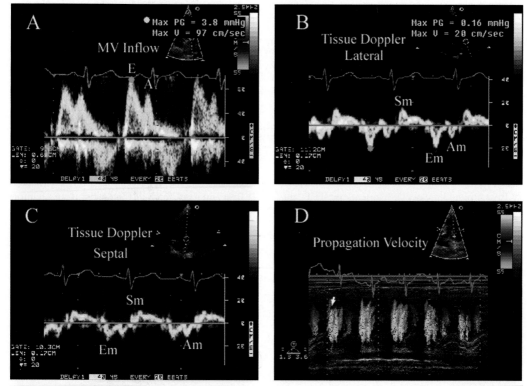

FIG. 1-4. Normal parameters of left ventricular diastolic function in a healthy 46-year-old. **A:** Mitral valve (MV) inflow pattern demonstrates predominant E wave velocity and an E/A ratio >1. **B:** Tissue Doppler of the basal lateral wall demonstrates systolic velocities (Sm), early diastolic (Em), and late diastolic (Am) velocities of 20 cm/sec, 18 cm/sec, and 10 cm/sec, respectively. The systolic velocity profile shows the velocities of biphasic ejection. **C:** Tissue Doppler of the basal septal wall demonstrates normal but lower corresponding velocities to those of the lateral wall (12 cm/sec, 12 cm/sec, and 10 cm/sec, respectively). **D:** Color M-mode flow propagation velocity of >80 cm/sec. Arrow depicts onset to peak of velocity.

sponding to the ejection phase (Figs. 1-3C and 1-4B,C).

■ Basal lateral and inferior wall velocities are higher than those of the septal and anterior walls.

■ Normal Sm velocities of 10 to 20 cm/sec predict normal systolic function (Table 1-7) (Figs. 1-3C and 1-4B,C).

Pitfalls

■ Simpson's rule for calculation of LVEF is time consuming and leads to overestimation of LVEF by underestimation of end-systolic volume.

■ Fractional shortening can be altered by changes in preload or afterload.

Diastolic Function

Diagnostic Methods

Isovolumic Relaxation Time

Time from aortic valve closure to beginning of mitral inflow (E wave) (8–12).

■ Best imaged from TTE apical or TEE mid-esophageal five-chamber views with the sample volume between the mitral inflow and LVOT to obtain both velocity patterns.

■ In normal subjects <20 years old, IVRT is <60 msec; in those 20 to 40 years old, IVRT is <75 msec; in those 40 to 60 years old, IVRT is <85 msec; and in those >60 years old, IVRT is <95 msec.

TABLE 1-7. *Normal Tissue Doppler Velocities of the Basal Ventricular Segments (cm/sec ± 1 SD)*

	Sm	Em	Am	Em/Am velocity ratio
Lateral	9–11 ± 2–3	13–18 ± 3–5	9–11 ± 2–4	1.3–1.5 ± 0.4–0.6
Septal	8.5–10 ± 2	9–11.5 ± 2–3	9–11 ± 1.5–2.5	1.0–1.1 ± 0.4–0.7
Anterior	9–11 ± 1–2	11–13 ± 3–4	10–11 ± 2–3	1.2 ± 0.4–0.7
Posterior/inferior	9–11 ± 2–3	11–14 ± 3–4	11–12 ± 2–3	1.1–1.3 ± 0.4–0.7
Right ventricular free wall	14–16 ± 2–4	13–19 ± 3–4	14–15 ± 3–4	1–1.4 ± 0.1–0.3

Am, late diastolic myocardial velocity; Em, early diastolic myocardial velocity; Sm, systolic myocardial velocity.

Mitral Inflow Pattern

- Best imaged from TTE apical or TEE mid-esophageal four-chamber views with sample volume placed within the LV and near the leaflets' coaptation point.
- Constituted by an early filling velocity (E wave) and atrial contraction velocity (A wave).
- Early left ventricular filling (E wave) is driven by the pressure gradient between left atria (LA) and left ventricle at the time of mitral valve opening.
- In normal subjects <40 years old, a rapidly relaxing LV causes an abrupt fall in left ventricular diastolic pressure, a transient high left atrial to left ventricular gradient, and a high E wave velocity.
- Therefore, E velocity is 50% to 100% higher than A velocity, and the E/A ratio is 1.5 to 2.0 (Figs. 1-3A and 1-4A).
    - After age 20 years, E peak velocity decreases by 2 to 6 cm/sec per decade of life.
    - After age 20 years, the A peak velocity increases by 2 to 9 cm/sec per decade of life.
    - After age 20 years, the E/A ratio decreases by 0.15 to 0.30 per decade of life.
- With aging (especially in subjects >60 years old), left ventricular relaxation slows, E wave velocity decreases, and A wave velocity predominates (Figs. 4-1 and 4-6 in Chapter 4).
    - Thus, in subjects 40 to 60 years old, the E/A ratio is 1.0 to 1.5, and in those >60 years of age, it is <1.
- The E deceleration time, measured from peak E velocity to its nadir, is a parameter of left ventricular relaxation and compliance.
    - In normal subjects <40 years old, it is 140 to 160 msec (Figs. 1-3A and 1-4A).
    - With aging, deceleration time increases to 160 to 200 msec in subjects 40 to 60 years old and >200 msec in those >60 years old.

Pulmonary Veins' Inflow Pattern

- Best imaged from TTE apical four-chamber view to assess right lower pulmonary vein. From TEE mid-esophageal short-axis view with a 20-degree to 40-degree clockwise and then counterclockwise rotation from the aortic valve to assess the left and right pulmonary veins, respectively.
- The pulmonary veins' inflow Doppler pattern (highest velocities obtained by placing the sample volume 0.5 to 1.0 cm into the pulmonary vein) include four components (Fig. 1-3B):
    - The first systolic forward flow (S1) occurs during atrial relaxation [after the P wave or before the initial portion of the QRS of the electrocardiogram (ECG)].
    - The second systolic forward flow (S2) occurs during left ventricular systolic descent of the base or annular displacement (its peak velocity corresponds to the T wave of the ECG and is higher than S1).
    - The third forward diastolic flow velocity (D) occurs during rapid filling of the left ventricle (after mitral valve opening), and its peak velocity corresponds to that of mitral E wave.
    - Flow reversal after atrial contraction is of smaller amplitude and shorter duration than mitral A wave.
- In healthy subjects <40 years old, because of the low left atrial pressure and low pulmonary veins' pressure gradient, the systolic velocities are normally lower than the diastolic velocities (Fig. 1-3B).
- In those >40 years old, as left ventricular relaxation decreases, left atrial diastolic velocities decrease and atrial reversal velocities increase in amplitude and duration.
- The sum of the VTI of S1 and S2 constitutes 60% to 70% of the sum of the VTI of systolic and diastolic velocities ("systolic fraction").

Tissue Doppler

- Pulsed wave myocardial diastolic velocities of the ventricular basal segments are reflective of left ventricular and right ventricular diastolic function.
- Best imaged from TTE and TEE four-chamber views.
- Em correlates inversely with the peak negative dP/dt or time constant of left ventricular or right ventricular relaxation (tau) and therefore is related to ventricular relaxation and elastic recoil and is less influenced by changes in preload.
- Normal velocities for Em and Am are >9 cm/sec, and the Em/Am ratio is normally >1 (Table 1-7) (Figs. 1-3C and 1-4B,C).
- As for the mitral velocities, an inverse relation exists between E' velocities and age.
- Tissue Doppler is also used to calculate the Tei index.

E Propagation Rate by Color M-Mode

- The M-mode cursor beam is placed parallel to the mitral inflow stream, and the Nyquist limit is set up at 50 to 60 cm/sec. The color M-mode flow propagation velocity is measured as the slope of the first aliasing velocity during early filling (from the mitral valve to 4 cm into the left ventricular cavity).
- The E propagation velocity is proportional to left ventricular systolic and diastolic function and is normally >40 cm/sec (Figs. 1-3D and 1-4D).

Pitfalls

- IVRT is not a true reflection of left ventricular relaxation in the presence of a high or low aortic diastolic pressure and/or the presence of MR or aortic regurgitation.
- Mitral inflow parameters lose specificity during tachycardia because A velocity increases and E/A ratio decreases.
- In the assessment of pulmonary veins' inflow pattern, early S1 and atrial reversal velocities are seen in only 30% to 40% of healthy subjects by TTE and ≥75% by TEE.
- Tissue Doppler and flow propagation velocity recordings are sometimes inadequate for reliable interpretation.

LEFT ATRIA

Size and Volume

During left ventricular systole, left atrial volume is highest and pressure is moderate; during atrial contraction, left atrial pressure is highest; and after atrial contraction, left atrial volume and pressure are lowest.

Best Imaging Planes

- TTE M-mode or 2D parasternal long-axis or short-axis views to obtain the anteroposterior diameter at end systole (end of T wave), and from trailing edge of anterior atrial wall to leading edge of posterior wall.
- By TEE, left atrial anteroposterior and mediolateral diameters are measured from the mid-esophageal four-chamber view from inner edge to inner edge of atrial walls.
- TTE or TEE orthogonal planes are used to measure atrial volumes and areas using Simpson's rule.

Normal Values

- By TTE, the maximal left atrial anteroposterior, mediolateral, and superoinferior diameters range from 2.2 to 4.1 cm, 2.5 to 6.0 cm, and 3.1 to 6.8 cm, respectively (13–15).
  - ◆ The anteroposterior diameter is the most commonly used to assess left atrial size.
- Another parameter of normal left atrial size is a left atrial to aortic root ratio <1.1 (Fig. 1-1).
- Left atrial volume and index range from 20 to 60 mL and 20 ± 6 mL/m², respectively.
  - ◆ Men, nonathletes, and subjects >50 years old have larger left atrial volumes than women, athletes, and younger subjects.
- Left atrial area ranges from 9 to 23 cm².
- Left atrial appendage anteroposterior and mediolateral diameters by TEE range from 1.5 to 4.3 cm and 1.0 to 2.8 cm, respectively.

Function

- Left atrial contractility and EF are dependent of atrial preload (pulmonary veins' flow) and afterload (left ventricular end-diastolic pressure before atrial contraction).

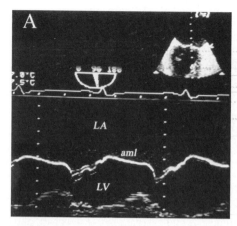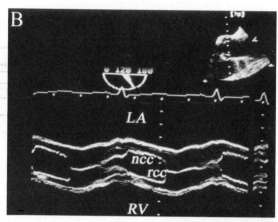

FIG. 1-5. Normal mitral and aortic valve thickness. **A:** M-mode echo from the mid-esophageal two-chamber view shows a uniformly thin (<2 mm) anterior mitral leaflet (aml). **B:** M-mode echo of normal aortic non (ncc) and right coronary cusps (rcc) obtained from the mid-esophageal longitudinal view of the aortic valve showing similar and uniform thickness (<2 mm) of the cusps. Also, note the normal mobility of the mitral leaflet and aortic cusps as well as the normal mobility and thickness of the aortic root. LA, left atrium; LV, left ventricle; RV, right ventricle.

■ Left atrial stroke volume is 20% to 40% of left ventricular stroke volume, and left atrial fractional emptying is approximately 60%.

Pressure

Definition

Left atrial pressure is a reflection of left ventricular filling pressure or diastolic function. Therefore, mitral and pulmonary vein inflow parameters used for assessment of left ventricular diastolic function apply to the assessment of left atrial pressure (8–12).

MITRAL VALVE

Best Imaging Planes

■ TTE M-mode or 2D parasternal long-axis and short-axis and apical four-chamber and two-chamber views.
■ TEE mid-esophageal four-chamber and two-chamber views at 0 degrees (exclude LVOT).

Leaflets

Thickness and Echoreflectance

■ Limited data are available regarding normal valve thickness values by TTE.

■ By TEE, normal mitral leaflets' thickness ranges from 0.7 to 3.0 mm (Fig. 1-5A) (16).
■ Using TEE-measured leaflet thickness as the standard, the specificity of visual assessment of mitral valve thickness is 87% by TEE and 83% by TTE.
■ Mitral leaflets have homogeneous soft tissue echoreflectance slightly higher than that of the myocardium.
■ **Pitfall**: Adequate measurement of leaflet thickness of any heart valve by TTE is infrequently accomplished and is commonly inaccurate.

Mobility and Length

■ Mobility of mitral leaflets is dependent on the primary structure, left ventricular preload, left atrial to left ventricular pressure gradient, and left ventricular contractility.
■ By M-mode TTE parasternal long-axis view, the anterior leaflet motion appears as an M shape, and the posterior leaflet appears as a blunted W (Fig. 1-1B,C). The initial opening of the anterior leaflet forms a ≥70-degree angle from the point of closure (D to E slope).
■ After rapid left ventricular filling, left ventricular volume and diastolic pressure increase,

and the anterior mitral leaflet partially closes and forms the E to F slope of ≥70 degrees.

◆ By 2D images, mitral leaflets show a parallel motion in relation to the interventricular septum (anterior leaflet) and posterior wall (posterior leaflet).

◆ The distance between the leaflets and respective left ventricular wall is <5 mm at their maximum excursion.

◆ Because the posterior leaflet is shorter and has a larger area of attachment to the mitral annulus, its mobility is less than that of the anterior leaflet.

Annulus

■ The mitral annulus diameter ranges from 2.0 to 3.8 cm.

■ It is measured from TTE or TEE four-chamber views, during early diastole (when mitral leaflets are at their most open position), and from the base of the anterior to the posterior leaflet (atrial side).

Subvalvular Apparatus

Chordae Tendinea

■ Insert at or near the free edges of the leaflets and, less commonly, into the body of leaflets and commissural portions.

■ Chordae from the posteromedial papillary muscle insert into the medial half of anterior and posterior leaflets, and those of the anterolateral papillary muscle insert into the lateral half of anterior and posterior leaflets.

■ Chordae appear as thin, linear, and homogeneously echoreflectant structures.

Papillary Muscles

■ By TTE, the posteromedial papillary muscle is best seen from the parasternal long-axis and short-axis, apical and subcostal views; the anterolateral papillary muscle is best seen from parasternal short-axis view.

■ By TEE, papillary muscles are best seen from transgastric short-axis and long-axis and mid-esophageal four-chamber and two-chamber views.

■ Papillary muscles are located in the posterior half of the LV and oriented parallel to mitral leaflets' closure line.

■ The posteromedial muscle is thicker than the anterolateral one, both muscles are of conic shape, and their maximum thickness is approximately 1.0 to 1.5 cm.

Regurgitation

MR in healthy subjects ranges from 38% to 45% by color Doppler, is mostly (70–80%) of trivial degree, and is characterized by early systolic, central, narrow, and small jets (<2 cm in length and <1 cm^2 in area).

AORTIC VALVE AND OUTFLOW TRACT

Best Imaging Planes

■ TTE parasternal long-axis and short-axis views and TEE mid-esophageal short-axis view at 30 to 60 degrees to assess commissures, cusp margins, and coronary sinuses.

■ TEE longitudinal view at 80 to 120 degrees assesses LVOT, noncoronary (sometimes left) and right coronary cusps, aortic annulus, and aortic root.

Cusps

Thickness and Echoreflectance

■ Normal thickness of aortic cusps ranges from 0.5 to 2.0 mm by TEE M-mode and 2D echo (Fig. 1-5B).

■ By quantitative TEE as standard, visual assessment of aortic cusps' thickness has a specificity of 92% by TEE and 87% by TTE (16).

■ Aortic cusps are homogeneously echoreflectant and of slightly higher echoreflectance than the myocardium.

Location

The right coronary cusp is located anteromedially; the noncoronary cusp is located posterior and in close proximity to the distal interatrial septum; and the left coronary cusp is laterally located.

Mobility and Length

■ Mobility of the aortic cusps is determined by left ventricular stroke volume and contractility.
■ Aortic cusps have a 90-degree systolic excursion from the aortic annulus, lie parallel and within a few millimeters from the aortic root walls, have a separation of ≥2 cm, and their length is 1.5 to 2.0 cm (Figs. 1-1D and 1-5B).

Annulus and Outflow Tract

■ The aortic annulus diameter at end-diastole ranges from 1.4 to 2.6 cm by TTE and 1.8 to 2.7 cm by TEE.
■ It is measured from the junction of the anterior aortic root wall with the interventricular septum and posterior root wall with the base of anterior mitral leaflet (intervalvular fibrosa).
■ The LVOT diameter ranges from 1.8 to 2.4 cm and is measured during mid-systole (end of ST segment) and within 1 cm of aortic annulus from the inner portion of proximal interventricular septum to the intervalvular fibrosa.

Valve and Outflow Tract Velocities

■ Normal valve and LVOT velocities are laminar, with an acceleration time shorter than the deceleration time. Normal valve and LVOT velocities range from 1.0 to 1.7 m/sec and 0.7 to 1.1 m/sec, respectively (Fig. 1-6).
■ Also, two preejection velocities can be seen in the LVOT (Fig. 1-6):
 ◆ The first, highest velocity (A wave) results from flow into the aortic valve caused by atrial contraction.
 ◆ The second velocity corresponds to flow produced by left ventricular isovolumetric contraction and mitral valve closure.
 ◆ By TEE, a parallel alignment of pulsed and continuous wave Doppler with the aortic valve can be accomplished from the transgastric view at 60 to 90 degrees.

Regurgitation

The prevalence of aortic regurgitation in healthy people aged 10 to 50 years ranges from 0% to 2%;

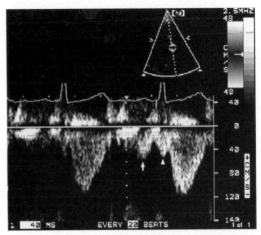

FIG. 1-6. Normal left ventricular outflow tract velocities. Pulsed Doppler recording at the left ventricular outflow demonstrates a normal laminar flow velocity of <1.2 m/sec during the ejection period with a short acceleration but a longer deceleration time. Two other preejection velocities are also noted. The first velocity or A wave (*arrow*) results from atrial contraction causing extension of flow into the outflow tract. The second velocity (*arrowhead*) results from flow produced by isovolumetric contraction and mitral valve closure.

in obese subjects, up to 7%; in subjects ≥70 years old, ≥10%; and is generally trivial to mild (17).

AORTA

Ascending Aorta

Extends for approximately 5 cm from the aortic annulus to its junction with the aortic arch and is subdivided into the sinuses and tubular portions.

Aortic Sinuses

■ The right, left, and noncoronary sinuses of Valsalva are located just above the aortic cusps. At this level, the aortic root diastolic diameter is 2.1 to 3.5 cm, 3 to 5 mm larger than the annulus and 1 to 3 mm larger than the sinotubular portion (Figs. 1-1D and 1-5B) (18).
■ By M-mode or 2D TEE, thickness of anterior and posterior aortic root walls is <2.2 mm (Figs. 1-1D and 1-5B) (19).

Tubular Aorta

- Extends for approximately 3 cm from the sino-tubular junction, and its diameter measured from the inner edge of anterior wall to leading edge of the posterior wall ranges from 1.7 to 3.4 cm.
- Thickness of aortic walls at this level is similar to that at the sinuses level (<2.2 mm).
- Aortic root motion is normally >1 cm or a 30-degree to 45-degree angle from end-diastole to its maximal systolic anterior excursion (Fig. 1-1D).

Aortic Arch

- From the suprasternal notch view, the arch and left subclavian, left common carotid, and innominate arteries are commonly visualized.
- By TEE, the distal portion and anterior wall are best visualized, but approximately 2 cm behind the trachea are not seen ("the blind spot").

Descending Aorta

- From TTE parasternal long-axis view, it is best seen posterior to the atrioventricular groove and distal portion of LA; from TTE apical four-chamber view, it is seen lateral to the LA; and from the apical two-chamber view, it is seen posterior to LA.
- Normal diameter ranges from 2.0 to 2.5 cm.

RIGHT VENTRICLE

Best Imaging Planes

- TTE parasternal long-axis and short-axis, parasternal RV long-axis, and apical and sub-costal four-chamber views.
- TEE transgastric short and longitudinal RV views and basal four-chamber view.

Size

- Assessment of right ventricular size is difficult and requires integration of all echo planes.
- TTE parasternal long and subcostal four-chamber views frequently transect the RV at its anterosuperior and posterolateral horns, respectively. Thus, right ventricular size is smallest from these views.

- The apical four-chamber view better reflects the right ventricular size, but it may transect the RV oblique to its long axis and overestimate its size.
- The right ventricular end-diastolic anteroposterior and mediolateral diameter at its mid-cavity should not exceed 3.5 cm and 4.2 cm, respectively (Fig. 1-1A).
- **Pitfalls:** In the assessment of right ventricular size, false positives occur if the transducer probe is not located over the left ventricular apex, and false negatives occur if LV is concurrently enlarged.

Wall Thickness

Best assessed by M-mode images, and ranges from 2 to 5 mm.

- **Pitfalls**
  - ◆ Assessment of right ventricular wall thickness is commonly inaccurate due to poor endocardial resolution of the right ventricular lateral wall from TTE apical four-chamber view.
  - ◆ In addition, right ventricular walls are lined up with multiple trabeculae carneae (small muscle bands) that can be misinterpreted as right ventricular hypertrophy.
  - ◆ Right ventricular wall thickness from subcostal four-chamber view may be overestimated because the ultrasound beam may be tangential to the posterolateral right ventricular wall.
  - ◆ Thus, visual assessment of right ventricular wall thickness lacks specificity.

Wall Motion

- Right ventricular wall motion is subjectively assessed by its inward motion rather than endocardial thickening.
- **Pitfall:** Assessment of right ventricular wall motion is limited due to difficulties in defining endocardial systolic thickening and lack of a standard.

Systolic Function

Key Diagnostic Features

- A systolic excursion of the tricuspid annulus toward the cardiac apex of ≥2 cm denotes normal right ventricular systolic function (normal RVEF is ≥40%).

- Using tissue Doppler imaging, a peak systolic tricuspid annular velocity of >11.5 cm/sec (normal range, 11.6 to 21.1 cm/sec) is predictive of normal RVEF (20–23).
- A time from onset of ECG QRS to peak systolic annular velocity of >200 msec predicts normal RVEF.
- **Pitfall:** Difficulties in measuring right ventricular volumes have made assessment of RVEF difficult and inaccurate.

Diastolic Function

- Assessed by similar methods used to assess left ventricular diastolic function (20–23).
- Right ventricular IVRT, tricuspid valve inflow, and inferior vena cava (IVC) or hepatic veins' Doppler flow patterns are similar to those of left ventricular IVRT and mitral and pulmonary veins' inflow patterns.

RIGHT ATRIA

Size

Best Imaging Planes

- TTE apical and subcostal four-chamber views.
- TEE transgastric long-axis view of the right ventricular and basal four-chamber view.

Normal Values

- The right atrial superoinferior and mediolateral dimensions at end-systole range from 3.4 to 4.9 cm and 3.0 to 4.6 cm, respectively.
- Right atrial area ranges from 8.3 to 19.5 cm² and should not exceed that of the LA.

Pressure

Inferior Vena Cava Dynamics

- A negative intrathoracic pressure generated by inspiration of 5 to 10 mm Hg causes IVC collapse. Therefore, IVC size in response to respiration provides an estimate of the mean right atrial pressure.

- Right atrial pressure is low (<5 mm Hg) if IVC is small (≤1.0 cm) and collapses with inspiration. Right atrial pressure is normal (5–10 mm Hg) if IVC is normal (1.0–1.5 cm) and collapses >50%.

Hepatic Veins' Flow

- Determined by the pressure gradient between these vessels and RA.
- The first predominant systolic flow of the hepatic veins is due to a decrease in right atrial pressure during atrial relaxation (after P wave of QRS) and systolic downward displacement of the tricuspid annulus.
- The second diastolic flow is related to a decrease in right atrial pressure during right ventricular filling.
- Minimal systolic and diastolic flow reversals are seen after the systolic and diastolic forward flows (Fig. 1-7A).
- During inspiration, systolic and diastolic flows increase, but reversal flow velocities decrease. Opposite changes occur during expiration and apnea.
- In healthy persons, the VTI of systolic flow of hepatic veins constitutes >50% of the sum of systolic and diastolic VTI (15,17).

Pitfalls

- A markedly negative intrathoracic pressure during inspiration causes IVC collapse despite an elevated right atrial pressure in obstructive airway disease, pleural effusions, or any respiratory distress.
- In patients on positive-pressure ventilation, IVC does not collapse despite a normal right atrial pressure.

TRICUSPID VALVE

Best Imaging Planes

- TTE parasternal long-axis view of the right ventricular inflow, parasternal short-axis view, and apical or subcostal four-chamber views to assess the anterior and posterior leaflets.

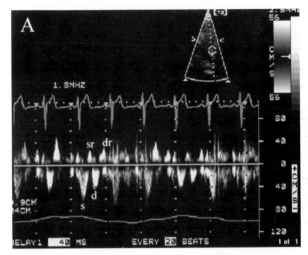 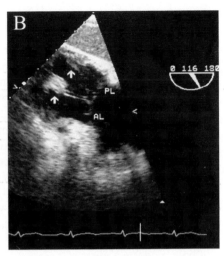

FIG. 1-7. Normal flow pattern of the hepatic veins and normal tricuspid valve apparatus. **A:** Pulsed Doppler recordings of the hepatic veins obtained from the subcostal view and recorded at 25 cm/sec paper speed demonstrates the normal predominance of the systolic (s) over the diastolic (d) velocities, more noticeable in this tracing at the end of inspiration. The respective systolic (sr) and diastolic (dr) flow reversals are noted. **B:** This transgastric longitudinal transesophageal echocardiographic view of the right ventricle demonstrates normal-appearing posterior (PL) and anterior (AL) tricuspid leaflets, thin chordae tendinea, and corresponding small posterior and large anterior papillary muscles (*arrows*).

- TEE transgastric long-axis view of the right ventricle allows detailed visualization of anterior and posterior leaflets, chordae, and corresponding papillary muscles (Fig. 1-7B).
- TEE transgastric short-axis view to assess all three tricuspid leaflets and mid-esophageal four-chamber view to assess anterior and septal leaflets.

Leaflets

Thickness

- By multiplane 2D TEE images, thickness of basal, mid-, and tip portions of the anterior and septal tricuspid valve leaflets can be measured from the mid-esophageal four-chamber view. The posterior leaflet can be measured from the transgastric right ventricular long-axis view.
- Normal thickness of the tricuspid leaflets ranges from 0.7 to 3.0 mm (16).
- Using quantitative TEE as standard, visual assessment of tricuspid valve thickness has a specificity of 99% by TEE and 97% by TTE.

Mobility and Length

- The anterior and posterior leaflets follow a similar mobility pattern to that of mitral leaflets. The septal leaflet is the shortest and least mobile.
- The largest anterior leaflet extends from the anterior to inferolateral portions of the tricuspid annulus. The septal leaflet extends from the muscular to the membranous interventricular septum and inserts up to 8 mm more apically than the anterior mitral leaflet. The posterior leaflet extends from the inferior septum to the inferolateral wall.

Annulus

The annulus' diameter by TTE or TEE ranges from 2.0 to 4.0 cm and is measured during early diastole from the base of the anterior leaflet to the base of the septal leaflet.

Subvalvular Apparatus

- From TTE parasternal long-axis view of the RV and from the subcostal four-chamber view, the anterior and posterior papillary muscles are partially visualized.

- From TEE transgastric long-axis view of the RV, the posterior and anterior papillary muscles and their chordal attachments are well defined (Fig. 1-7B).
- The largest anterior papillary muscle is located behind the commissures of the anterior and posterior leaflets and attaches to the right ventricular anterolateral wall and to the moderator band.
- The posterior papillary muscle lies behind the commissure of the posterior and septal leaflets.
- The smallest septal papillary muscle tethers the anterior and septal leaflets against the infundibular wall.

Regurgitation

- Tricuspid regurgitation (TR) by color Doppler ranges from 15% to 78% and is highest (60–65%) in subjects 10 to 30 years old and lowest (15–35%) in those 30 to 50 years old.
- TR is seen in up to 90% of athletes, in contrast to <25% of sedentary subjects.
- Regurgitation is mostly (>80%) of trivial degree, with central small jets (areas <1.5 cm^2).

PULMONIC VALVE

Best Imaging Planes

- TTE parasternal and subcostal short-axis views and TEE transgastric and mid-esophageal short-axis views with the imaging plane parallel to the right ventricular outflow tract (RVOT) to assess the anterior and right posterior cusps, RVOT, annulus, and main PA.
- TEE mid-esophageal short-axis view (0–30 degrees) and slightly above the aortic valve cusps to assess all three cusps.

Cusps

- By TEE 2D, leaflets' thickness measured at their mid-portion from the mid-esophageal short-axis and longitudinal views ranges from 0.7 to 2.0 mm (16). TTE data are not available.
- Using quantitative TEE as standard, the visual assessment of the pulmonic valve thickness has a specificity of 97% by TEE and 94% by TTE.

- Reflectance, mobility, and length of pulmonic cusps are similar to those of the aortic cusps.
- Flow velocities across the pulmonic valve in normal adults range from 0.6 to 0.9 m/sec.

Right Ventricular Outflow Tract and Pulmonic Valve Annulus

- By TTE 2D images, RVOT diameter (measured within 1 cm from the annulus) and pulmonic valve annulus range from 1.8 to 3.4 cm and 1.8 to 2.2 cm, respectively.
- By TEE, RVOT diameter ranges from 1.6 to 3.6 cm.

Regurgitation

Pulmonic regurgitation in healthy persons ranges from 28% to 88%; it is highest in patients <30 years old and lowest in those 30 to 50 years old. It is usually trivial and has central jets with areas ≤1 cm^2.

PULMONARY ARTERY

Best Imaging Planes

- TTE parasternal and subcostal short-axis views.
- TEE mid-esophageal short-axis view of the pulmonic valve with the imaging plane parallel to the RVOT (approximately 30–45 degrees).
- Also, the right and left PAs can be seen from TTE suprasternal or supraclavicular views.

Diameters

By TTE, the diameter of the main, right, and left PAs range from 0.9 to 2.9 cm, 0.7 to 1.7 cm, and 0.6 to 1.4 cm, respectively. By TEE, the right PA diameter ranges from 1.2 to 2.2 cm.

Flow

PA flow gradually accelerates and decelerates and increases by 15% during inspiration. Peak velocities in adults range from 0.6 to 0.9 m/sec and acceleration time (onset to peak velocity) is >110 msec.

Systolic Pressure

- The right ventricular and PA systolic pressures are equal in the absence of pulmonic stenosis. PA systolic pressure is estimated by using the modified Bernoulli equation as $4V^2$ (V = peak TR velocity) + right atrial pressure.
- A normal PA systolic pressure is ≤30 mm Hg.
- The correlation between Doppler-derived and catheter-measured PA pressure is 0.96, with an interobserver and intraobserver variability of <2 mm Hg.
- **Pitfalls**
  - Underestimation or overestimation of PA systolic pressure by Doppler echo is generally related to errors in estimating right atrial pressure and poorly defined TR peak velocity.
  - PA pressure cannot be estimated in most healthy subjects because of difficulties in recording peak trivial TR velocities.

Diastolic Pressure

PA diastolic pressure can be estimated as $4V^2$ (V = pulmonic regurgitation end-diastolic velocity by continuous wave Doppler) + right atrial pressure.

PERICARDIUM

Best Imaging Planes

TTE long parasternal and subcostal four chamber views and TEE transgastric short-axis and long-axis views of LV and RV to assess pericardial layers and their sliding motion.

Normal Features

- The cavity between the visceral and parietal pericardium contains approximately 20 to 30 mL of fluid that allows pericardial layers to slide over each other during cardiac motion.
- The pericardial cavity extends anterosuperiorly just above the origin of the great vessels and posteriorly to the insertion of the pulmonary veins and vena cava.
- In diastole, the pericardium appears as a single, highly reflective linear structure best noticed posterior to the LV. In systole, a few millimeters of pericardial layer separation can be noted.
- To improve visualization of the pericardium, the transmitted pulse or gain can be decreased to attenuate the echoreflectance of endocardial and myocardial surfaces (Fig. 1-1A–C).
- Normal pericardial thickness by TEE is 1.2 ± 0.8 mm.
- Normal negative intrapericardial pressure of –1 to –3 mm Hg, especially during inspiration, allows a positive transmural pressure gradient and increased heart chamber filling and stroke volume, especially of the right heart.

NORMAL VARIANTS OF THE LEFT HEART

Bridging Trabeculations or False Tendons

- Linear or band-like fibromuscular structures traversing the left ventricular cavity in variable directions, more echoreflectant than the myocardium, more frequently seen in the distal third of the LV, single or multiple, and extending from apical lateral wall to interventricular septum or from basal to mid- and distal septum (Fig. 1-8A).
- Rarely, trabeculations connect papillary muscles or a papillary muscle to the septum or free wall.
- With harmonic and digital imaging, trabeculations are seen in >30% of studies.
- Their separation from the endocardium during systole (forming a systolic slack) and underlying normal inward wall motion and endocardial thickening help to differentiate them from thrombi (see Figs. 2-4 and 14-2).

Pectinate Muscles

- Muscle ridges that extend from the lateral to medial wall of left atrial appendage. They appear as nonmobile linear projections or indentations of the appendage wall with similar echoreflectance to that of the appendage wall and are commonly seen traversing the entire appendage (Fig. 1-8B).
- Best seen by TEE mid-esophageal short-axis view.
- Similar muscle ridges are occasionally seen on the lateral wall of right atrial appendage.

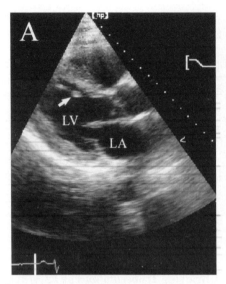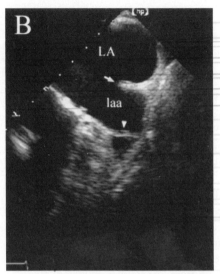

FIG. 1-8. Left ventricular bridging trabeculation and atrial appendage pectinate muscle and ridge. **A:** This parasternal long-axis view of the left ventricle (LV) demonstrates a prominent bridging trabeculation (*arrow*) with a similar echoreflectance to that of the myocardium and extending from the basal to the distal anteroseptal wall. **B:** This transesophageal echocardiographic view of the left atrial appendage (laa) demonstrates a prominent pectinate muscle (*arrowhead*) with similar echoreflectance to that of the atrial wall and traversing the appendage from its lateral to medial wall. Also note a prominent ridge (*arrow*) at the most superior aspect of the appendage. This ridge is formed by the junction of the anterior wall of the left upper pulmonary vein and the lateral wall of the laa. LA, left atrium.

Left Upper Pulmonary Vein Ridge

■ Formed by the junction of the anterior wall of left upper pulmonary vein and lateral wall of left atrial appendage, more noticeable in its most medial and superior portion, and frequently protrudes into the left atrial cavity and mimics an left atrial mass (Fig. 1-8B).

■ Best seen by TEE mid-esophageal short-axis view of left atrial appendage and infrequently from TTE apical four-chamber view.

Valve Excrescences

■ Result from constant bending and buckling of the leaflets, leading to tearing of subendocardial collagen and elastic fibers, which subsequently endothelialize.

■ Are thin (0.6–2.0 mm in width), elongated (4–16 mm in length), and hypermobile structures seen at the coaptation point of the aortic or mitral leaflets and rarely on the right-sided valves (24).

■ Those on the aortic valve prolapse to the LVOT during diastole (Fig. 1-9A).

■ Those on the mitral valve prolapse into the LA during systole.

■ Are detected almost exclusively by TEE in up to 35% to 40% of healthy subjects, persist unchanged over time, and are probably not associated with cardioembolic risk.

Nodes of Aranti

Tiny nodules at the tip of each of the aortic cusps, more noticeable with aging, and almost exclusively seen by TEE, but the proportion of subjects with these nodes is unknown.

Transverse Sinus

■ A pericardial fold creating a small triangular space between the LA, ascending aorta, and PA. It is generally filled with fluid, but it can also accumulate fatty tissue.

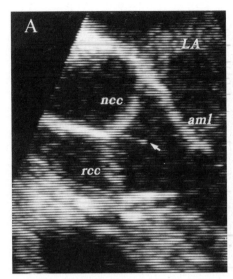
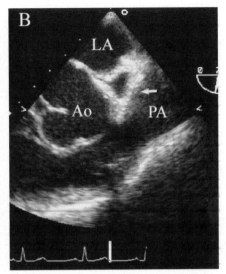

FIG. 1-9. Aortic valve excrescence and transverse sinus. **A:** This longitudinal close-up transesophageal echocardiographic (TEE) view of the aortic valve demonstrates a thin and elongated valve excrescence located at the coaptation point of the noncoronary cusp (ncc) and right coronary cusp (rcc) prolapsing into the left ventricle during diastole (*arrow*). **B:** This TEE basal view longitudinal to the main pulmonary artery (PA) demonstrates the transverse sinus (*arrow*), an echolucent structure of triangular appearance located between the left atrial anterolateral wall, the posterolateral wall of the ascending aorta, and the posterior wall of the PA. aml, anterior mitral leaflet; Ao, aorta; LA, left atrium.

- Although this is a normal variant common to left and right heart, it can be mistaken as part of the atrial appendage, with the atrial wall portion or its fatty tissue content misinterpreted as an atrial mass (Fig. 1-9B).
- Best visualized from the TEE basal short-axis view just above the aortic valve cusps.

NORMAL VARIANTS OF THE RIGHT HEART

Moderator Band

A large muscle bundle that extends from the anterolateral right ventricular wall and base of the anterior papillary muscle to the distal third of the interventricular septum. It is seen in approximately two-thirds of healthy persons by TTE or TEE (Fig. 1-10A).

Eustachian Valve

- A fold or ridge of right atrial endocardium that originates from the inferior portion of the crista terminalis and extends from the IVC to the interatrial septum above the fosa ovale.
- Appears as a linear, nonmobile echodensity that originates from the inferior aspect of the IVC junction with the RA (behind the tricuspid annulus), runs through the most posterior aspect of the atrial wall, and extends to the proximal portion of the fosa ovale (Fig. 1-10A).

Chiari's Network

- A remnant of the embryonic sinus venosus and a variant of the Eustachian valve that extends from the inferior inlet of the IVC through the posterior right atrial wall into the fosa ovale.
- Best visualized by TTE apical and subcostal four-chamber views or TEE four-chamber view.
- Appears as thin, filamentous, and undulating hypermobile structure with a prevalence of <2% by TTE and ≥10% by TEE (Fig. 1-10B).

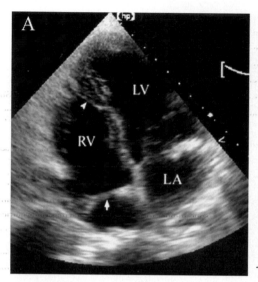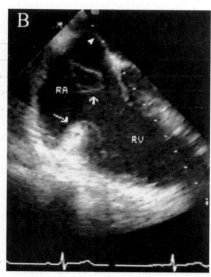

FIG. 1-10. Moderator band, Eustachian valve, Chiari's network, and epicardial fat. **A:** This transthoracic echocardiographic four-chamber view demonstrates a prominent moderator band (*arrowhead*) extending from the mid-distal septum to the apical lateral wall. Also note in this view a prominent Eustachian valve appearing as a band-like structure extending from the inferolateral aspect of the right atrial wall (area of junction with the inferior vena cava) to the fossa ovale area (*arrow*). **B:** This transesophageal echocardiographic four-chamber view demonstrates a Chiari's network (*short arrow*) appearing as a homogeneously echoreflectant, thin or linear, and hypermobile or waving (rope-like) structure extending from the superior to the inferior aspect of the right atrium (RA). This view also demonstrates prominent epicardial fat deposition on the lateral atrioventricular groove of the tricuspid valve (*long arrow*). LA, left atrium; LV, left ventricle; RV, right ventricle.

NORMAL VARIANTS COMMON TO THE LEFT AND RIGHT HEART

Interatrial Septal Aneurysm

- Outpouching of the interatrial septum of >15 mm that moves 11 to 15 mm toward either or both atria, most commonly involving the fosa ovale area and, rarely, the entire interatrial septum (see Figs. 14-6 through 14-8).
- Its prevalence in healthy persons is <1% by TTE and 3% to 8% by TEE, and it is frequently associated with a patent foramen ovale (up to 77%).
- Although its prevalence in patients with suspected cardioembolism increases to 15%, a causal relationship has not been established.

Patent Foramen Ovale

- A small gap in the foramen ovale from failure of the secundum and primum septum to fuse,

forming a one-way valve allowing flow from RA to LA.
- Its prevalence in healthy persons is up to 10% by TTE and up to 30% by TEE, and it is commonly (40%) associated with an atrial septal aneurysm. A higher prevalence has been reported in patients with suspected cardioembolism, but a causal relationship has not been established.
- The diagnosis is confirmed by demonstration of a small amount of saline contrast or bubbles entering the LA within three cardiac cycles. Valsalva maneuver increases its detection (Fig.14-6).
- Appearance of bubbles in the LA after four cycles suggests a pulmonary arteriovenous fistula.

Epicardial Fat

- Best seen by TTE long parasternal and subcostal views.

- More prevalent in the elderly, patients who are obese, patients with diabetes, and women.
- Predominantly located anteroapical and posterolateral to the RV as well as at the atrioventricular groove of the tricuspid valve (this last potentially mistaken as extracardiac mass) (Fig. 1-10B). Posterior located epicardial fat is rare (<7%) in a general population (25).
- Has a characteristic speckled or granular echoreflectance.

Lipomatous Hypertrophy of the Interatrial Septum

- Characterized by varying degrees of fatty infiltration of the proximal and distal portions of the septum with sparing of the fossa ovale area, giving the septum the typical appearance of a dumbbell, doughnut, or hourglass. Rarely, the entire interatrial septum is involved.
- Fatty infiltration can be significant and predominant on the right atrial side. Therefore, it can be mistaken with a right atrial lipoma, myxoma, or thrombus. TEE is helpful in these cases.
- It is generally incidentally detected and currently of undefined clinical significance.
- Its true prevalence is unknown, but with current harmonic and digital imaging, it is probably detected in at least 5% of patients referred for echocardiography.

REFERENCES

1. Cheitlin MD, Armstrong WF, Aurigemma GP, et al. ACC/AHA/ASE guideline update for the application of echocardiography—summary article: a report of the American College of Cardiology/American Heart Association Task Force on Practice Guidelines (ACC/AHA/ASE Committee to Update the 1997 Guidelines for the Clinical Application of Echocardiography). *J Am Coll Cardiol* 2003;42:954–970.
2. Triulzi M, Gillam L, Gentile F, et al. Normal adult cross-sectional echocardiographic values: linear dimensions and chamber areas. *Echocardiography* 1994;1:403–426.
3. Celentano A, Palmieri V, Arezzi E, et al. Gender differences in left ventricular chamber and midwall systolic function in normotensive and hypertensive adults. *J Hypertens* 2003;21:1415–1423.
4. Cohen G, White M, Sochowski R, et al. Reference values for normal adult transesophageal echocardio-

graphic measurements. *J Am Soc Echocardiogr* 1995;8:221–230.
5. Myerson SG, Montgomery HE, World MJ, et al. Left ventricular mass: reliability of M-mode and 2-dimensional echocardiographic formulas. *Hypertension* 2002;40:673–678.
6. Armstrong WF, Pellikka PA, Ryan T, et al. Stress echocardiography: recommendations for performance and interpretation of stress echocardiography. *J Am Soc Echocardiogr* 1998;11:97–104.
7. Massie BM, Schiller NB, Ratshin RA, et al. Mitral-septal separation: a new echocardiographic index of left ventricular function. *Am J Cardiol* 1997;39:1008–1016.
8. Waggoner AD, Bierig MS. Tissue Doppler imaging: a useful echocardiographic method for the cardiac sonographer to assess systolic and diastolic ventricular function. *J Am Soc Echocardiogr* 2001;14:1143–1152.
9. Tekten T, Onbasili AO, Ceyhan C, et al. Novel approach to measure myocardial performance index: pulse wave tissue Doppler echocardiography. *Echocardiography* 2003;20:503–510.
10. Yamada H, Goh PP, Sun JP, et al. Prevalence of left ventricular diastolic dysfunction by Doppler echocardiography: clinical application of the Canadian Consensus Guidelines. *J Am Soc Echocardiogr* 2002;15: 1238–1244.
11. Yamamoto K, Nishimura RA, Burnett JC, et al. Assessment of left ventricular end-diastolic pressure by Doppler echocardiography: Contribution of duration of pulmonary venous versus mitral flow velocity curves at atrial contraction. *J Am Soc Echocardiogr* 1997;10:52–59.
12. Garcia MJ, Smedira NG, Greenberg NL, et al. Color M-mode Doppler flow propagation velocity is a preload insensitive index of left ventricular relaxation: animal and human validation. *J Am Coll Cardiol* 2000;35:201–208.
13. Thomas L, Levett K, Boyd A, et al. Compensatory changes in atrial volumes with normal aging: is atrial enlargement inevitable? *J Am Coll Cardiol* 2002;40: 1630–1635.
14. Thomas L, Levett K, Boyd A, et al. Changes in regional left atrial function with aging. Evaluation by Doppler tissue imaging. *Eur J Echocardiogr* 2003;4:92–100.
15. Poutanen T, Jokinen E, Sairanen H. Left atrial and left ventricular function in healthy children and young adults assessed by three-dimensional echocardiography. *Heart* 2003;89:544–549.
16. Crawford MH, Roldan CA. Quantitative assessment of valve thickness in normal subjects by transesophageal echocardiography. *Am J Cardiol* 2001;87:1419–1423.
17. Shively BK, Roldan CA, Gill EA, et al. Prevalence and determinants of valvulopathy in patients treated with dexfenfluramine. *Circulation* 1999;100:2161–2167.
18. Poutanen T, Tikanoja T, Sairanen H, et al. Normal aortic dimensions and flow in 168 children and young adults. *Clin Physiol Funct Imaging* 2003;23:224–229.

19. Roldan CA, Chavez J, Weist P, et al. Aortic root disease and valve disease associated with ankylosing spondylitis. *J Am Coll Cardiol* 1998;32:1397–1404.

20. Meluzin J, Spinarova L, Bakala J, et al. Pulse Doppler tissue imaging of the velocity of tricuspid annular systolic motion. *Eur Heart J* 2001;22:340–348.

21. Spencer KT, Weinert L, Lang RM. Effect of age, heart rate and tricuspid regurgitation on the Doppler echocardiographic evaluation of right ventricular diastolic function. *Cardiology* 1999;92:59–64.

22. Ozer N, Tokgozoglu L, Coplu L, et al. Echocardiographic evaluation of left and right ventricular diastolic function in patients with chronic obstructive pulmonary disease. *J Am Soc Echocardiogr* 2001;14: 557–561.

23. Arce OX, Knudson OA, Ellison MC, et al. Longitudinal motion of the atrioventricular annuli in children: reference values, growth related changes, and effects of right ventricular volume and pressure overload. *J Am Soc Echocardiogr* 2002;15:906–916.

24. Roldan CA, Shively BK, Crawford MH. Valve excrescences: prevalence, evolution and risk for cardioembolism. *J Am Coll Cardiol* 1998;30:1308–1314.

25. Iacobellis G, Assael F, Ribaudo MC, et al. Epicardial fat from echocardiography: a new method for visceral adipose tissue prediction. *Obes Res* 2003;11:304–310.

2

Coronary Artery Disease

Carlos A. Roldan

- The history and physical examination remain the cornerstone for the initial assessment of patients with known or suspected coronary artery disease (CAD).
- History in patients with CAD can be atypical, however. Up to 25% of elderly or diabetic patients have a silent myocardial infarction (MI); the magnitude of symptoms does not correlate with extent of CAD; with typical symptoms, <30% of admitted patients have an acute coronary syndrome (ACS); and the predictive value for CAD of classic angina is ≥50% in women.
- Most patients with an ACS have a normal physical examination.

- Electrocardiography (ECG) may mimic ischemic injury in acute pericarditis, left ventricular aneurysm, and early repolarization. In addition, approximately 15% to 20% of patients with ACS have a normal ECG.
- Finally, of the 5 million Americans presenting to emergency rooms with chest pain, 85% do not have ACS, but 3% to 5% with acute myocardial infarction (AMI) are discharged home.

PREVALENCE

- CAD is the most prevalent clinical problem in adult cardiology; it affects more than 12 million Americans and is the leading cause of death in the United States.

- There are at least 5 million emergency department visits per year for chest pain, and >1 million Americans experience a new or recurrent AMI each year (1,2).

ECHOCARDIOGRAPHY

Class I Indications for Use in Coronary Artery Disease

Echocardiography (echo) is of important complementary diagnostic and prognostic value to the history and physical examination and ECG in patients presenting with chest pain, ACS [ST-segment elevation MI (STEMI), non–ST-segment elevation MI (NSTEMI), and unstable angina (USA)] and in those with known chronic CAD (Table 2-1) (1–4).

Diagnosis of Coronary Artery Disease: Methods and Key Diagnostic Features

Resting Echocardiography

- Wall motion abnormalities are the *sine qua non* of myocardial ischemia or MI.
- The left ventricle (LV) is divided into 16 myocardial segments with a specific arterial supply (Table 2-2; see Chapter 1, Fig. 1-2) (4,5).
- Each segment is graded based on inward wall motion and endocardial thickening on a scale of 1 to 5, where 1 = normal, 2 = hypokinetic, 3 = akinetic, 4 = dyskinetic, and 5 = aneurysmal (Table 2-3).
- An overall wall motion score and index are the sum of each wall segment score divided by the total of segments scored. Thus, a normal overall wall motion score and index are 16 and 1, respectively. The higher the score and index, the worse the extent and severity of ischemia or MI.
- Independent of wall motion abnormalities, aortic valve sclerosis (especially if mixed nodular and diffuse sclerosis) and mitral annular sclerosis are predictive of underlying CAD (6).

Stress Echocardiography

- Comparison of resting with peak stress wall motion results in four types of wall motion

TABLE 2-1. *Class I Indications for Echocardiography in Coronary Artery Disease*

In patients with chest pain

And suspected acute myocardial ischemia, when baseline ECG is nondiagnostic and study can be obtained during pain or shortly thereafter

And severe hemodynamic instability

And clinically evident or suspected aortic valve stenosis, mitral valve prolapse, hypertrophic cardiomyopathy, or pericarditis

In patients with acute coronary syndromes for diagnosis and risk stratification

To diagnose acute myocardial ischemia or MI not evident by standard means

To assess MI size or extent of jeopardized myocardium, or both

To measure global and regional left ventricular function

Inferior MI with bedside evidence suggesting complicating right ventricular MI

To assess post-MI mechanical complications (TEE when TTE not diagnostic)

To assess the presence/extent of inducible ischemia when abnormal baseline ECG (stress echo) is present

In patients with chronic coronary artery disease

To diagnose myocardial ischemia in symptomatic individuals (stress echo)

To assess functional significance of coronary lesions for planning percutaneous coronary intervention (stress echo)

To assess restenosis after revascularization in patients with atypical recurrent symptoms (stress echo)

To assess myocardial viability (hibernating myocardium) for planning revascularization (dobutamine stress echo)

To assess ventricular function to guide institution and modification of drug therapy

ECG, electrocardiography; MI, myocardial infarction; TEE, transesophageal echocardiography; TTE, transthoracic echocardiography.

Modified from Cheitlin MD, Armstrong WF, Aurigemma GP, et al. ACC/AHA/ASE guideline update for the clinical application of echocardiography: summary article. *J Am Coll Cardiol* 2003;42:954–970.

response and corresponding clinical scenarios: (a) absent or low likelihood of CAD, (b) ischemia without MI, (c) ischemic viable myocardium (stunned or hibernating), or (d) MI with nonviable myocardium (Table 2-4) (7).

- The diagnostic accuracy of stress echo in the detection of CAD increases as (a) the severity and extent of CAD increase, (b) the severity of wall motion or number of asynergic seg-

TABLE 2-2. *Left Ventricular Wall Segments and Corresponding Coronary Artery Supply*

Left ventricular wall segment	Coronary artery supply
Basal, mid-, and apical anterior	LAD
Basal, mid-, and apical anterior septum	LAD
Apical lateral	LAD
Basal and mid-anterolateral	LAD/LCX
Basal and mid-inferior	RCA
Basal and mid-inferior septum	RCA
Apical inferior	RCA/LAD
Basal and mid-inferolateral	LCX

LAD, left anterior descending artery; LCX, left circumflex artery; RCA, right coronary artery.

ments increases, and (c) the predicted maximal heart rate is achieved or exceeded.

Assessment of Myocardial Viability

- Dobutamine echo is the most commonly used technique for assessment of myocardial viability (8).
- A resting hypokinetic or akinetic segment that improves in wall motion and endocardial thickening with low dose dobutamine ($\leq$10 µg/kg/min) but deteriorates at higher dose ("biphasic response") indicates *"viable ischemic myocardium with a flow limiting coronary artery stenosis."*
- A resting hypokinetic or akinetic wall that shows sustained (low-dose and high-dose) improvement in wall motion and endocardial thickening indicates *"viable nonischemic myocardium with a nonflow limiting coronary artery stenosis."*
- An akinetic, thin, and hyperreflectant segment with no change with dobutamine indicates *"nonviable myocardium."*

Resting Echocardiography in Patients with Suspected Acute Coronary Syndromes

Key Diagnostic Features

- Segmental wall motion abnormalities occur within 30 minutes of a coronary artery occlusion and before chest pain, ischemic ECG changes, and elevation of myocardial isoenzymes.
- In patients with chest pain, a new or worsening (transient or persistent) wall motion abnormality indicates myocardial ischemia or MI with high sensitivity, specificity, and predictive value (9,10).
- Resting echo detects wall motion abnormalities in 90% to 100% of patients with STEMI and identifies the culprit coronary artery (concordance with angiography of >80%) in 75% to 85% of those with NSTEMI, and only in 20% of patients with USA (11). Thus, absence of wall motion abnormalities during chest pain indicates low likelihood of AMI.
- In patients with suspected ACS and technically difficult echo images, cavity-enhancing contrast agents are of important value in the recognition of wall motion abnormalities (Fig. 2-1).

Key Prognostic Features

- In patients with USA, new or worsening left ventricular systolic dysfunction predicts severe CAD with extensive areas of jeopardized ischemic myocardium (9,10).
- A wall motion score index >1.5 or $\geq$4 abnormal segments in the distribution of an MI-related artery or in remote areas are highly predictive of large MI or multivessel CAD, respectively.
- A wall motion score index >1.5 or left ventricular ejection fraction (LVEF) $\leq$40% indi-

TABLE 2-3. *Scoring System for Grading Left Ventricular Wall Motion*

Score	Wall motion	Systolic wall motion	Endocardial thickening
1	Normal	Normal	Normal (>30%)
2	Hypokinesis	Reduced	Reduced (<30%)
3	Akinesis	Absent or reduced if dragged by other normal walls	Absent; thinning and hyperreflectance are common
4	Dyskinesis	Outward	Thinning and hyperreflectance in most cases
5	Aneurysmal	Diastolic deformity	Absent and thinning

TABLE 2-4. *Patterns of Left Ventricular Wall Motion on Stress Echocardiography and Clinical Implications*

Wall motion at rest	Wall motion at peak stress	Clinical implication
Normal wall excursion and endocardial thickening	Hyperdynamic and symmetric wall thickening	Absent or very low likelihood of coronary artery disease
Normal wall excursion and endocardial thickening	Hypokinetic, akinetic, uncommonly dyskinetic	Ischemia without MI
Wall hypokinesis or akinesis with partial or full endocardial thickening	Augmented, hypokinetic, akinetic or dyskinetic	Viable stunned (if augmented), ischemic (if worsens), or hibernating myocardium (if a biphasic response noted)
Akinetic and thinned wall	Akinetic or dyskinetic	Transmural MI and no viability

MI, myocardial infarction.

cates higher in-hospital post-MI angina, MI extension or expansion, post-MI mechanical complications, ventricular arrhythmias, heart failure, cardiogenic shock, and death.

- Patients with moderate to severe left ventricular systolic dysfunction have three times higher mortality than those with normal left ventricular function, even in the presence of a similar extent of CAD.

- Thus, resting echo in patients with ACS identifies those who would benefit from aggressive medical therapy, urgent cardiac catheterization, and percutaneous or surgical coronary revascularization.

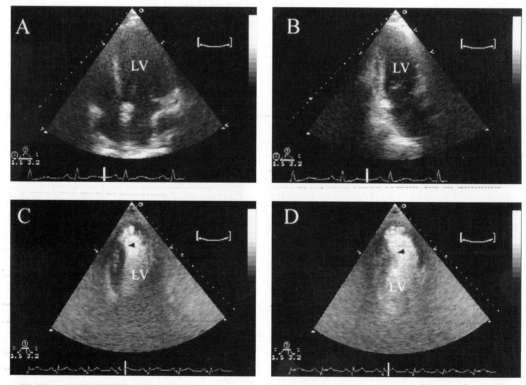

FIG. 2-1. Cavity-contrast agents and wall motion abnormalities. **A,B:** Technically difficult transthoracic echocardiographic apical four-chamber and two-chamber views, precluding detection of wall motion abnormalities in a patient with unstable angina. Corresponding panels **C** and **D** with a cavity-enhancing contrast agent demonstrate a hinge point (*arrowheads*) and akinesis of apical septum, apical inferior, and apical segments. LV, left ventricle.

Resting Echocardiography for Post–Myocardial Infarction Patients: Key Diagnostic Features

Salvaged or Jeopardized Myocardium

- The comparison of resting wall motion abnormalities or perfusion defects by myocardial contrast echo before and after reperfusion interventions determines the extent of salvaged myocardium at risk for recurrent ischemia or MI.
- Post–reperfusion therapy, myocardial stunning can resolve within 3 to 5 days. Thus, improvement of left ventricular wall motion and function on predischarge echo after an anterior MI may indicate no need for long-term anticoagulation.
- Persistent significant wall motion abnormalities with thinning or hyperreflectance, left ventricular aneurysm, or LVEF ≤35% suggest large MI. In these patients, aggressive afterload reduction therapy for left ventricular remodeling is needed.

Post–Myocardial Infarction Ischemia, Extension, or Expansion

- *Post-MI angina:* transient or persistent worsening of wall motion abnormalities in the MI or non-MI–related artery distribution without myocardial isoenzymes re-elevation.
- *Post-MI extension:* re-elevation of myocardial isoenzymes in addition to new or worse wall motion abnormalities.
- *Post-MI expansion:* an increased area of wall thinning in the infarct zone; it is progressive within 7 days post-MI. That may lead to aneurysm and/or thrombus formation, wall rupture, recurrent ischemia, heart failure, and ventricular arrhythmias.

Right Ventricular Infarction

- Right ventricular MI occurs in 25% to 30% of patients with posteroinferior MI.
- Echo findings include right ventricular dilatation and dysfunction, abnormal motion of the right ventricular free wall, tricuspid regurgitation of variable severity, paradoxical septal motion, plethoric inferior vena cava (right atrial hypertension), and, rarely, shunting from the right atrium to the left atrium through a patent foramen ovale.

- Patients with right ventricular MI have an increased incidence of heart failure, mechanical complications, and mortality independent of the extent of left ventricular dysfunction (12).

Left Ventricular Diastolic Dysfunction

In patients with ACS with or without clinical heart failure, left ventricular diastolic dysfunction ranges from impaired relaxation to decreased left ventricular compliance.

Impaired Left Ventricular Relaxation

Impaired left ventricular relaxation manifests as a decrease in E wave velocity, prolongation of E deceleration time (>160 msec), E/A ratio <1, and prolongation of the isovolumic relaxation time (IVRT) to >90 msec.

Decreased Left Ventricular Compliance

- Pseudonormal mitral inflow pattern: E velocity increase, A velocity decrease, E deceleration time shortens (140 to 160 msec), and E/A ratio is 1.0 to 1.5.
- Restrictive mitral inflow pattern: high E/A ratio (>1.5), short E deceleration time (<140 msec), and short IVRT (<110 msec).
- Abnormal pulmonary veins' inflow:
  - A decreased or absent pulmonary vein systolic inflow, a predominant diastolic inflow, and an atrial reversal velocity of longer duration than the mitral A velocity.
  - The restrictive mitral and pulmonary vein inflows are predictive of high left ventricular filling pressure or pulmonary capillary wedge >20 mm Hg and are independent predictors of cardiac death (13).
- Tissue Doppler:
  - A decrease in the pulsed wave systolic and diastolic myocardial velocities of the basal lateral and septal walls has been shown to correlate with left ventricular systolic and diastolic dysfunction in post-MI patients.
  - A lack of increase in systolic velocities from baseline to peak dobutamine dose or peak exercise has demonstrated high sensitivity and specificity for detection of ischemia and is probably superior to the development of wall motion abnormalities (14,15).

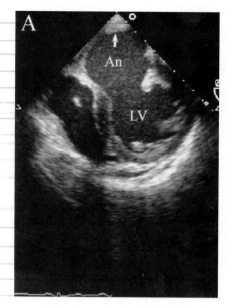 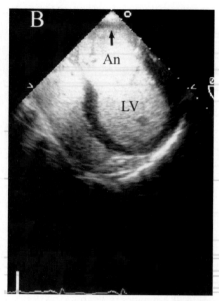

FIG. 2-2. Left ventricular aneurysm with thrombi. **A:** Transesophageal echocardiographic (TEE) short-axis view of the left ventricle in a patient post–inferior wall myocardial infarction with a stroke and a technically difficult transthoracic echocardiography demonstrates marked inferior and inferoseptal walls' outward diastolic deformity diagnostic of an aneurysm (An) with a highly suspected well-layered or flat thrombi (*arrow*). **B:** Similar TEE view with a cavity-enhancing contrast agent confirms the left ventricular aneurysm and delineates a flat-filling defect in the inferior wall consistent with thrombi (*arrow*). LV, left ventricle.

■ Color M-mode propagation velocity: Color M-mode propagation velocity of the left ventricular filling is decreased (normal range, 40–80 cm/sec) in patients with ischemic left ventricular diastolic dysfunction (see Chapter 4, Figs. 4-5 and 4-6).

Left Ventricular Aneurysm

■ Left ventricular aneurysm is defined as an outward diastolic and systolic deformity of the thinned and scarred infarcted area (Fig. 2-2). Its incidence ranges from 8% to 22%; it occurs predominantly (>90%) at the apex and after anterior MI; and it generally occurs within the first week post-AMI.

■ Patients with a left ventricular aneurysm have a high risk for thrombus formation and are at increased risk for in-hospital and 1-year mortality.

■ Transthoracic echocardiography (TTE) has a sensitivity of >90% for detecting a left ventricular aneurysm.

Left Ventricular Thrombus

■ Left ventricular thrombi occur most commonly (>90%) within the first week after a STEMI, with a higher incidence in anterior than in inferior or lateral MI (>20% vs. 1%, respectively); they most commonly occur at the left ventricular apex and are almost always associated with an apical aneurysm or apical wall akinesis or dyskinesis (Fig. 2-3).

■ Predictors of left ventricular thrombus formation include a high (>1.5) wall motion score index, high left ventricular end-systolic and end-diastolic volumes, and an EF ≤40% (16).

■ A left ventricular thrombus appears as a distinct mass that protrudes into the left ventricular cavity and can be sessile and of oval shape; pedunculated and mobile; or flat, mimicking left ventricular endocardium (Figs. 2-2, 2-3, and 14-1).

■ A recently formed thrombus has echoreflectance similar to that of the myocardium. An

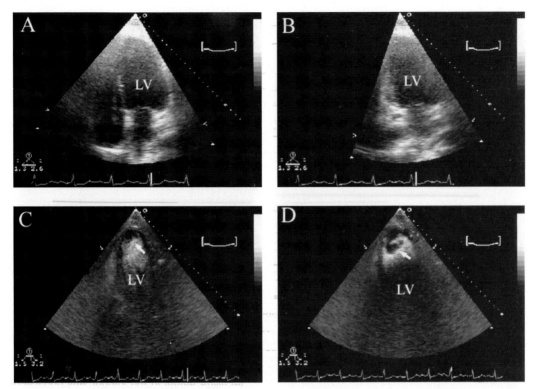

FIG. 2-3. Left ventricular thrombi. Technically difficult transthoracic echocardiographic apical four-chamber **(A)** and two-chamber views **(B)** in a patient post–anterior myocardial infarction and peripheral embolism precluding adequate assessment of wall motion abnormalities and the exclusion of left ventricular thrombi. Corresponding panels **C** and **D** with the use of a cavity-enhancing contrast agent demonstrate left ventricular apical segments' akinesis with a large, irregular, multilobar, apical-filling defect consistent with an apical thrombi (*arrows*). LV, left ventricle.

old thrombus has a heterogeneous, increased echoreflectance and rarely can be calcified.

- A mobile thrombus is associated with higher risk of cardioembolism.
- TTE has a sensitivity of 90% to 95% and a specificity of 85% to 95% for detection of left ventricular thrombus and is higher with the use of 3.5-MHz and 5-MHz transducers, harmonic imaging, and left ventricular cavity-enhancing contrast agents.
- Current use of cavity-enhancing contrast agents has improved the sensitivity and especially the specificity of echo for detection of left ventricular thrombi.
- With the use of a cavity-enhancing contrast, a thrombus appears as a discrete filling defect in continuity with abnormal (akinetic or dyskinetic) endocardium, whereas a bridging tra-

beculation surrounded by contrast appears as a linear filling defect that separates from a normal or abnormal endocardium during systole (Figs. 2-4 and 14-2).

Pericarditis

- Pericarditis occurs within 3 to 10 days post-MI, with an incidence up to 25% in large STEMI (lower in patients treated with thrombolytic therapy or primary angioplasty or stenting) and is associated with small-sized to moderate-sized and generally loculated effusions.
- Pericarditis ≥2 weeks post-MI suggests Dressler's syndrome, which is associated with small to large circumferential pericardial effusions and, rarely, cardiac tamponade.

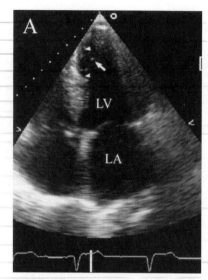 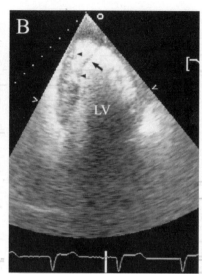

FIG. 2-4. Anteroseptal myocardial infarction and suspected apical thrombi. **A:** This apical transthoracic echocardiographic four-chamber view demonstrates akinesis with thinning and hyperreflectance of the apical septum and apex (*arrowheads*). An ill-defined apical structure, a portion of which is seen in this figure (*arrow*), could not be clearly differentiated as thrombi or an apical trabeculation. **B:** With the use of a cavity-enhancing contrast agent, a linear or band-like structure (*arrow*) is seen traversing the left ventricle from the akinetic (*arrowheads*) mid-distal septum to the apex. These findings are consistent with an apical bridging trabeculation rather than a thrombi. LA, left atrium.

■ Echo is highly sensitive for detection of post-MI loculated or circumferential pericardial effusions (17).

Detection of Mechanical Complications of Post–Myocardial Infarction: Key Diagnostic Features

Ischemic Mitral Regurgitation and Papillary Muscle Rupture

■ The incidence of ischemic mitral regurgitation (MR) in post-MI patients is approximately 20%, is similar in anterior and inferior MI, and is most commonly mild to moderate, but it is associated with an increased short-term and long-term mortality.

■ In inferior MI, the ischemic or infarcted posteromedial papillary muscle causes tethering and decreased mobility of the medial half, predominantly of the posterior mitral leaflet, leading to leaflet malcoaptation, relative anterior leaflet prolapse or pseudoprolapse, and an eccentric, posterolaterally directed MR jet (Fig. 2-5).

■ In anterior MI, left ventricular dilatation and dysfunction lead to downward and lateral displacement of both papillary muscles, incomplete but symmetric leaflets malcoaptation, and central MR.

■ When papillary muscle rupture is partial, prolapse of one or both mitral leaflets can be demonstrated. When rupture is complete, MR is severe, and the involved mitral leaflet with a portion of its papillary muscle becomes flail or prolapses freely into the left atrium (Fig. 2-6).

■ TTE underestimates the severity of eccentric MR jets; therefore, TEE is the test of choice if significant MR is suspected clinically or by TTE.

Ventricular Septal Defect

■ Ventricular septal defects (VSDs) occur most commonly in the apical posterior and apical anterior septum, frequently with a serpiginous course. They are most commonly single defects.

■ VSDs are best visualized from TTE parasternal short-axis view below the level of the papillary muscles and from apical or subcostal

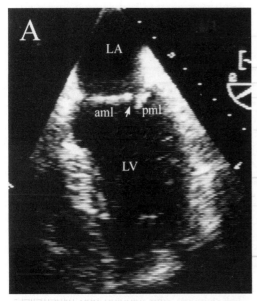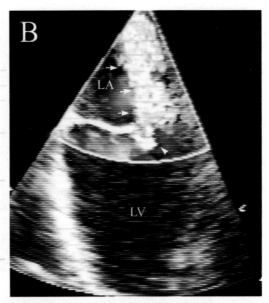

FIG. 2-5. Ischemic mitral valve pseudoprolapse and mitral regurgitation. **A:** This transesophageal echocardiographic four-chamber view shows tethering of the posterior mitral leaflet (pml) and asymmetric and incomplete leaflets' malcoaptation (*arrow*), leading to pseudoprolapse of the anterior mitral leaflet (aml). **B:** Severe mitral regurgitation was demonstrated by color Doppler with a highly eccentric and posterolaterally directed jet extending to the pulmonary veins (*arrows*). Also, note the large flow convergence zone (*arrowhead*). LA, left atrium; LV, left ventricle.

four-chamber views with anterior or posterior angulation for anterior and posterior defects, respectively (Fig. 2-7).

- The associated acute right ventricular volume overload leads to right ventricular dilatation and dysfunction, paradoxical septal motion, and right atrial hypertension and dilatation (18).
- The sensitivity of TTE and TEE color Doppler for VSD detection ranges from 86% to 95% and >95%, respectively. The width of the color Doppler jet correlates with the defect size at surgery or pathology.

Free Wall Rupture

- Free wall rupture occurs more commonly in patients with a posterolateral MI (circumflex artery occlusion) and in those with unsuccessful thrombolytic therapy (5.9% vs. 0.5%) (19).
- It manifests as a hemopericardium (frequently with intrapericardial densities or clots) and cardiac tamponade, with frequent compression of the left heart chambers.

Pseudoaneurysm

- Pseudoaneurysm is a myocardial rupture contained by pericardial adhesions, which form a pouch that communicates with the LV (Fig. 2-8).
- Pseudoaneurysm is characterized by a narrow neck, with a neck to maximum diameter ratio of <0.5, flow in and out of the pericardial space, abnormal swirling flow within the pseudoaneurysm, and an infrequently visualized myocardial tear.
- Echo is highly sensitive for detection of left ventricular free wall rupture and left ventricular pseudoaneurysm (19).

Resting and Stress Echocardiography after Treatment of Acute Coronary Syndromes: Key Diagnostic and Prognostic Features

- In patients with chest pain seen in the emergency room or admitted for further evaluation, a positive exercise or dobutamine echo is predictive of increased early and 6-month rates of recurrent nonfatal MI, USA, coronary

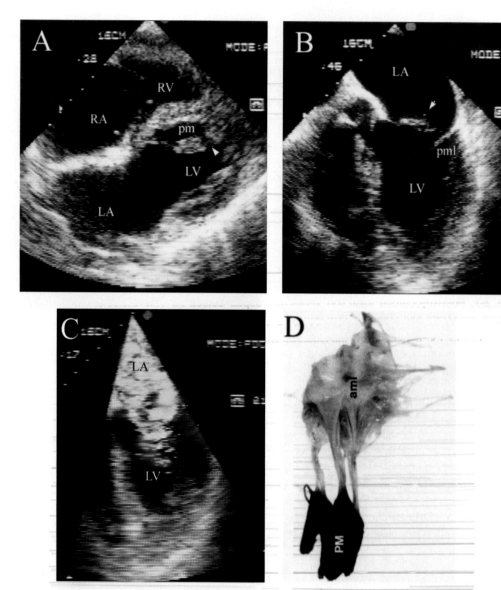

FIG. 2-6. Post–myocardial infarction papillary muscle rupture. **A:** This transthoracic echocardiography subcostal four-chamber view shows complete rupture of the posteromedial papillary muscle (pm) (*arrowhead*). **B:** This transesophageal echocardiographic four-chamber view demonstrates a flail anterior mitral leaflet with a portion of the posteromedial papillary muscle attached (*arrow*). **C:** Severe mitral regurgitation by color Doppler. **D:** Completely transected posteromedial papillary muscle (PM) with a normal morphology of the anterior mitral leaflet. aml, anterior mitral leaflet; LA, left atrium; LV, left ventricle; pml, posterior mitral leaflet; RA, right atrium; RV, right ventricle.

revascularization, and cardiac death (Table 2-5) (5,20).

- In patients with AMI or USA, a wall motion score index ≥1.5, EF ≤45%, or MR severity >2 on resting echo have increased risk of car-

diac death, recurrent USA, and nonfatal MI or congestive heart failure over a 2-year follow-up period (Table 2-5) (9,11).

- In post-MI patients, a left atrial volume index of >32 mL/m² (normal 20 ± 6 mL/m²) is a

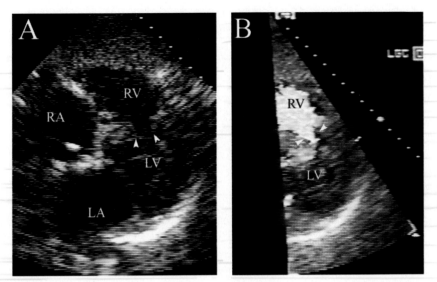

FIG. 2-7. Post–myocardial infarction ventricular septal defect. **A:** This transthoracic echocardio-graphic subcostal four-chamber view shows a large (>1 cm) ventricular septal defect located at the basal–mid-inferior septum (*arrowheads*). **B:** Color Doppler confirms a left to right communication (*arrowheads*). LA, left atrium; LV, left ventricle; RA, right atrium; RV, right ventricle.

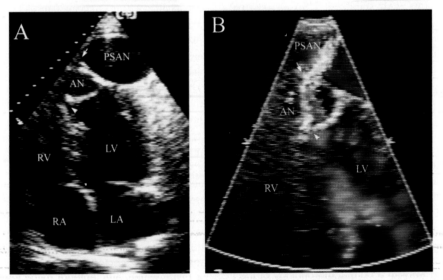

FIG. 2-8. Post–myocardial infarction left ventricular pseudoaneurysm (PSAN). **A:** This transthoracic echocardiographic apical four-chamber view shows dehiscence (*arrowhead*) of a patched apical aneu-rysm (AN) with subsequent rupture (*arrow*) and the formation of a PSAN. **B:** Color Doppler demon-strates bidirectional flow between the left ventricle (LV) and AN (*arrowhead*) and the AN and PSAN (*arrow*). LA, left atrium; RA, right atrium; RV, right ventricle.

TABLE 2-5. *Diagnostic Value of Echocardiography for Myocardial Ischemia or Viability and Future Cardiac Events in Patients with Chest Pain, Unstable Angina, and Myocardial Infarction*

Clinical scenario/technique	Sensitivity (%)	Specificity (%)	PPV (%)	NPV (%)
Unstable angina/pacing TTE	88–95	87–91	95–97	67–87
Chest pain or acute MI/resting echo	47–94	53–99	31–91	90–99
Post-MI ischemia/exercise echo	55–82	67–95	44–94	83–100
Post-MI ischemia/dipyridamole	63–93	78–92	43–95	84–97
Post-MI ischemia/DSE	68–82	80–98	65–86	85–88
Post-MI viability/DSE	74–97	73–96	67–91	77–94
Post-MI viability/low level exercise	81	92	95	73
Prognosis/resting or stress echo[a]: WMSI >1.5–2.0, ≥4 abnormal segments, myocardial viability (biphasic response), remote asynergy, LVEF <45%, or MR >2	79–97	17–90	24–89	82–98

DSE, dobutamine stress echocardiography; LVEF, left ventricular ejection fraction; MI, myocardial infarction; MR, mitral regurgitation; NPV, negative predictive value; PPV, positive predictive value; TTE, transthoracic echocardiography; WMSI, wall motion score index.

[a]Predicts death, recurrent unstable angina or MI, heart failure, cardiogenic shock, arrhythmias, or revascularization.

---

powerful predictor of all-cause mortality and remains an independent predictor after adjustment for clinical factors, left ventricular systolic function, and Doppler parameters of diastolic dysfunction (21).

■ In patients with stabilized USA, a positive predischarge exercise echo predicts a 20% risk of cardiac death, nonfatal MI, or late (>3 months) revascularization over a 2-year period, as compared to a <5% rate of events among those with a negative test (22).

■ A stress echo 1 to 3 weeks after an uncomplicated NSTEMI or STEMI identifies the following three groups:

   ◆ Sixty percent of patients with viable but ischemic myocardium: Unless revascularized, these patients have a 5% to 10% rate of cardiac death or MI; a 10% to 30% rate of USA; and a 20% to 40% rate of revascularization over a 1-year to 2-year follow-up period (23,24).

   ◆ Twenty percent to 30% of patients with myocardial viability but no ischemia: A sustained improvement in wall motion has high sensitivity (>80%), specificity (>75%), and predictive value (>80%) for a patent artery (TIMI 2 or 3 antegrade flow with <30% residual stenosis), and recovery of regional wall motion and LVEF at 1-month and 6-month follow-up (8,24).

   ◆ Ten percent to 20% of patients with no viability and no ischemia have the best prognosis.

Stress Echocardiography in Chronic Coronary Artery Disease

Key Diagnostic Features

■ In patients with chronic stable angina, stress echo can localize a *de novo* native stenosed vessel and restenosis of a native coronary artery after angioplasty or stent placement; it can also detect disease of a saphenous vein or arterial bypass graft and define the severity and extent of ischemia.

■ The overall sensitivity, specificity, and predictive value of stress echo is >80%. The diagnostic accuracy of the test varies, however, according to the clinical characteristics of the population studied, degree and extent of CAD, stress modality used, target heart rate achieved, time of imaging, use of harmonic imaging, and the severity of test positivity.

■ The overall sensitivity, specificity, and predictive value of treadmill or bicycle exercise, dobutamine, adenosine, and high-dose dipyridamole echo are similar (Table 2-6).

   ◆ If one segment is involved or a wall motion deteriorates by one grade, the positive predictive value for CAD is ≤85% as compared to ≥95% if four or more segments are involved or if wall motion deteriorates two or more grades.

   ◆ The sensitivity of the test is <70% or >85% if the maximum heart rate achieved is <75% or >85%, respectively (22); when a major vessel

TABLE 2-6. *Diagnostic Value of Stress Echocardiography in Chronic Ischemic Heart Disease*

Test	Overall sensitivity (%)	Sensitivity 1VD (%)	Sensitivity MVD (%)	Specificity (%)	PPV (%)	NPV (%)
TM	73–97	59–93	73–100	64–100	90–100	44–87
SBE	76–93	70–84	80–100	80–94	90–96	58–85
UBE	71–93	61–93	80–95	78–96	86–97	50–93
DSE	54–96	50–95	77–96	66–100	65–96	52–88
Dipyridamole	55–93	33–88	76–93	76–96	44–72	84–99
Adenosine	45–85	39–80	74–85	76–100	—	—
Pacing TTE	83–95	75–80	88–95	76–91	95–97	67–87
Pacing TEE	86–93	69–85	82–93	89–100	—	—

1VD, one-vessel disease; DSE, dobutamine stress echocardiography; MVD, multivessel disease; NPV, negative predictive value; PPV, positive predictive value; SBE, supine bicycle exercise; TEE, transesophageal echocardiography; TM, treadmill; TTE, transthoracic echocardiography; UBE, upright bicycle exercise.

stenosis is >70% and proximally located; or when multivessel CAD is present (25,26).

♦ With supine or upright bicycle exercise, the detection and extent of ischemia are also slightly higher than with treadmill exercise because images are obtained at peak exercise and at maximum heart rate achieved (27).

♦ The sensitivity of dipyridamole echo is higher with high-dose (0.84 mg/kg) as compared to low-dose (0.56 mg/kg) dipyridamole. Similarly, adenosine echo using 0.18 mg/kg/min and atropine has higher sensitivity and specificity for detecting CAD as compared to 0.14 mg/kg/min.

♦ Second harmonic imaging as compared to fundamental imaging and cavity-enhancing contrast agents during stress echo improves endocardial resolution, especially of the lateral and anterior walls; improves interobserver agreement in assessing wall motion; and increases the sensitivity of the test without affecting its specificity (28,29).

♦ The diagnostic value of harmonic imaging is further improved when used with intravenous contrast agents containing perfluorocarbon (29,30).

Key Prognostic Features

■ Development on stress echo of multiple (two or more) wall motion abnormalities at a low workload, transient left ventricular dilatation, and decrease in global left ventricular function suggests severe multivessel or left main CAD and a higher likelihood of future cardiac events.

■ In patients with chronic stable angina, a positive stress echo predicts a 10% to 20% rate/year of USA, MI, need for percutaneous or surgical revascularization, heart failure, or cardiac death as compared to 1% to 5% in those with a negative test (31).

■ A positive pharmacologic stress echo in patients with known or suspected CAD undergoing vascular surgery bears a >20% operative risk of angina, MI, CABG, or death as compared to <7% in those with a negative test.

♦ Patients with the highest risk (>40% postoperative events) are those with ischemia at <60% of predicted maximum heart rate; at intermediate risk (<10% events) are those with ischemia at >60% of predicted heart rate; and at low risk (0% events) are those with no ischemia (31,32).

Ischemic Cardiomyopathy: Key Diagnostic Features

■ Ischemic cardiomyopathy manifests on echo with multiple regional wall motion abnormalities corresponding to a single (e.g., left anterior descending artery) or multiple coronary artery distributions.

■ Wall akinesis or dyskinesis with thinning and hyperreflectance is highly specific for CAD.

■ In patients with global left ventricular hypokinesis without wall thinning or hyperreflectance, resting echo cannot distinguish an ischemic from a nonischemic or a mixed cardiomyopathy.

■ With low-dose dobutamine echo (5–10 µg/kg/min), a biphasic response or continuous wall thickening and contraction (myocardial contractile reserve) indicates a chronically ischemic (hibernating) myocardium.

■ Patients with myocardial contractile reserve in five or more segments who undergo revascularization have a >90% survival at 2 to 3 years as compared to 50% to 80% if treated medically.

■ Patients with no myocardial viability who undergo revascularization have a similarly high 2-year mortality (approximately 20%) when compared to those treated medically (33).

■ A resting end-diastolic wall thickness of >0.6 cm has a sensitivity of 94% and a specificity of 48% for recovery of wall motion after revascularization. The combination of wall thickness and contractile reserve during dobutamine infusion improves the specificity of the test to 77% (34).

■ A sustained and global contractile improvement with dobutamine (>10 µg/kg/min) may indicate a nonischemic cardiomyopathy and a better outcome than an ischemic or biphasic response (35).

■ Patients with ischemic cardiomyopathy with left ventricular systolic dysfunction and a blunted or no contractile reserve have the worst prognosis.

Pitfalls of Resting and Stress Echocardiography in Coronary Artery Disease

■ Approximately 5% to 10% of patients undergoing resting echo and up to 15% of those undergoing stress echo may have limited visualization of myocardial segments for accurate interpretation.

■ The sensitivity of resting echo for detecting wall motion abnormalities progressively decreases as the amount of time between resolution of chest pain and acquisition of images increases.

■ Resting echo lacks sensitivity for detection of wall motion abnormalities when a subendocardial infarction involves <20% of the myocardial thickness.

■ Resting echo cannot accurately separate acute ischemia or MI from a recent or old MI or from myocarditis or nonischemic cardiomyopathy.

■ In patients with conduction disturbances (left bundle-branch block or ventricular-paced rhythm), the associated paradoxical septal motion may be misclassified as ischemic wall motion abnormality.

■ Endocardial thinning and scarring are specific (but not sensitive) signs of infarction or ischemia.

■ Exercise echo may fail to detect wall motion abnormalities if there is a significant delay (>1 min) in performing the peak stress study.

   ◆ Dobutamine or exercise echo have lower sensitivity in women than in men, especially in patients with single-vessel disease (35).

   ◆ The sensitivity of stress echo is low for single-vessel CAD (especially for circumflex disease), in patients with left ventricular hypertrophy, and in those with small LV.

REFERENCES

1. Ryan TJ, Anderson JL, Antman EM, et al. ACC/AHA guidelines for the management of patients with acute myocardial infarction. *J Am Coll Cardiol* 1999;34:890–911.

2. Braunwald E, Antman EM, Beasley JW, et al: ACC/AHA guidelines for the management of patients with unstable angina and non-ST-segment elevation myocardial infarction. *J Am Coll Cardiol* 2000;36:970–1062.

3. Gibbons RJ, Chatterjee K, Daley J, et al. ACC/AHA/ACP-ASIM guidelines for the management of patients with chronic stable angina. *J Am Coll Cardiol* 1999;33:2092–2197.

4. Cheitlin MD, Armstrong WF, Aurigemma GP, et al. ACC/AHA/ASE guideline update for the clinical application of echocardiography: summary article. *J Am Coll Cardiol* 2003;42:954–970.

5. Yao SS, Qureshi E, Sherrid MV, et al. Practical applications in stress echocardiography: risk stratification and prognosis in patients with known or suspected ischemic heart disease. *J Am Coll Cardiol* 2003;42:1084–1090.

6. Tolstrup K, Crawford MH, Roldan CA. Morphologic characteristics of aortic valve sclerosis by transesophageal echocardiography: importance for the prediction of coronary artery disease. *Cardiology* 2002;98:154–158.

7. Colon PJ 3rd, Guarisco JS, Murgo J, et al. Utility of stress echocardiography in the triage of patients with atypical chest pain from the emergency department. *Am J Cardiol* 1998;82:1282–1284.

8. Bolognese L, Buonamicic P, Cerisano G, et al. Early dobutamine echocardiography predicts improvement in regional and global left ventricular function after reperfused acute myocardial infarction without residual stenosis of the infarct-related artery. *Am Heart J* 2000;139:153–163.

9. Stein JH, Neumann A, Preston LM, et al. Improved risk stratification in unstable angina: identification of patients at low risk for in-hospital cardiac events by

admission echocardiography. *Clin Cardiol* 1998;21: 725–730.

10. Mohler ER 3rd, Ryan T, Segar DS, et al Clinical utility of troponin T levels and echocardiography in the emergency department. *Am Heart J* 1998;135:253–260.

11. Carluccio E, Tommasi S, Bentivoglio M, et al. Usefulness of the severity and extent of wall motion abnormalities as prognostic markers of an adverse outcome after a first myocardial infarction treated with thrombolytic therapy. *Am J Cardiol* 2000;85:411–415.

12. Mehta SR, Eikelboom JW, Natarajan MK, et al. Impact of right ventricular involvement on mortality and morbidity in patients with inferior myocardial infarction. *J Am Coll Cardiol* 2001;37:37–43.

13. Moller JE, Sondergaard E, Poulsen SH, et al. Pseudonormal and restrictive filling patterns predict left ventricular dilation and cardiac death after a first myocardial infarction: a serial color-M-mode Doppler echocardiographic study. *J Am Coll Cardiol* 2000;36: 1841–1846.

14. Madler CF, Payne N, Wilkenshoff U, et al. Non-invasive diagnosis of coronary artery disease by quantitative stress echocardiography: optimal diagnostic models using off-line tissue Doppler in the MYDISE study. *Eur Heart J* 2003;24:1584–1594.

15. Pasquet A, Armstrong G, Beachler L, et al. Use of segmental tissue Doppler velocity to quantitate exercise echocardiography. *J Am Soc Echocardiogr* 1999;12: 901–912.

16. Neskovic AN, Marinkovic J, Bojic M, et al. Predictors of left ventricular thrombus formation and disappearance after anterior wall myocardial infarction. *Eur Heart J* 1998;19:908–916.

17. Nagahama Y, Sigiura T, Takehana K, et al. The role of infarction-associated pericarditis on the occurrence of atrial fibrillation. *Eur Heart J* 1998;19:287–292.

18. Crenshaw BS, Granger LB, Brinbaum Y, et al. Risk factors, angiographic patterns and outcomes in patients with ventricular septal defects complicating acute myocardial infarction. GUSTO-I (Global Utilization of Streptokinase and TPA for Occluded Coronary Arteries) Trial Investigators. *Circulation* 2000;101:27–32.

19. Purcaro A, Costantini C, Ciampani N, et al. Diagnostic criteria and management of subacute ventricular free wall rupture complicating acute myocardial infarction. *Am J Cardiol* 1997;80:397–405.

20. Geleijnse M, Elhendy A, Kasprzak J, et al. Safety and prognostic value of early dobutamine-atropine stress echocardiography in patients with spontaneous chest pain and a non-diagnostic electrocardiogram. *Eur Heart J* 2000;21:397–406.

21. Moller JE, Hillis GS, Oh JK, et al. Left atrial volume. A powerful predictor of survival after acute myocardial infarction. *Circulation* 2003;107:2207–2212.

22. Lin SS, Lauer MS, Marwick TH. Risk stratification of patients with medically treated unstable angina using exercise echocardiography. *Am J Cardiol* 1998;82: 720–724.

23. Franklin KB, Marwick TH. Use of stress echocardiography for risk assessment of patients after myocardial infarction. *Cardiol Clin* 1999;17:521–538.

24. Previtali M, Fetiveau R, Lanzarini L, et al. Prognostic value of myocardial viability and ischemia detected by dobutamine stress echocardiography early after acute myocardial infarction treated with thrombolysis. *J Am Coll Cardiol* 1998;32:380–386.

25. Hoffmann R, Lethen H, Kuhl H, et al. Extent and severity of test positivity during dobutamine stress echocardiography. Influence on the predictive value for coronary artery disease. *Eur Heart J* 1999;20:1485–1492.

26. Tousoulis D, Loukianos R, Cokkinos P, et al. Relation between exercise and dobutamine stress-induced wall motion abnormalities and severity and location of stenosis in single-vessel coronary artery disease. *Am Heart J* 1999;138:873–879.

27. Badruddin SM, Ahmad A, Mickelson J, et al. Supine bicycle versus post-treadmill exercise echocardiography in the detection of myocardial ischemia: a randomized single-blind crossover trial. *J Am Coll Cardiol* 1999;33:1485–1490.

28. Franke A, Hoffmann R, Kuhl HP, et al. Non-contrast second harmonic imaging improves interobserver agreement and accuracy of dobutamine stress echocardiography in patients with impaired image quality. *Heart* 2000;83:133–140.

29. Mor-Avi V, Lang RM. Use of contrast enhancement for the assessment of left ventricular function. *Echocardiography* 2003;20(7):637–642.

30. Cwajg J, Xie F, O'Leary E, et al. Detection of angiographically significant coronary artery disease with accelerated intermittent imaging after intravenous administration of ultrasound contrast material. *Am Heart J* 2000;139:675–683.

31. Krivokapich J, Child JS, Walter DO, et al. Prognostic value of dobutamine stress echocardiography in predicting cardiac events in patients with known or suspected coronary artery disease. *J Am Coll Cardiol* 1999;33:708–716.

32. Das M, Pellikka P, Mahoney D, et al. Assessment of cardiac risk before nonvascular surgery: dobutamine stress echocardiography in 530 patients. *J Am Coll Cardiol* 2000;35:1647–1653.

33. Duncan AM, Francis DP, Gibson DG, et al. Differentiation of ischemic from nonischemic cardiomyopathy during dobutamine stress by left ventricular long-axis function: additional effect of left bundle-branch block. *Circulation* 2003;108:1214–1220.

34. Cwajg JM, Cwajg E, Nagueh SF, et al. End-diastolic wall thickness as a predictor of recovery of function in myocardial hibernation: relation to rest-redistribution T1–201 tomography and dobutamine stress echocardiography. *J Am Coll Cardiol* 2000;35:1152–1161.

35. Lewis JF, Lin L, McGorray S, et al. Dobutamine stress echocardiography in women with chest pain. Pilot phase data from the National Heart, Lung and Blood Institute Women's Ischemia Syndrome Evaluation (WISE). *J Am Coll Cardiol* 1999;33:1462–1468.

3

Ventricular Systolic Dysfunction

William A. Zoghbi and Juan Carlos Plana

- Evaluation of left ventricular and right ventricular systolic function is an essential part of an echocardiographic examination.
- Ventricular function can be evaluated qualitatively or quantitatively.
- Left ventricular systolic function has been more extensively evaluated and is more readily amenable to quantitation compared to right ventricular function.
- Global and regional ventricular function is assessed by evaluating endocardial motion and wall thickening. Doppler echo complements cardiac imaging by quantitating cardiac output (CO), regional function, and rate of pressure generation.

- The degree of left ventricular and right ventricular dysfunction is a powerful predictor of clinical outcomes.

DEFINITION AND ETIOLOGIES

- The most commonly used index of global ventricular systolic function is left ventricular ejection fraction (LVEF).
  - ◆ Several studies have shown that EF is among the most important prognostic parameters in cardiovascular disease.
  - ◆ A normal LVEF is ≥50%.
- Stroke volume (SV), CO, and rate of rise of left ventricular systolic pressure (dP/dt) are

also measures of systolic function and can be derived with echo and Doppler techniques.

- EF, similar to other measures of systolic or diastolic function, is load dependent.
  - ◆ For example, EF is higher than expected in significant chronic mitral regurgitation (reduced afterload), whereas EF may be reduced in acute hypertension.
  - ◆ Finally, EF alone may be misleading in conditions of severe focal regional dysfunction, such as a large left ventricular apical aneurysm with otherwise preserved regional function.
- Common etiologies of left ventricular systolic dysfunction (LVSD) include ischemic heart disease, hypertensive heart disease, valvular heart disease, primary nonischemic cardiomyopathy, infiltrative cardiomyopathy, and congenital heart disease.

ECHOCARDIOGRAPHY AND DOPPLER METHODS

- Echo with Doppler is an ideal noninvasive imaging tool to evaluate ventricular function. Indications for echo in patients with suspected or known ventricular dysfunction are listed in Table 3-1.
- Transthoracic echocardiography (TTE) is used in the majority of cases. In technically difficult studies, contrast agents improve echo images.
- With the advent of contrast, transesophageal echocardiography (TEE) is rarely performed for the sole evaluation of ventricular function.
- Various methods have been used to evaluate and quantitate ventricular systolic function (Table 3-2). Currently, the most commonly used methods are those of two-dimensional (2D) echocardiography (echo), either qualitatively or quantitatively.
- Doppler examination complements the overall evaluation by providing an independent method for quantifying SV and CO. A detailed evaluation of commonly used methods follows, with emphasis on technique, features, and pitfalls.

M-Mode

- Although M-mode echo can be used for the evaluation of ventricular function, it should be

TABLE 3-1. *Indications for Echocardiography in Patients with Suspected Systolic Dysfunction*

Valvular heart disease
Chest pain/angina/unstable angina
Risk assessment, prognosis, and assessment of therapy in acute myocardial infarction
Diagnosis, prognosis, and assessment of intervention in coronary heart disease
Suspected heart failure
Cardiomyopathies
Systemic hypertension
Screening for the presence of cardiovascular disease (genetically transmitted disease or potential heart donors)
Pulmonary disease
Critically ill patients
Critically injured patients
Congenital heart disease

used with extreme caution to evaluate global left ventricular function. This is because the limited regional function evaluation is extrapolated to global function.

- Thus, in general, M-mode can be used in conditions of normal regional function or global regional dysfunction inferred from 2D imaging.

Best Imaging Planes

- TTE: Parasternal long-axis and short-axis views.
- TEE: Transgastric long-axis and short-axis views.

TABLE 3-2. *Parameters Used in the Assessment of Regional and Global Systolic Function*

Cardiac imaging (M-mode/two-dimensional/three-dimensional)
  Left ventricular volumes/left ventricular mass
  Stroke volume/cardiac output
  Ejection fraction
  Fractional shortening/fractional area change
  Left ventricular wall stress
  Mitral E point septal separation
  Descent of the cardiac base
Echocardiography and Doppler techniques
  Stroke volume/cardiac output
  dP/dt
  Systolic time intervals
  Tei index
  Tissue Doppler (velocity, strain, and strain rate)

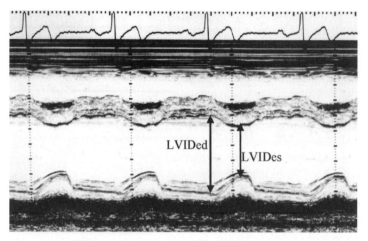

FIG. 3-1. M-mode echocardiogram showing measurements of left ventricular internal diameter at end-diastole (LVIDed) and end-systole (LVIDes). M-mode echocardiography can be used for determination of global left ventricular function only in situations of normal regional function or diffuse hypokinesis, as determined by two-dimensional echocardiography.

Diagnostic Methods

- M-mode echo allows measurement of wall thickness and ventricular internal dimensions during the cardiac cycle.
- Its high resolution facilitates tracking and recognition of the endocardial borders.
- Measurement of the left ventricle (LV) is made by positioning the ultrasound beam just beyond the mitral leaflet tips (chordal level) and as perpendicular as possible to the ventricular long axis, centering it in the short-axis view.
- Left ventricular wall thickness and dimensions are measured from leading edge to leading edge of each interface in question (1).
- Other information about systolic function can be derived with M-mode, including E point septal separation and the degree of anteroposterior motion of the aortic root.
  - ◆ With normal systolic function, the anterior mitral leaflet opens during diastole, nearly touching the interventricular septum, with a resultant small E point septal separation (<5 mm).

Diagnostic Formulas

- Fractional shortening (%) = 100 × (LVIDed – LVIDes)/LVIDed, where LVIDed and LVIDes

are the left ventricular internal diameters at end-diastole and end-systole, respectively (Fig. 3-1).
- LVEF = fractional shortening × 1.7, to be used only in normal regional function or in ventricles with diffuse hypokinesis.

Key Diagnostic Features

- In systolic dysfunction, the E point septal separation increases as a result of a combination of left ventricular dilatation and reduced motion of the anterior leaflet of the mitral valve in the setting of a reduced transmitral flow.
- The anteroposterior motion of the aortic annulus also decreases as the CO diminishes in patients with LVSD.

Pitfalls

- Overestimation of the internal diameter of the LV occurs if the M-mode ultrasound beam is oblique to the long axis of the ventricle.
- Underestimation of diameters can occur if the beam is not centered in the ventricular chamber.
  - ◆ 2D-guided imaging should be used to assure the adequate positioning of the ultrasound beam.
- With diseases that affect the symmetry of the chamber and regional function, the measurements obtained at the base of the

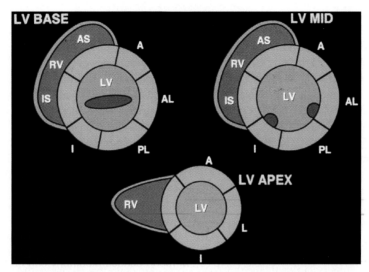

FIG. 3-2. Diagrams depicting the segmentation of the left ventricle into 17 cardiac segments. The very tip of the left ventricular apex, as the seventeenth segment, is not shown in this picture. A, anterior wall; AL, anterolateral wall; AS, anterior septum; I, inferior wall; IS, inferior septum; L, lateral wall; LV, left ventricle; PL, posterolateral wall; RV, right ventricle.

heart may not be representative of the left ventricular dimensions and function, hence altering the possibility of estimating EF based on diameters.

- E point septal separation may not reflect left ventricular function; it is increased in the presence of aortic regurgitation or reduced in acute systolic dysfunction with preserved left ventricular size.
- Because of M-mode limitations, it is highly recommended to use 2D echo and, in the near future, 3D echo to calculate ventricular dimensions, volumes, and EF.

Two-Dimensional Echocardiography

Best Imaging Planes

Transthoracic Echocardiography

- LV: parasternal long-axis and short-axis views, apical two-chamber and four-chambers views, apical long-axis view, subcostal views.
- Right ventricle (RV): parasternal long-axis and short-axis views, right ventricular inflow, apical four-chamber and subcostal views.

Transesophageal Echocardiography

- LV: four-chamber and two-chamber and long-axis from mid-esophageal view; transgastric long-axis and short-axis views.
- RV: Mid-esophageal four-chamber view; transgastric right ventricular inflow view and short-axis view.

Diagnostic Methods and Formulas

Left Ventricular Systolic Function

Qualitative and Semi-Quantitative Evaluation

- Estimation of global ventricular function is accomplished by evaluating the degree of endocardial motion and ventricular wall thickening for each myocardial segment and integrating the information from multiple tomographic planes.
- For evaluation of regional function, the LV is divided into 17 segments (2): six segments at the cardiac base (mitral valve level), six at the mid ventricle (papillary muscle level), four at the apical portion of the ventricle (no papillary muscles), and one at the very apex (Fig. 3-2).
- Regional wall motion is scored according to the recommendations of the American Society

of Echocardiography (1) as: normal or hyperdynamic function = 1, hypokinesis = 2, akinesis = 3, dyskinesis = 4, and aneurysmal = 5.

- ◆ A wall motion score index (WMSI) is an index of global left ventricular function and is derived as the sum of segmental scores divided by the number of segments evaluated. A normal WMSI is therefore 1.
- ◆ Increasing WMSI denotes worse global dysfunction and carries a poor prognosis (usually >1.4).
- ◆ A WMSI of 2 usually corresponds to an LVEF in the range of 30% to 39%.

■ Requirements for successful estimation of EF or WMSI include adequate endocardial definition, adequate visualization of the cardiac apex, and recognition and avoidance of foreshortening of the ventricle. The same principles apply during TEE examination (3); however, the cardiac apex during TEE is more difficult to image appropriately.

■ Additional parameters to consider in estimating left ventricular function also include the size and shape of the ventricle and the descent of the cardiac base. For example, for the same extent of endocardial excursion, a small ventricle has a higher EF than a large ventricle.

■ Descent of the cardiac base during systole is an index of global ventricular function. The magnitude of this motion reflects the extent of left ventricular longitudinal shortening.

- ◆ Healthy subjects have a descent of the base of >8 mm (mean, 12 ± 2 mm).
- ◆ A mitral annulus descent of <8 mm identifies patients with EF <50%, with a sensitivity of 98% and a specificity of 82% (4).

■ The degree of systolic left ventricular dysfunction is usually reported as follows:

- ◆ Mild when EF is 40% to 49%.
- ◆ Moderate when EF is 30% to 39%.
- ◆ Severe when EF <30%.
- ◆ An experienced observer can estimate EF in incremental intervals of 5% to 10%.

Pitfalls and Challenges

■ Interpreter's experience.

- ◆ The accuracy of the qualitative estimation of EF is largely dependent on the experience of the reader.

- ◆ Derivation of WMSI is more reproducible than qualitative estimation of LVEF.

■ Inadequate endocardial border definition.

- ◆ The accuracy of assessment of EF depends on adequate visualization of the endocardium.
- ◆ In technically difficult studies (e.g., in patients with chronic obstructive pulmonary disease or in intensive care units), the use of contrast for left ventricular opacification improves endocardial border delineation, estimation, and quantitation of LVEF (Fig. 3-3) (5,6).

■ Foreshortening.

- ◆ Foreshortening is a limitation in tomographic imaging in which the imaging plane does not transect the ventricle through its center. Although this can be seen from any view, it occurs frequently with apical imaging.
- ◆ The true cardiac apex may not be seen, and the ventricle then appears smaller than observed from other windows. This may lead to overestimation of global function.
- ◆ Apical foreshortening can be suspected and avoided by using a combination of apical four-chamber and two-chamber imaging—to better locate the cardiac apex—and several short-axis views.
- ◆ On TEE examination, because the true apex may not be adequately visualized, a limited TTE, focused on apical views, would complete a thorough evaluation if apical motion or pathology is in question.

■ Asynchrony and asymmetry of contraction.

- ◆ The integration of wall motion obtained from multiple tomographic views is challenging in the presence of asynchrony (e.g., intraventricular conduction delay or ventricular paced rhythm) and asymmetry of contraction (localized or multiple regional abnormalities).

Evaluation of Right Ventricular Function

■ Evaluation of right ventricular systolic function includes integration of information on right ventricular size, endocardial motion, and descent of the tricuspid annulus in systole.

■ Because the geometry of the RV is complex, evaluation of right ventricular size and function from multiple tomographic planes is recommended.

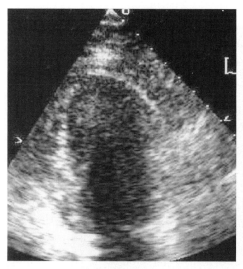 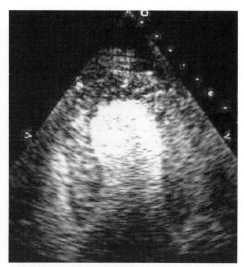

FIG. 3-3. Example of enhancement of left ventricular endocardium and definition of the endocardial border with contrast echocardiography.

◆ There is no accepted method for quantitation of right ventricular function.

◆ Available methods are those of modified Simpson's rule or fractional area change from the four-chamber window (see Method of Discs).

■ Septal motion gives a clue to the etiology of right ventricular dilatation.

  ◆ A flattened septum in both diastole and systole supports the presence of systolic pressure overload.

  ◆ Flattening of the septum in diastole only, with resolution of the deformation in systole, supports other etiologies, such as volume overload or states of elevated right ventricular diastolic pressure (e.g., right ventricular infarction), or both.

Quantitative Evaluation of Systolic Performance

Quantitative evaluation of systolic performance is performed by calculating the change in estimated left ventricular volumes or areas from end-diastole to end-systole.

Method of Discs

■ Left ventricular volumes can be calculated using the modified Simpson's rule or method of discs from orthogonal apical views (apical four-chamber and two-chamber views) (1).

■ In the method of discs, the LV is cut into a number (n) of cylinders or discs of equal height, perpendicular to the long axis of the ventricle (Fig. 3-4).

■ The volume of each cylinder is calculated as

$$V = \pi \, (ai \times bi) \, L/4n$$

where L/n is the height of the cylinder, and ai and bi are the diameters of the cylinder from the two orthogonal views.

■ Ventricular volume is then derived as the sum of the volumes of the cylinders. EF (%) is therefore derived as

$$EF = 100 \times (EDV - ESV)/EDV$$

where EDV and ESV are the end-diastolic and end-systolic volumes, respectively.

■ If only one apical view is available, a single plane method is used.

■ The left ventricular endocardial borders can be traced manually or detected automatically using acoustic quantification (Fig. 3-5).

■ Care should be taken to ensure adequate tracking of the endocardium, however, as automatic border delineation currently is still gain dependent.

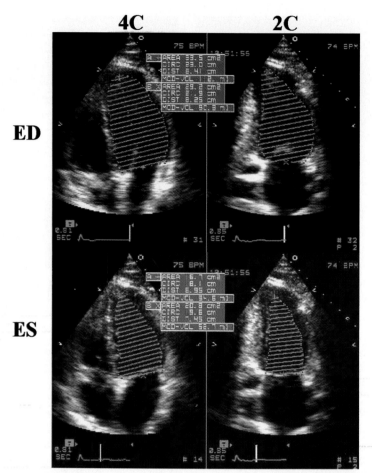

FIG. 3-4. Use of the method of discs or modified Simpson's rule in determination of left ventricular volumes and ejection fraction from the four-chamber (4C) and two-chamber (2C) views at end-diastole (ED) and end-systole (ES). This example is from a healthy individual with an ejection fraction of 56%.

Multiple Diameter Method

- The multiple diameter method is based on a simplification of the area length method (5,7) and has the advantage of using all available tomographic longitudinal views, including the parasternal views (Fig. 3-6), and avoiding areas of endocardial dropout.
- Equidistant internal diameters at the proximal third, mid-, and distal third of the LV (when available) are measured at end-diastole and end-systole, and shortening of the long axis is estimated from apical function.
- Calculation of EF is derived by computer. In the case of normal regional function or diffuse hypokinesis, derivation of EF from one

diameter (e.g., from the parasternal long axis) suffices.
- Another advantage of this method is its feasibility with TEE (8).

Diagnostic Formulas

- The mathematical basis for the simplified method for determining EF by measuring left ventricular internal dimensions is as follows (7):

$$EF = (\%\Delta D^2) + ([1 - \Delta D^2]\,[\%\Delta L])$$

where $\%\Delta D^2 = 100 \times (LVED^2 - LVES^2)/LVED^2$; $\%\Delta D^2$ = fractional shortening of the square of the minor axis; and $\%\Delta L$ = fractional shortening of the long axis, mainly

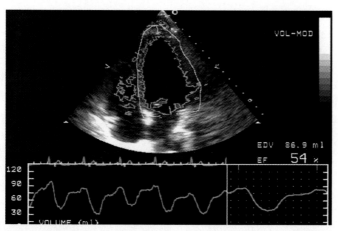

FIG. 3-5. Example of automated border detection and determination of ventricular volume and ejection fraction (EF) in a healthy individual with small end-diastolic volume (EDV). EF is 54%.

related to apical contraction as follows: 15% for normal, 5% for hypokinetic apex, 0% for akinetic, –5% for dyskinetic apex, and –10% for apical aneurysm.

■ From a practical standpoint, after delineation of representative diameters, one is prompted to estimate apical contraction as above, after which EF is determined.

Three-Dimensional Echocardiography

■ 3D echo has gradually evolved from a tedious reconstruction of tomographic images to real-time 3D imaging (9).

■ 3D echo provides a promising modality to evaluate right and left ventricular function by providing a full set of data for volume and EF calculation.

■ With this technique, tomographic cuts for evaluation of regional function and calculation of volumes and EF are sequential and parallel to each other from any window, improving the accuracy of interpretation of regional and global function.

■ Thus, limitations such as adequate evaluation of the apex and foreshortening are overcome more easily.

■ Similar to 2D, 3D echo can be combined with contrast administration for enhanced endocardial definition in difficult cases.

■ Pitfalls:
 ◆ Real-time 3D echo is still in its infancy and will undoubtedly improve in several domains.

◆ Review and processing of the information currently requires off-line processing for quantitation of volumes and EF.

◆ Image resolution is not yet similar to 2D echo.

Pulsed and Continuous Wave Doppler

■ Pulsed Doppler and continuous wave Doppler provide various parameters of systolic ventricular function. These include measurements of SV and CO, determination of dP/dt in the presence of regurgitant valvular lesions, and measurements of timing intervals of contraction and relaxation.

■ Best imaging plans: These include in TTE and TEE, all views that combine 2D imaging and Doppler flow at or close to the valve annuli.

Pulsed Doppler: Determination of Stroke Volume and Cardiac Output

■ SV and CO can be determined by evaluating cross-sectional area (CSA) of flow by 2D echo and flow velocity by Doppler.

■ Because flow area in the heart varies with the cardiac cycle, SV determination is best performed at or just proximal to a valve annulus.

■ The most accurate and reproducible site for measurement of SV is the left ventricular outflow tract (LVOT). The second best site is the

END-DIASTOLE   END-SYSTOLE

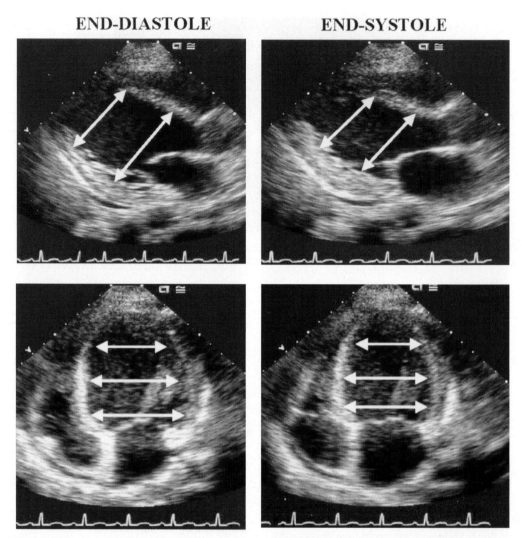

FIG. 3-6. Example of the multiple diameter method in determination of left ventricular ejection fraction. The advantage of this method is the incorporation of parasternal windows, particularly if the apical views are technically difficult. This method can also be used with transesophageal echocardiography.

mitral annulus, followed by the pulmonic annulus.

Diagnostic Methods and Formulas

- SV at any valve annulus—the least variable anatomic area of a valve apparatus—is derived as the product of CSA and the velocity time integral (VTI) of flow at the annulus (Fig. 3-7) (10).
- Assumption of a circular geometry has worked well clinically for most valves, with the exception of the tricuspid annulus. The annular diameter (d) is measured in early systole for the aortic and pulmonic annulus and in mid-diastole for the mitral annulus. Thus,

$$SV = CSA \times VTI$$
$$= \pi d^2/4 \times VTI$$
$$= 0.785 \ d^2 \times VTI$$

- CO is then derived by multiplying SV by heart rate as CO = SV × heart rate.
- Cardiac index is calculated as CO divided by body surface area in m^2 as cardiac index = CO/body surface area.

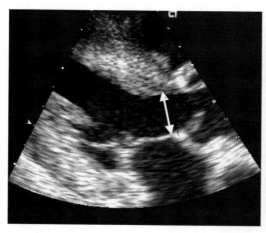 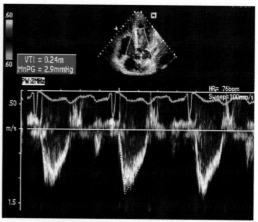

A   B

Stroke Volume = CSA X VTI

FIG. 3-7. Determination of cardiac output at the left ventricular outflow tract (LVOT). Measurement of diameter is performed from the parasternal long axis just below the aortic valve annulus in early systole **(A)**. **B:** Pulsed Doppler recording in the LVOT from the apical window is performed, and a velocity time integral (VTI) is measured. Stroke volume is determined as cross-sectional area × VTI or $\pi d^2/4$ × VTI. In this case, the stroke volume is (3.14 × 24) or 75 mL. HR, heart rate.

■ Having calculated SV, LVEF can also be calculated using a combination of Doppler and 2D measurements as

$$EF = SV/EDV$$

■ EDV can be calculated by using the method of discs (described in the section Method of Discs) or by using a simple diameter method, such as (11)

$$EDV = [\text{maximal long-axis diameter} \times \text{maximal short-axis diameter} \times 3.44] - 6$$

■ Using the principles described above, SV can be calculated for the different valves.

■ In a healthy heart, the SV measured through the different valves is equal.

■ In the presence of valvular regurgitation or an intracardiac shunt, however, calculation of volumes at two different valves also allows quantitation of the degree of regurgitation or shunting (12).

Pitfalls

Several situations can interfere with the accurate determination of the SV by Doppler echo.

■ Annulus measurement.
  ◆ The mathematic equation to calculate the area of the annulus is based on the assumption of a circular geometry. This assumption is best for the LVOT.
  ◆ Furthermore, small errors in the measurement of the diameter result in larger errors because of the quadratic relationship of the variables.

■ Placement of the Doppler sample in the LVOT.
  ◆ Caution must be exerted in the placement of the Doppler sample in the LVOT (13).
  ◆ To ensure that the Doppler sample was adequately placed, only the closing click of the aortic valve should be visualized.
  ◆ If the opening click is recorded, the Doppler sample volume is too far into the aortic valve and should be moved more apical.

■ Angle of incidence of the Doppler beam.
  ◆ Because of dependency of the Doppler shift on the angle of incidence with flow, increasing angulation (of significance if >20 degrees) leads to substantially lower estimated velocities and, hence, smaller calculated SV.

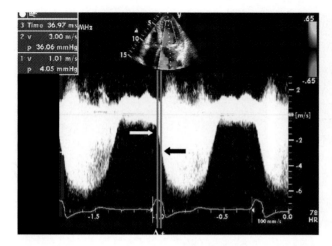

FIG. 3-8. Determination of the rate of rise of left ventricular systolic pressure (dP/dt) from the mitral regurgitation jet recording by continuous wave Doppler from the apical window in a patient with depressed systolic function. Measurement of the velocity and respective determination of pressure using the simplified Bernoulli equation is performed at 1 m/sec and 3 m/sec (*arrows*). The time duration (in seconds) between these two measurements is determined. dP/dt is derived as 32/time duration; in this case, it is 32 mm Hg/0.037 sec = 865 mm Hg/sec. HR, heart rate.

- ◆ Repositioning the transducer and ultrasound beam to yield the highest velocity at the desired site decreases this error.

Acceleration Time of Aortic Flow

- The shape of the Doppler curve in the LVOT provides important information about ventricular function.
- When systolic function is normal, the isovolumic contraction period is short, the acceleration rate of blood in early systole is fast, and the time interval from onset of flow to maximum velocity is short.
- Conversely, when left ventricular function is depressed, the isovolumic contraction period (also known as the *preejection period*) is prolonged, the acceleration of blood in early systole diminishes, and the time to peak velocity increases.

Rate of Rise of Left Ventricular Systolic Pressure

- When mitral regurgitation is present, the continuous wave Doppler velocity curve relates to the instantaneous pressure difference between the LV and the left atrium in accordance with the Bernoulli principle (14).
- dP/dt, an index of global ventricular systolic function, can therefore be estimated.

- Using the modified Bernoulli equation ($\Delta P = 4V^2$), pressure is estimated at two time points of the onset of the mitral regurgitation jet—at 1 m/sec ($\Delta P = 4$ mm Hg) and at 3 m/sec ($\Delta P = 36$ mm Hg)—and the time interval between these points is measured. $\Delta P/\Delta t$, a measure of dP/dt, is then derived using the following formula (Fig. 3-8):

$$\Delta P/\Delta t = (\text{gradient at V3} - \text{gradient at time interval/V1})$$
$$= (36-4)/\text{time interval}$$
$$= 32/\text{time interval}$$

- Qualitatively, in a ventricle with normal systolic function, the mitral regurgitant velocity rises rapidly during early systole.
- In contrast, in patients with left ventricular dysfunction, the rate of rise in ventricular pressure and, hence, the slope of rise of regurgitant velocity is reduced (14).
- A normal $\Delta P/\Delta t$ by Doppler is >1,200 mm Hg/sec.
- **Pitfalls:**
  - ◆ A requirement for this method is the presence and adequate recording of a mitral regurgitation jet by continuous wave Doppler.
  - ◆ Adequate alignment of the ultrasound beam with the jet is necessary to minimize errors in velocity.
  - ◆ Because the time interval between the two velocities is quite short in duration, a small error in measurement significantly impacts the derived parameter.

Tei Index

- In 1995, Tei et al. evaluated a new Doppler index of combined systolic and diastolic function (Tei index, or myocardial performance index) to separate patients with normal systolic function from patients with heart failure (15).
- The index is calculated with the following formula:

  Tei index = (isovolumic contraction time + isovolumic relaxation time)/ejection time

- Separation between healthy individuals and patients with dilated cardiomyopathy using the Tei index was superior to other available indexes (15). Furthermore, other studies have indicated a prognostic value of the Tei index after acute myocardial infarction (16).
- **Pitfalls:**
  - ◆ Further experience is needed with the Tei index to define its role and limitations in the evaluation of cardiac systolic function.
  - ◆ Load dependency of time intervals of ejection, isovolumic contraction, and relaxation is another pitfall.

Tissue Doppler

- Tissue Doppler, in contrast to Doppler evaluation of blood velocity, emphasizes the low velocities with high amplitude that emanate from contraction and relaxation of the heart muscle.
- Tissue Doppler can be recorded as color Doppler in the 2D imaging plane or as a pulsed spectral Doppler, at a particular site of the myocardium, or as a color M-mode.
- This methodology can be used to evaluate regional systolic and diastolic function, as well as timing of contraction and relaxation (Fig. 3-9) (17).
- Tissue Doppler technology can be used to evaluate myocardial velocities or can be processed to perform strain and strain rate imaging.
- Strain (as a percentage) is a measure of tissue deformation during the cardiac cycle ($\Delta L/Lo$), where Lo is the length of the myocardial segment at baseline and ΔL is the change in length along the axis of imaging.

- Strain rate (in sec^{-1}) is the fractional rate of deformation ($\Delta L/Lo/dt$).
- Tissue velocity in the long axis of the heart normally decreases from the cardiac base to the apex and is affected by cardiac motion and tethering.
- An advantage of strain and strain rate imaging is that they are less influenced by cardiac motion or tethering, and they change less from base to apex.
- Currently, however, a limitation of strain rate imaging is its signal to noise ratio.
- A clinical application of tissue Doppler is the evaluation of asynchronous cardiac contraction for selection of patients for and assessment of resynchronization therapy (18).

PROGNOSTIC VALUE OF SYSTOLIC DYSFUNCTION IN DIFFERENT CLINICAL SETTINGS

Asymptomatic Patients

- Congestive heart failure is a progressive disorder that begins with LVSD and culminates with symptoms from fluid overload and poor end-organ perfusion.
- Individuals in the early stages of LVSD are typically asymptomatic due to compensatory mechanisms, including the activation of the autonomic nervous systems and the release of neurohormones (19).
- Asymptomatic LVSD dysfunction has an estimated prevalence of 3% to 6%, and it is at least as common in the community as systolic heart failure (19,20).
- Because it often occurs in the absence of known cardiovascular disease, this condition may go unrecognized and undertreated.
- In randomized trials, individuals with asymptomatic LVSD have high rates of heart failure and death.
- However, very little is known about the prognosis of this condition in the community in which a substantially lower prevalence of myocardial infarction, milder degrees of systolic dysfunction, and older individuals are likely present, as compared to those enrolled in clinical trials.

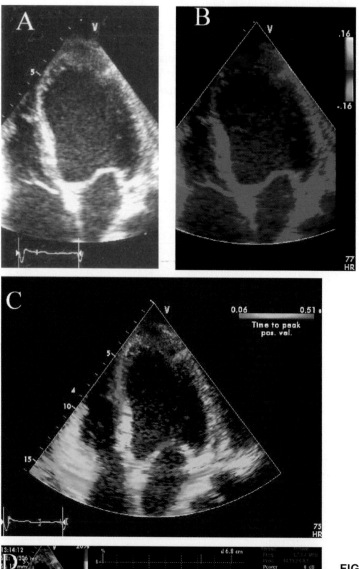

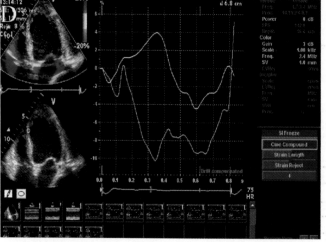

FIG. 3-9. Composite showing application of tissue Doppler imaging in the evaluation of regional function. **A:** A regular two-dimensional echocardiogram. **B:** Tissue velocity by color tissue Doppler with an area of abnormal systolic velocity in the apical septum (*blue*). **C:** Asynchrony in ventricular function depicted by delayed contraction in the apical septal area in red. **D:** Strain imaging during the cardiac cycle at two sites: normal basal septum in green, and abnormal dyskinetic apical septum in yellow. HR, heart rate.

- Current evidence is inadequate to support community-wide screening for asymptomatic LVSD; however, an effort should be made to recognize asymptomatic left ventricular dysfunction in selected high-risk populations (e.g., prior treatment with cardiotoxic agents and a strong family history of cardiomyopathy).
- Randomized, controlled trials have established that therapy with angiotensin-converting enzyme inhibitors for selected patients with left ventricular dysfunction can delay or prevent the onset of overt congestive heart failure (21,22).

Dilated Cardiomyopathy

- Dilated cardiomyopathy is characterized by a global decline in systolic function.
- 2D echo in conjunction with Doppler parameters has been used to assess prognosis in these patients.
- There is a relationship between LVEF and the deceleration time (DT) of the mitral E wave by Doppler, with mortality at 2 years (23).
  - An LVEF <25% and DT <130 msec yielded a 2-year survival of 35%.
  - Patients with LVEF <25% and a DT >130 msec had a 2-year survival of 72%.
  - Patients with an EF >25% had a 95% survival at 2 years.
- The presence of right ventricular dysfunction inevitably adds morbidity and mortality to the prognosis of patients with dilated cardiomyopathy at any point in the course of the disease.

Hypertensive Heart Disease

- Hypertension is a major risk factor for the development of heart failure.
- After adjustments for age and other risk factors, the hazard for developing heart failure in hypertensive patients is twofold in men and threefold in women (24).
- The two main mechanisms through which hypertension causes heart failure are (a) accelerated atherosclerosis and (b) elevated left ventricular wall stress, with secondary neurohormonal activation and left ventricular hypertrophy.

- 2D echo is a helpful tool to follow the progression of hypertensive cardiovascular disease.
- 2D echo allows assessment of left ventricular hypertrophy and quantitation of left ventricular mass (1).
- Left ventricular hypertrophy is a well-known risk factor for death, major cardiovascular events, and heart failure, both in normotensive and, to a higher extent, hypertensive patients.
- In addition, an increased left ventricular mass is an independent predictor of worse outcomes in asymptomatic and symptomatic left ventricular dysfunction (25).

USE IN THERAPEUTIC INTERVENTIONS

Medical Therapy

- As mentioned in Prognostic Value of Systolic Dysfunction in Different Clinical Settings, left ventricular mass and the presence of left ventricular hypertrophy are independent predictors of adverse cardiovascular events.
- The goal in the selection of an antihypertensive agent is to pick one that would normalize systolic and diastolic blood pressures and revert, at least in part, the increased left left ventricular mass when present, thereby improving prognosis.

Cardiomyoplasty

- In the case of the right dynamic cardiomyoplasty, the left latissimus dorsi muscle is placed anteriorly to the right ventricular free wall and fixed distally to the diaphragm (26). The muscle is paced in synchronization with two sensing epicardial leads that are inserted in the left ventricular wall.
- Echo is used to evaluate changes in right ventricular diameter and EF.
- Recently published 10-year follow-up indicates that there are hemodynamic and functional improvements after right ventricular cardiomyoplasty, without perioperative mortality, long-term malignant arrhythmias, or right ventricular function-related deaths.

■ Right ventricular cardiomyoplasty associated with tricuspid valve surgery, when required, could be an effective treatment for severe right ventricular failure.

■ The right ventricular myocardial wall and chamber appeared better adapted than the left ventricle when assisted by an electro-stimulated latissimus dorsi. The anatomic and hemodynamic characteristics and thickness of the RV can be more easily compressed during systole by the paced latissimus dorsi muscle.

Biventricular Pacing

■ Cardiac resynchronization therapy has emerged as an effective treatment for patients with persistent moderate to severe heart failure on medical therapy who have a ventricular dyssynchrony.

■ Cardiac resynchronization therapy has been shown to improve functional class, exercise capacity, and quality of life.

■ Cardiac resynchronization therapy is associated with reverse left ventricular remodeling, improved systolic and diastolic function, and decreased mitral regurgitation.

■ Left ventricular remodeling contributes to the symptomatic improvement and may herald an improved long-term survival (27).

■ Not every patient benefits from having just a wide QRS complex on the electrocardiogram or from the initial "out of the box" settings for the biventricular pacemaker, however.

■ There is growing evidence and interest in the need to "optimize" the atrioventricular delay and LV–RV pacing delay with the new generation of pacemakers.

■ Tissue Doppler techniques are poised to provide the methodology to evaluate the efficacy and optimize the use of this new therapeutic modality (18).

REFERENCES

1. Schiller NB, Shah PM, Crawford M, et al. Recommendations for quantitation of the left ventricle by two-dimensional echocardiography. American Society of Echocardiography Committee on Standards, Subcommittee on Quantitation of Two-Dimensional Echocardiograms. *J Am Soc Echocardiogr* 1989;2:358–367.

2. Cerqueira MD, Weissman NJ, Dilsizian V, et al. Standardized myocardial segmentation and nomenclature for tomographic imaging of the heart: a statement for healthcare professionals from the Cardiac Imaging Committee of the Council on Clinical Cardiology of the American Heart Association. *J Nucl Cardiol* 2002;9:240–245.

3. Smith MD, MacPhail B, Harrison MR, et al. Value and limitations of transesophageal echocardiography in the determination of left ventricular volumes and ejection fraction. *J Am Coll Cardiol* 1992;19:1213–1222.

4. Simonson JS, Schiller NB. Descent of the base of the left ventricle: an echocardiographic index of left ventricular function. *J Am Soc Echocardiogr* 1989;2:25–35.

5. Hundley WG, Kizilbash AM, Afridi I, et al. Administration of an intravenous perfluorocarbon contrast agent improves echocardiographic determination of left ventricular volumes and ejection fraction: comparison with cine magnetic resonance imaging. *J Am Coll Cardiol* 1998;32:1426–1432.

6. Yong Y, Wu D, Fernandes V, et al. Diagnostic accuracy and cost-effectiveness of contrast echocardiography on evaluation of cardiac function in technically very difficult patients in the intensive care unit. *Am J Cardiol* 2002;89:711–718.

7. Quiñones MA, Waggoner AD, Reduto LA, et al. A new, simplified and accurate method for determining ejection fraction with two-dimensional echocardiography. *Circulation* 1981;64:744–753.

8. Doerr HK, Quiñones MA, Zoghbi WA. Accurate determination of left ventricular ejection fraction by transesophageal echocardiography utilizing a non-volumetric method. *J Am Soc Echocardiogr* 1993;6:476–481.

9. Sugeng L, Weinert L, Thiele K, et al. Real-time three-dimensional echocardiography using a novel matrix array transducer. *Echocardiography* 2003;20:623–635.

10. Lewis JF, Kuo LC, Nelson JG, et al. Pulsed Doppler echocardiographic determination of stroke volume and cardiac output: clinical validation of two new methods using the apical window. *Circulation* 1984;70:425–431.

11. Tortoledo FA, Quiñones MA, Fernandez GC, et al. Quantification of left ventricular volumes by two-dimensional echocardiography: a simplified and accurate approach. *Circulation* 1983;67:579–584.

12. Zoghbi WA, Enriquez-Sarano M, Foster E, et al. Recommendations for evaluation of the severity of native valvular regurgitation with two-dimensional and Doppler echocardiography. *J Am Soc Echocardiogr* 2003;16:777–802.

13. Fisher DC, Sahn DJ, Friedman MJ, et al. The effect of variations on pulsed Doppler sampling site on calculation of cardiac output: an experimental study in open-chest dogs. *Circulation* 1983;67:370–376.

14. Chung N, Nishimura RA, Holmes DR, et al. Measurement of left ventricular dP/dt by simultaneous Doppler echocardiography and cardiac catheterization. *J Am Soc Echocardiogr* 1992;5:147–152.

15. Tei C, Ling LH, Hodge DO, et al. New index of combined systolic and diastolic myocardial performance:

a simple and reproducible measure of cardiac function: a study in normal and dilated cardiomyopathy. *J Cardiol* 1995;26:357–366.

16. Poulsen SH, Jensen S, Ielsen JC, et al. Serial changes and prognostic implications of a Doppler derived index of combined left ventricular systolic and diastolic myocardial performance in acute myocardial infarction. *Am J Cardiol* 2001;85:19–25.

17. Miyatake K, Yamagishi M, Tanaka N, et al. New method for evaluating left ventricular wall motion by color coded tissue Doppler imaging. In vitro and in vivo studies. *J Am Coll Cardiol* 1995;25:717–724.

18. Sogaard P. Sequential versus simultaneous biventricular resynchronization of severe heart failure: evaluation by tissue Doppler imaging. *Circulation* 2003;106:2078–2084.

19. Wang T, Levy D, Benjamin E, et al. The epidemiology of "asymptomatic" left ventricular systolic dysfunction: implications for screening. *Ann Intern Med* 2003;138:7–16.

20. Hunt SA, Baker DW, Chin MH. ACC/AHA guidelines for the evaluation and management of chronic heart failure in the adult: executive summary. A report of the American College of Cardiology/American Heart Association Task Force on Practice Guidelines (Committee to revise the 1995 Guidelines for the Evaluation and Management of Heart Failure). *J Am Coll Cardiol* 2003;38:2101–2113.

21. The SOLVD Investigators. Effect of enalapril on mortality and the development of heart failure in asymptomatic patients with reduced left ventricular ejection fractions. *N Engl J Med* 1992;327:685–691.

22. Pfeffer MA, Braunwald E, Moye LA. Effect of captopril on mortality and morbidity with left ventricular dysfunction after myocardial infarction. Results of the survival and ventricular enlargement trial. The SAVE Investigators. *N Engl J Med* 2003;327:669–677.

23. Rihal CS, Nishimura RA, Hatle LK. Systolic and diastolic dysfunction in patients with clinical diagnosis of dilated cardiomyopathy. Relation to symptoms and prognosis. *Circulation* 1994;90:2772–2779.

24. Levy D, Larson MG, Vasan RS. The progression from hypertension to congestive heart failure. *JAMA* 2003;275:1557–1562.

25. Quiñones MA, Greenberg BH, Kopelen HA, et al. Echocardiographic predictors of clinical outcome in patients with left ventricular dysfunction enrolled in the SOLVD registry and trials: significance of left ventricular hypertrophy. Studies of Left Ventricular Dysfunction. *J Am Coll Cardiol* 2000;35:1237–1244.

26. Chacques JC, Argyriadis PG, Fontaine G. Right ventricular cardiomyoplasty: 10-year follow-up. *Ann Thoracic Surg* 2003;75:1464–1468.

27. St. John Sutton M, Abraham WT, Smith AL. Effect of cardiac resynchronization on left ventricular size and function in chronic heart failure. *Circulation* 2003;107:1985–1990.

4

Ventricular Diastolic Dysfunction

Robert A. Taylor

- Ventricular filling (diastolic function) is dependent on elastic recoil, ventricular energy-dependent relaxation, compliance, and atrial pressure.
- Ventricular filling is influenced by volume status or preload, diastolic filling time, wall tension, and contractility.
- Elevated right ventricular and left ventricular filling pressures are related to reduced contractility (systolic dysfunction) or increased chamber stiffness (diastolic dysfunction).
- Diastolic dysfunction is a state of increased ventricular stiffness that prevents adequate filling of the ventricles at normal atrial pressures and is

due to impaired relaxation, decreased compliance, or both. These abnormalities occur over a continuum.
- Diastolic dysfunction is the cause of heart failure in 30% to 40% of patients.
- Asymptomatic diastolic dysfunction is common and is a poor prognostic indicator.
- The history and physical examination in patients with heart failure is inaccurate in distinguishing systolic from diastolic dysfunction. Also, the physical examination is limited in the detection of diastolic dysfunction of any degree.

TABLE 4-1. *Causes of Left Ventricular Diastolic Dysfunction*

Isolated diastolic dysfunction
Hypertension with and without left ventricular hypertrophy
Valvular disease before systolic dysfunction
  Mitral or tricuspid regurgitation
  Aortic or pulmonic stenosis
  Aortic or pulmonic regurgitation
Aging
Hypertrophic cardiomyopathy
Restrictive cardiomyopathy
  Infiltrative diseases
    Hemochromatosis
    Amyloidosis
    Glycogen storage disease
    Sarcoidosis
  Carcinoid
  Radiation
  Endomyocardial disease (with and without eosinophilia)
  Scleroderma
  Endomyocardial fibrosis
Constrictive pericarditis
Post–heart transplant inflammation
Mixed systolic and diastolic dysfunction
Ischemic cardiomyopathy
Hypertensive cardiomyopathy
Valvular disease with ventricular systolic dysfunction
Other nonischemic cardiomyopathies
  Toxins (e.g., alcohol, amphetamines, cocaine)
  Tachycardia-induced cardiomyopathy
  Viral (including human immunodeficiency virus)
  Peripartum cardiomyopathy
  Obesity
  Amyloidosis
  Restrictive cardiomyopathy

TABLE 4-2. *Causes of Right Ventricular Diastolic Dysfunction*

Diseases of the pulmonary arteries
Primary pulmonary hypertension
Toxin-induced (i.e., anorexic agents)
Vasculitides
Congenital heart disease (atrial or ventricular septal defects and patent ductus arteriosus)
Infection
  Human immunodeficiency virus
Diseases of the pulmonary parenchyma
Chronic obstructive lung disease
Restrictive lung diseases
Infiltrative/granulomatous diseases
Cystic fibrosis
Upper airway obstruction
Arteriovenous fistulas within the lung
Diseases of the thoracic cage and neuromuscular system
Obesity-hypoventilation/sleep apnea
Pharyngeal-tracheal obstruction
Kyphoscoliosis
Pleural fibrosis
Neuromuscular disorders
Diseases causing left atrial or pulmonary venous hypertension
Elevated left ventricular diastolic pressure
Aortic valve disease
Mitral valve disease
Congenital pulmonary vein stenosis
Pulmonary venoocclusive disease
Nonvasculitic diseases resulting in pulmonary artery obstruction
Acute and chronic thromboembolism
Hemoglobinopathies (e.g., sickle cell disease)
Primary or metastatic malignancies
Peripheral pulmonic stenosis
Congenital pulmonary hypoplasia

COMMON ETIOLOGIES

■ Diastolic dysfunction may be caused by systolic dysfunction, may be isolated to diastolic abnormalities, or may be mixed (Table 4-1).
■ *Isolated diastolic dysfunction*: The most common causes are aging, hypertension with and without left ventricular hypertrophy, and coronary artery disease.
■ *Mixed systolic and diastolic dysfunction*: All disease processes causing left ventricular systolic dysfunction cause some degree of diastolic dysfunction due to the effects of ventricular dilatation on left ventricular compliance. Hypertension and coronary artery disease are the predominant causes.
■ The most common causes of right ventricular diastolic dysfunction are pulmonary hypertension of any etiology (Table 4-2), and right ventricular ischemia or infarction.

ECHOCARDIOGRAPHY

Indications for Echocardiography in Patients with Diastolic Dysfunction

The American College of Cardiology/American Heart Association guidelines do not specifically delineate indications for echocardiography (echo) in diastolic dysfunction; however, guidelines for echo in patients with suspected cardiomyopathy or heart failure apply to diastolic dysfunction (1).

M-Mode and Two-Dimensional Echocardiography: Assessment of the Morphology of the Left and Right Heart Chambers

Best Imaging Planes

- Transthoracic echo (TTE) parasternal long- and short-axis and apical views.
- Transesophageal echo (TEE) transgastric long- and short-axis and mid-esophageal views.

Diagnostic Methods

- Measurements of left ventricular dimensions are made between the mitral valve and papillary muscles at the mitral valve leaflet tips.
- Measurements of the interventricular septum (IVS) and posterior wall (PW) thicknesses are made at the mitral valve tips at end-diastole.
- Measurements of IVS, PW, and left ventricular end-diastolic dimension (LVEDD) are used to calculate left ventricular mass as = $0.80 \times 1.05 \times (IVS + PW + LVEDD)^3 - (LVEDD)^3$.
- Two-dimensional (2D) imaging is essential for proper sample placement of pulsed and continuous wave, tissue, and color Doppler.

Key Diagnostic Features of Specific Conditions

- Coronary artery disease and ischemic cardiomyopathy.
  - ◆ Wall motion abnormalities associated with thinning or scarring are highly specific for ischemic heart disease as a primary or contributing factor to left ventricular diastolic dysfunction.
  - ◆ Acute or chronic myocardial ischemia results in diastolic dysfunction ranging from impaired left ventricular relaxation to restrictive filling.
  - ◆ Symptoms of congestive heart failure in ischemic cardiomyopathies correlate with

echo measures of elevated left ventricular end-diastolic pressure (LVEDP).
  - ◆ Left atrial dimension of >4.5 cm provides evidence of left ventricular diastolic dysfunction independent of left ventricular ejection fraction.
- Hypertensive heart disease.
  - ◆ Echo evidence of left ventricular hypertrophy, increased left ventricular mass, and diastolic dysfunction occurs well in advance of systolic dysfunction.
  - ◆ Increases in left ventricular wall thickness (>1.2 cm in men and 1.1 cm in women) or left ventricular mass (>294 g for men and >198 g for women) indicate left ventricular hypertrophy due to systemic hypertension, hypertrophic cardiomyopathy, or infiltrative diseases.
- Restrictive cardiomyopathy.
  - ◆ Characteristic echo findings include normal ventricular dimensions, biatrial enlargement, and usually preserved systolic function.
  - ◆ Findings are almost exclusively of severe diastolic dysfunction.
- Infiltrative heart diseases.
  - ◆ Amyloidosis.
    - • Normal systolic function without dilatation of the right ventricle (RV) or left ventricle (LV).
    - • Pronounced speckling and hypertrophy of the myocardium (often referred to as having a "ground glass" appearance) is seen. The valvular structures may demonstrate similar findings.
    - • Pericardial effusions may also be present.
  - ◆ Sarcoidosis.
    - • Infiltration of the myocardium with non-caseating granulomas produces left ventricular dilatation and regional wall motion abnormalities (especially of the mid- and basal segment), commonly misinterpreted as coronary artery disease.
  - ◆ Endomyocardial fibrosis.
    - • Fibrotic and thrombotic (echodense) thickening of the endocardium, particularly at the left ventricular and/or right ventricular apices.
    - • The degree of diastolic dysfunction is usually severe with restrictive features.

■ Hypertrophic cardiomyopathy.
  ◆ Asymmetric hypertrophy with normal to hyperdynamic left ventricular systolic function and dynamic subaortic outflow obstruction manifested by systolic anterior motion of the mitral valve.
■ Pulmonary hypertension and cor pulmonale.
  ◆ Chronic moderate or worse (>45 mm Hg) pulmonary hypertension leads to right ventricular hypertrophy, dilatation, and diastolic dysfunction.
  ◆ Flattening of septum (D-shaped septum) in late systole and early diastole is characteristic.
  ◆ Concavity of the IVS toward the LV with a dilated, hypertrophied, and hypocontractile RV.
  ◆ Right ventricular size ≥ LV suggests right ventricular dilatation. Quantitatively, right ventricular size in the anteroposterior dimension from the parasternal view (by either M-mode or 2D) should not exceed 3.5 cm.
  ◆ The downward systolic excursion of the tricuspid annulus (toward the cardiac apex) in the four-chamber view <2 cm indicates right ventricular systolic dysfunction.
  ◆ Right atrial dilatation is present if the maximal lateral dimension (parallel to the tricuspid annulus) exceeds 4 cm. Right atrial size should not exceed that of the left atrium.
  ◆ Right atrial pressure is >10 mm Hg if there is dilatation (>1.5) of the inferior vena cava (IVC) and IVC shows <50% collapse with inspiration.
■ Valvular heart disease.
  ◆ Stenotic or regurgitant lesions must be at least moderate to cause diastolic dysfunction.
  ◆ Left-sided valvular diseases may cause right ventricular diastolic dysfunction by causing pulmonary hypertension.
■ Constrictive pericarditis.
  ◆ The thickened and calcified pericardial sac causes a physical constraint to ventricular filling.
  ◆ Septal motion is paradoxical, and the IVC is plethoric.
  ◆ Respiratory variation of ≥25% and ≥40% in transmitral and transtricuspid E velocities are diagnostic features of constriction.

■ Age-related changes.
  ◆ Healthy elderly patients often display ≥ mild atrial dilatation on 2D and M-mode images in association with impaired left ventricular relaxation.
■ Cardiac transplant rejection.
  ◆ The increase in myocardial stiffness results from myocyte necrosis.
  ◆ Abnormal left ventricular and right ventricular filling can be identified at an early stage in acute rejection using Doppler echo.
  ◆ 2D and M-mode echoes are usually unremarkable.

Pitfalls

■ 2D echo does not allow for the functional assessment of diastolic function.
■ M-mode echo does not allow characterization of myocardial diseases or functional assessment of ventricular filling.

Doppler Echocardiography: Assessment of the Severity of Diastolic Function

Pulsed Wave Doppler

Transmitral and Tricuspid Inflow Patterns

See Figure 4-1.

Best Imaging Planes

■ TTE apical and TEE mid-esophageal four-chamber views with the sample volume at the leaflet tips.
■ TTE apical or TEE five-chamber views with the sample volume between leaflet tips and left ventricular outflow tract for imaging mitral inflow and aortic valve closure clicks to measure isovolumic relaxation time (IVRT) (period from aortic valve closure to mitral valve opening).

Key Diagnostic Features

■ Impaired relaxation.
  ◆ Prolonged deceleration time (DT) (>240 msec) of early filling (E velocity), prolonged IVRT (≥110 msec), reduced E velocity, dominant atrial (A) velocities, and decreased E/A ratio (<1) are characteristic (2) (Fig. 4-1).
  ◆ Indicates usually normal or nearly normal ventricular end-diastolic pressure (EDP).

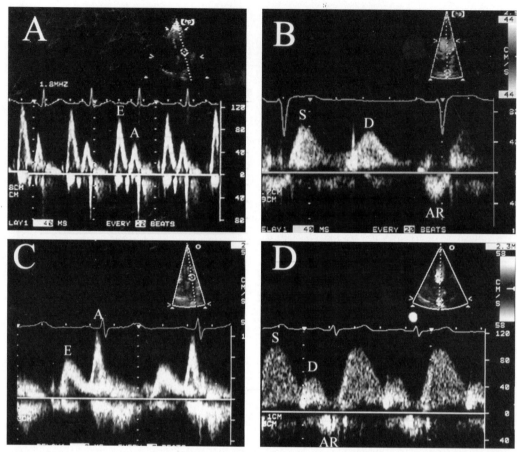

FIG. 4-1. Mitral and pulmonary veins' inflows in healthy subjects. **A,B:** Normal mitral valve and pulmonary vein inflows in a healthy 43-year-old man with an early diastolic transmitral velocity (E wave)/atrial filling transmitral velocity (A wave) (E/A) ratio >1.5, a short E deceleration time, predominant systolic (S) over diastolic (D) pulmonary vein velocities, and, in the same time scale, a pulmonary vein atrial reversal (AR) velocity of shorter duration than the mitral A velocity. **C,D:** Mitral and pulmonary vein inflows in a healthy 65-year-old man with abnormal ventricular relaxation as manifested by an E/A ratio <1 and a prolonged deceleration time of >240 msec. The normal pulmonary vein inflow with a predominant S velocity and a short-lasting AR predict normal left atrial pressure.

■ Pseudonormalization.
  ◆ Decreased ventricular compliance and increased EDP cause an increase in left atrial pressure to preserve transvalvular (mitral or tricuspid) gradient resembling a normal diastolic filling pattern.
  ◆ Increased E velocity, decreased A velocity, pseudonormalized E/A ratio (1.0–1.5), shortened DT (160–240 msec), and shortened IVRT (<90 msec) (Figs. 4-2, 4-3, and 4-4).
  ◆ This pattern indicates moderate diastolic dysfunction.

■ Restrictive filling pattern.
  ◆ Indicates severe diastolic dysfunction and high EDP.
  ◆ Characterized by high E wave velocity and small A wave velocity, E/A ratio >1.5, shortening of DT (<160 msec) and IVRT (<70 msec) (Fig. 4-5) (2–4).

Pitfalls
■ Velocities are dependent on heart rate and ventricular loading conditions, ventricular relaxation properties, and atrial filling pressure.

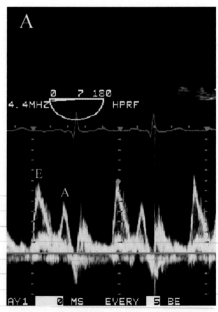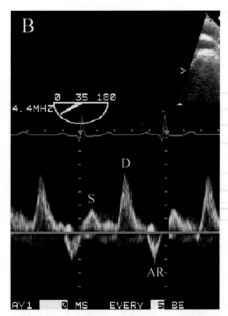

FIG. 4-2. Left atrial hypertension in a patient with symptomatic severe aortic stenosis. These transesophageal echocardiographic mitral **(A)** and pulmonary vein **(B)** inflow patterns demonstrate pseudonormalization of the mitral inflow (E/A ratio >1.5), short E deceleration time (<160 msec), a blunted systolic (S) velocity, a predominant diastolic (D) velocity, and an atrial reversal (AR) of slightly longer duration than the mitral A velocity. E/A, early diastolic transmitral velocity (E wave)/ atrial filling transmitral velocity (A wave).

- Tachycardia and first-degree atrioventricular block cause merging of E and A waves, obscuring filling patterns.
- Atrial fibrillation and flutter decrease diagnostic accuracy of velocities.
- Significant mitral regurgitation or tricuspid regurgitation may produce pseudonormalized inflow patterns.
- Diagnostic accuracy is also lower in the presence of normal ventricular systolic function.

Pulmonary Veins' Inflow Patterns

See Figures 4-2, 4-3, 4-4.

Best Imaging Planes

- TTE apical four-chamber view to assess the right lower pulmonary vein.
- TEE basal short-axis view to assess the left upper and right upper pulmonary veins.
- Sample volume is placed within 1 cm of pulmonary veins.

Key Diagnostic Features

- Include assessment of systolic velocity (S wave), diastolic velocity (D wave), and atrial flow reversal peak velocity and duration.
- Pulmonary veins' inflow patterns provide similar information about left ventricular filling as mitral inflow and complement the assessment of diastolic dysfunction (2–4).
- Normally, S wave is greater than D wave, and atrial reversal velocity is of smaller amplitude and shorter duration than the mitral A velocity.
- Impaired left ventricular relaxation is characterized by diminished D wave, predominant S wave, and increased atrial reversal velocity (Figs. 4-1 and 4-6).
- Pulmonary vein inflow helps in distinguishing between normal and pseudonormal mitral inflow patterns. In the normal pattern, the S wave is dominant. With pseudonormalization, D wave predominates, and the DT of the D wave is <150 msec and correlates well with

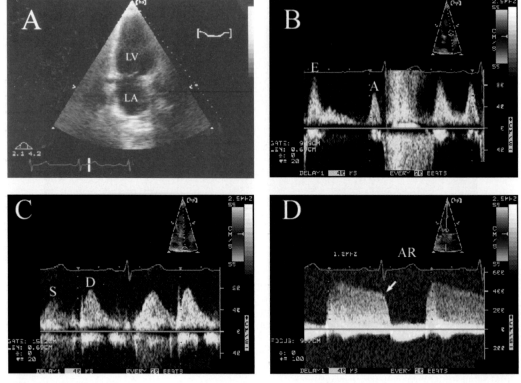

FIG. 4-3. Elevated left ventricular end-diastolic pressure in a patient with coronary artery disease and mild aortic regurgitation. **A:** Left atrial enlargement on transthoracic echocardiographic two-chamber view. **B:** Pseudonormalization of mitral inflow (E/A >1.5 and short E deceleration time). **C:** Blunted systolic (S) and predominant diastolic (D) velocities of the pulmonary vein inflow. **D:** End-diastolic peak velocity of aortic regurgitation of 3.7 m/sec (*arrow*) and equivalent to an end-diastolic gradient of 55 mm Hg by the Bernoulli equation. The patient's diastolic pressure was 80 mm Hg. Therefore, the patient's left ventricular end-diastolic pressure was 25 mm Hg (80 mm Hg – 55 mm Hg). E/A, early diastolic transmitral velocity (E wave)/atrial filling transmitral velocity (A wave); LA, left atrium; LV, left ventricle.

moderate elevation of LVEDP (Figs. 4-1, 4-2, 4-3, and 4-4).

■ High LVEDP as reflected by a restrictive mitral inflow is equivalent to a restrictive pulmonary vein inflow characterized by dominant D wave, diminished S wave, and atrial reversal flow reversal peak velocity ≥0.35 m/sec and of longer duration than the mitral A wave (Fig. 4-5).

■ Therefore, an accurate assessment of left ventricular diastolic dysfunction integrates mitral inflow and pulmonary veins according to the Canadian Consensus Guidelines (Table 4-3) (4).

Pitfalls

Physiologic factors affecting mitral inflow (preload, heart rate, atrial fibrillation, and mitral regurgitation) also alter pulmonary vein inflows.

Hepatic Veins' Flow Patterns

Best Imaging Planes

TTE subcostal view with sample volume 1 to 2 cm proximal to IVC/right atrium junction.

Key Diagnostic Features

■ The hepatic veins' flow patterns include a systolic (S wave), diastolic (D wave), and systolic and diastolic reversal waves.

■ The flow patterns of the hepatic veins mirror those of the pulmonary veins and reflect the right atrial pressure and diastolic properties of the RV.

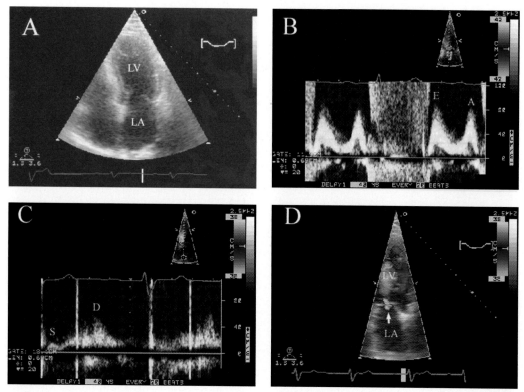

FIG. 4-4. Left atrial hypertension and diastolic mitral regurgitation in a patient with severe hypertensive heart disease. **A:** This transthoracic echocardiographic four-chamber view demonstrates severe left ventricular hypertrophy and moderate left atrial enlargement. **B:** Pseudonormalization of the mitral inflow. **C:** Absent systolic (S) velocities and predominant diastolic (D) velocities of the pulmonary vein inflow. **D:** Diastolic mitral regurgitation (*arrow*) in this patient with severely elevated left ventricular end-diastolic pressure and prolonged PR interval. E/A, early diastolic transmitral velocity (E wave)/atrial filling transmitral velocity (A wave); LA, left atrium; LV, left ventricle.

- Normally, the S wave predominates, and the reversal velocities are low.
- With decreased compliance and increased RVEDP, the D-wave velocity becomes larger than the S wave and the reversal velocities increase (Fig. 4-7).
- These changes can be seen with tricuspid regurgitation, tamponade, constriction, restriction, and cor pulmonale.
- Increase of reversal flows in the hepatic vein (>20%) during apnea suggests increased right atrial pressure and RVEDP.

Pitfall

Imaging of the hepatic veins and Doppler recordings are limited in the absence of significant right atrial hypertension.

Tei or Myocardial Performance Index

- Defined as the sum of isovolumic contraction and IVRT divided by left ventricular ejection time.

Tei index = (IVRT + isovolumic contraction)/ ejection time

- It is a sensitive measure of left ventricular systolic and diastolic function.
- The normal value is 0.39 ± 0.05. The higher the index, the worse the diastolic and systolic dysfunction (5).
- The Tei index is independent of heart rate, blood pressure, and severity of mitral regurgitation, and it has a low degree of interobserver and intraobserver variability.

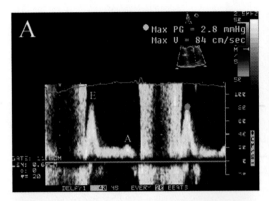
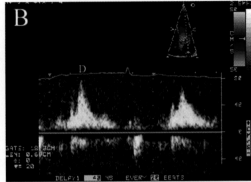
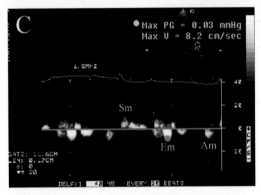
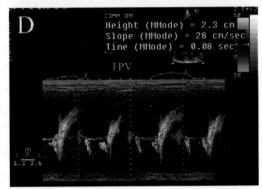

FIG. 4-5. Severe left atrial hypertension in a patient with dilated cardiomyopathy. **A:** Restrictive mitral valve inflow pattern with an early diastolic transmitral velocity (E wave)/atrial filling transmitral velocity (A wave) (E/A) ratio >2 and E deceleration time <140 msec. **B:** Pulmonary vein inflow with basically absent systolic velocities, predominant diastolic (D) velocities, and an atrial reversal velocity of longer duration than the mitral A velocity. **C:** Tissue Doppler of the basal lateral wall demonstrates decreased systolic (Sm) and significantly decreased early (Em) and late (Am) diastolic myocardial velocities. The E/Em ratio was >10. **D:** Color M-mode flow propagation velocity (FPV) demonstrated a velocity of <30 cm/sec.

■ **Pitfall:** The Tei index incorporates both systolic and diastolic factors and therefore cannot be used to measure or distinguish diastolic from systolic dysfunction.

Tissue Doppler Imaging

Best Imaging Planes

■ TTE apical or TEE mid-esophageal four-chamber views.
■ Basal septal and left ventricular or right ventricular basal lateral segments (at the annulus level) are sampled.

Diagnostic Methods

■ Tissue Doppler imaging (TDI) measures the mitral or tricuspid annulus or basal ventricular myocardial velocities.
■ TDI of these regions demonstrate systolic (Sm), early diastolic (Em), and late diastolic (Am) velocities (Figs. 4-5, 4-6, and 4-7).
■ Spectral gain settings must be reduced to optimally record low-velocity and high-intensity signals from the myocardium and eliminate blood flow signals.
■ Pulsed TDI is relatively independent of loading conditions and superior to conventional

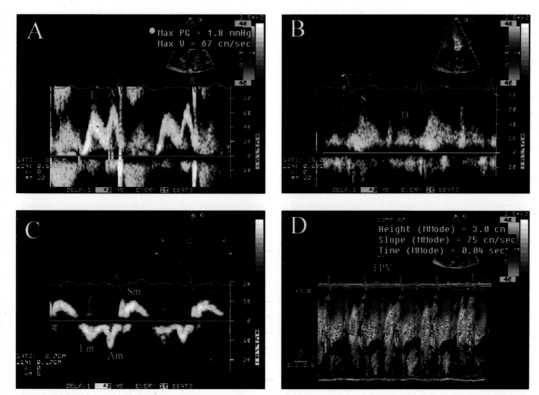

FIG. 4-6. Abnormal left ventricular relaxation in a patient with mild hypertrophic cardiomyopathy. **A:** Mitral inflow with an early diastolic transmitral velocity (E wave)/atrial filling transmitral velocity (A wave) (E/A) ratio <1.0. **B:** Normal pulmonary vein inflow with predominance of the systolic velocities (S). **C:** Normal (>10 cm/sec) systolic (Sm) and diastolic (Em and Am) tissue Doppler velocities. The E/Em ratio was <8. **D:** Normal color M-mode flow propagation velocity (FPV) of 75 cm/sec.

TABLE 4-3. *Canadian Consensus Guidelines for Classifying Diastolic Dysfunction by Pulsed Wave Doppler*

	TMF			PVF	
Grade of function	E/A	DT (msec)	AR − A (msec)	AR (m/sec)	S/D
Normal	1–2	150–200	<20	<0.35	≥1
Mild dysfunction	<1	>200	<20	<0.35	≥1
Mild/moderate dysfunction	<1	>200	≥20	≥0.35	≥1
Moderate dysfunction	1–2	150–200	≥20	≥0.35	0.5–<1
Severe dysfunction	>2	<150	≥20	≥0.35	<0.5

AR, peak atrial systolic pulmonary venous reversal flow velocity; AR − A, difference between the duration of the transmitral A wave and the peak atrial systolic pulmonary venous reversal flow wave; DT, deceleration time of the E wave; E/A, early diastolic transmitral velocity (E wave)/atrial filling transmitral velocity (A wave); PVF, pulmonary vein flow velocity; S/D, peak systolic pulmonary vein flow velocity/peak diastolic pulmonary venous flow velocity; TMF, transmitral flow velocity.

Adapted from Yamada H, Goh PP, Sun JP, et al. Prevalence of left ventricular diastolic dysfunction by Doppler echocardiography: clinical application of the Canadian Consensus Guidelines. *J Am Soc Echocardiogr* 2002;15: 1238–1244.

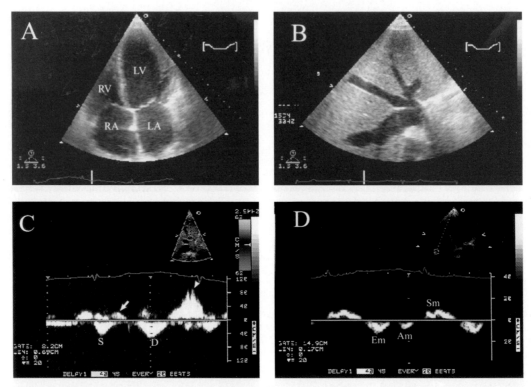

FIG. 4-7. Right atrial hypertension in a patient with dilated cardiomyopathy. **A:** Apical transthoracic echocardiographic (TTE) four-chamber view illustrating severe left and right heart chambers' enlargement. **B:** Subcostal TTE demonstrating severe plethora with no respiratory collapse of the inferior vena cava and hepatic veins ("deer head sign"). **C:** Hepatic veins' flow with blunting of the systolic (S) velocity, predominant diastolic (D) velocity, increased systolic reversal (*arrow*), and marked diastolic reversal (*arrowhead*). **D:** Tissue Doppler of the basal right ventricular free wall with decreased systolic (Sm) and diastolic (Em and Am) myocardial velocities. LA, left atrium; LV, left ventricle; RV, right ventricle.

mitral inflow indexes in the assessment of left ventricular and right ventricular diastolic dysfunction (6–8).

Key Diagnostic Features

- TDI measures contraction and relaxation velocities of myocardium.
- Peak Em has been shown to inversely correlate with the time constant of left ventricular isovolumic relaxation (*tau*).
- Normal values for the basal segments are generally >10 cm/sec. With diastolic dysfunction, Em velocity decreases (Figs. 4-5, 4-6, and 4-7).
- Abnormalities in TDI velocities correlate well with standard mitral and pulmonary vein inflow patterns of diastolic dysfunction (Table 4-4).
- Em correlates with the rate in change of the left ventricular long axis during early filling, providing information related to left ventricular relaxation.
- Em velocities decrease with age and left ventricular hypertrophy.
- The ratio of Em/Am is normally >1 as seen with the mitral E/A ratio.
- Pulsed TDI is superior to conventional pulsed Doppler of mitral inflow velocities in distinguishing restrictive cardiomyopathy from constrictive pericarditis. A reduction in Em is seen in restrictive cardiomyopathy but not in constrictive pericarditis.

Pitfalls

- Measurements of myocardial velocities are done at selected sites, limiting full evaluation of diastolic dysfunction in patients with segmental wall motion abnormalities.

TABLE 4-4. *Tissue Doppler Velocities Corresponding to the Standard Classification of Diastolic Function by Transmitral and Pulmonary Vein Parameters*

	Normal	Abnormal relaxation	Pseudonormal	Restrictive
Em (cm/sec)	16.0 ± 3.8	7.5 ± 2.2	7.6 ± 2.2	8.1 ± 3.5
Am (cm/sec)	11.0 ± 2.1	11.7 ± 2.4	8.5 ± 2.7	3.9 ± 1.3
Sm (cm/sec)	9.7 ± 1.9	6.5 ± 1.8	6.2 ± 1.7	4.0 ± 1.2

■ Alignment of the ultrasound beam parallel to the moving heart muscle may be difficult.

Color M-Mode Propagation Velocity

Color M-mode Doppler recorded across the mitral valve during diastole allows measurement of the flow propagation velocity (Vp) as the slope of flow wave front at the transition of the no color and color (manually) or the first aliasing velocity (45 cm/sec) during early left ventricular filling (9).

Best Imaging Planes

■ TTE apical two-chamber and four-chamber views.
■ TEE long-axis view at mid-esophagus.
■ Recordings are obtained from the plane of the mitral valve to 4 cm into the left ventricular cavity (automated).

Key Diagnostic Features

■ Vp correlates with invasive measurements of left ventricular relaxation and compliance and relates inversely with *tau* (10–12).
■ Vp is relatively preload independent in comparison to mitral valve and pulmonary vein inflows.
■ Vp has been reported to be between 55 and 100 cm/sec in normal subjects. Lower velocities qualitatively relate to diastolic dysfunction (Figs. 4-5 and 4-6).
■ Combining Vp with some mitral inflow parameters correlates more accurately to pulmonary artery wedge pressures (PAWPs) than mitral inflow parameters alone (Table 4-5) (12,13).
■ The ratio of E/Vp provides an estimate of PAWP as follows:

$$PAWP = 5.27 \times (E/Vp) + 4.6 \ (r = 0.80)$$

■ Also, IVRT can be combined with Vp to estimate PAWP as:

$$PAWP = 1,000/(2 \times IVRT) + Vp \ (r = 0.88)$$

Pitfall

The manual calculation of the Vp slope is subjective with interobserver and intraobserver variability. Automated methods may decrease these problems.

Diagnostic Accuracy for Detection of Diastolic Dysfunction

■ M-mode and 2D echo are highly accurate in characterizing the diseases associated with diastolic dysfunction. Except for identifying left atrial dilatation, however, M-mode and 2D echo are poor predictors of the presence or severity of diastolic dysfunction.
■ Although each of the different Doppler echocardiography parameters are moderately to highly sensitive but quite specific in predicting elevated PAWP, when used in combination they are highly sensitive, specific, and predictive of high filling pressures (Table 4-5) (4,10,12,13).

Prognostic Value in Diastolic Dysfunction

■ Diastolic dysfunction in many clinical settings (even in the asymptomatic patient) portends an increased cardiovascular risk (Table 4-6) (13–19).
■ The cardiovascular risk is especially high with findings of restrictive physiology.

Indicators for Therapeutic Interventions in Diastolic Dysfunction

■ Symptoms of heart failure in patients with systolic dysfunction are caused primarily by elevations of ventricular filling pressures (restrictive

TABLE 4-5. *Doppler Echocardiography Diagnostic Accuracy for Detection of Elevated Left Ventricular Filling Pressures*

Variable	PAWP (mm Hg)	Sensitivity (%)	Specificity (%)	PPV (%)	NPV (%)
E/A >1.2	>10	92	95	—	—
E/A >1.6	>15	50	94	75	84
DT <140 msec	>15	52	89	75	76
IVRT <60 msec	>15	52	85	86	77
SFPV <50%	>10	85	95	—	—
SFPV <50%	>20	96	72	—	—
SFPV <35%	>18	90	85	—	—
PV$_A$ – MV$_A$ >0	>15	82–88	80–99	—	—
E/Vp >2.6	>15	74	95	89	86
E/Em >8	>15	87	66	61	89
1,000/ [(2 × IVRT) + Vp] >5.5	>15	87	97	95	93
1,000/ [(2 × IVRT) + Em] >7.25	>15	65	92	83	81

DT, deceleration time of the E wave; E/A, early diastolic transmitral velocity (E wave)/atrial filling transmitral velocity (A wave); E/Em, early diastolic transmitral velocity/early diastolic myocardial velocity; E/Vp, early diastolic transmitral velocity/flow propagation velocity; Em, early diastolic velocity; IVRT, isovolumic relaxation time; MV$_A$, transmitral valve A wave; NPV, negative predictive value; PAWP, pulmonary artery wedge pressure; PPV, positive predictive value; PV$_A$, pulmonary vein A wave; SFPV, systolic fraction of pulmonary veins' flow; Vp, propagation velocity.

or pseudonormalized filling patterns). Treatment with diuretic therapy and nitrates in this clinical setting is well established.

- In patients with left ventricular diastolic dysfunction, angiotensin-converting enzyme inhibitors and beta-blockers have been shown to improve symptoms, functional capacity, and long-term survival.

- Diastolic dysfunction in ischemic heart disease, infiltrative disorders, or valve disease suggests the need for more aggressive intervention.
- In patients with hypertrophic obstructive cardiomyopathy, diastolic dysfunction indicates the need for aggressive beta-blockers or calcium channel blockers.

TABLE 4-6. *Prognostic Value of Right Ventricular or Left Ventricular Diastolic Dysfunction in Different Clinical Settings*

Asymptomatic patients	In a population-based sample of middle-aged and elderly adults, mitral E/A >1.5 at baseline is associated with twofold increased all-cause mortality and threefold increased cardiac mortality independent of covariates.
Heart failure with normal EF	Increased risk with isolated diastolic dysfunction, especially if restrictive pattern, although not as elevated risk as with reduced EF <45%. E deceleration time <125 msec has a 2.4 risk for death or hospitalization and a 45% mortality at 4 years.
Heart failure with low EF	Increasing risk with worsening levels of diastolic dysfunction.
Acute MI	Doppler-derived mitral E wave DT <140 msec and Tei index >0.46 are independent risk factors after acute MI. The prognosis worsens with increasing quartiles of the Tei index.
Ischemic cardiomyopathy	Worsening prognosis with worsening diastolic dysfunction.
Hypertensive heart disease	Survival analysis shows cardiovascular risk increased from the lowest to the highest quintile of left ventricular mass.
Hypertrophic cardiomyopathy	Left ventricular diastolic dysfunction at rest is a strong independent predictor of progression to heart failure and death.
Restrictive cardiomyopathy	A restrictive filling pattern predicts an extremely poor prognosis.
Post–cardiac transplant	Diastolic dysfunction, especially if restrictive, is recognized to carry a poor clinical implication for the long-term progress of cardiac allograft recipients.

DT, deceleration time; E/A, early diastolic transmitral velocity (E wave)/atrial filling transmitral velocity (A wave); EF, ejection fraction; MI, myocardial infarction.

Use in the Pregnant Patient
with Diastolic Dysfunction

■ Few data exist on the occurrence of right ventricular and left ventricular diastolic dysfunction in the pregnant patient.

■ In a small series, pregnant women evaluated by TTE were found to have increased left ventricular mass, decreased fractional shortening, and abnormal relaxation (20).

■ In pregnant women with hypertension, mitral and pulmonary vein inflow evidence of diastolic dysfunction (high E/A ratio, pulmonary vein D wave predominance, and high pulmonary vein atrial reversal velocity) was found. These women also demonstrated color M-mode and TDI changes consistent with diastolic dysfunction (21).

■ Diastolic dysfunction resolves 1 to 2 months after delivery.

Follow-Up in Patients
with Diastolic Dysfunction

■ Impaired relaxation identifies patients with early stages of heart disease. Appropriate therapy may avert progression of diastolic dysfunction as well as functional disability. Follow-up echo may be necessary in these patients to initiate or evaluate response to therapy.

■ Pseudonormalization of the mitral inflow pattern is associated with decreased compliance and increased filling pressures. Echo plays an important role in identifying reversible causes for intervention.

■ A restrictive mitral inflow identifies advanced diastolic dysfunction with a poor prognosis, regardless of underlying cause. Echo can assist in the evaluation of response to therapy.

REFERENCES

1. Cheitlin MD, Armstrong WF, Aurigemma GP, et al. ACC/AHA/ASE guideline update for the application of echocardiography. Summary article. *J Am Coll Cardiol* 2003;42:954–970.

2. Appleton CP, Jensen JL, Hatle LK, et al. Doppler evaluation of left and right ventricular diastolic function: a technical guide for obtaining optimal flow velocity recordings. *J Am Soc Echocardiogr* 1997;10:271–291.

3. Garcia MJ, Ares MA, Asher C, et al. An index of early left ventricular filling that combined with pulsed Doppler peak E velocity may estimate capillary wedge pressure. *J Am Coll Cardiol* 1997;29:448–454.

4. Yamada H, Goh PP, Sun JP, et al. Prevalence of left ventricular diastolic dysfunction by Doppler echocardiography: clinical application of the Canadian Consensus Guidelines. *J Am Soc Echocardiogr* 2002;15:1238–1244.

5. Tei C, Ling LH, Hodge DO, et al. New index of combined systolic and diastolic myocardial performance: a simple and reproducible measure of cardiac function—a study in normals and dilated cardiomyopathy. *J Cardiol* 1995;26:357–366.

6. Farias CA, Rodriguez L, Garcia MJ, et al. Assessment of diastolic function by tissue Doppler echocardiography: comparison with standard transmitral and pulmonary venous flow. *J Am Soc Echocardiogr* 1999;12:609–617.

7. Oki T, Tabata T, Yamada H, et al. Clinical application of pulsed Doppler tissue imaging for assessing abnormal left ventricular relaxation. *Am J Cardiol* 1997;79:921–928.

8. Rodriguez L, Garcia M, Ares M, et al. Assessment of mitral annular dynamics during diastole by Doppler tissue imaging: comparison with mitral Doppler inflow in subjects without heart disease and in patients with left ventricular hypertrophy. *Am Heart J* 1996;131:982–987.

9. Brun P, Tribouilloy C, Duval AM, et al. Left ventricular flow propagation during early filling is related to wall relaxation: a color M-mode Doppler analysis. *J Am Coll Cardiol* 1992;20:420–432.

10. Garcia MJ, Smedira NG, Greenberg NL, et al. Color M-mode Doppler flow propagation velocity is a preload insensitive index of left ventricular relaxation: animal and human validation. *J Am Coll Cardiol* 2000;35:201–208.

11. Chamoun AJ, Xie T, Trough M, et al. Color M-mode flow propagation velocity versus conventional Doppler indices in the assessment of diastolic left ventricular function in patients on chronic dialysis. *Echocardiography* 2002;6:467–474.

12. Gonzalez-Vilchez F, Ayuela J, Ares M, et al. Comparison of Doppler echocardiography, color M-mode Doppler, and Doppler tissue imaging for the estimation of pulmonary capillary wedge pressure. *J Am Soc Echocardiogr* 2002;15:1245–1250.

13. Gonzalez-Vilchez F, Ares M, Ayuela J, et al. Combined use of pulsed and color M-mode Doppler echocardiography for the estimation of pulmonary capillary wedge pressure: an empirical approach based on an analytical relation. *J Am Coll Cardiol* 1999;34:515–523.

14. Bella JN, Palmieri V, Roman MJ, et al. Mitral ratio of peak early to late diastolic filling velocity as a predictor of mortality in middle-aged and elderly adults: the Strong Heart Study. *Circulation* 2002;105:1928–1933.

15. Xie G, Berk MR, Smith MD, et al. Prognostic value of Doppler transmitral flow pattern in patients with congestive heart failure. *J Am Coll Cardiol* 1994;24:132–139.

16. Wang M, Yip GW, Wang AY, et al. Peak early diastolic

mitral annulus velocity by tissue Doppler imaging adds independent and incremental prognostic value. *J Am Coll Cardiol* 2003;1:820–826.

17. Pinamonti B, Zecchin M, Li Lenarda A, et al. Persistence of restrictive left ventricular filling pattern in dilated cardiomyopathy: an ominous prognostic sign. *J Am Coll Cardiol* 1997;29:604–612.

18. Verdecchia P, Carini G, Circo A, et al. Left ventricular mass and cardiovascular morbidity in essential hypertension: the MAVI study. *J Am Coll Cardiol* 2001;38: 1829–1835.

19. Maron MS, Olivotto I, Betocchi S, et al. Effect of left ventricular outflow tract obstruction on clinical outcome in hypertrophic cardiomyopathy. *N Engl J Med* 2003;348:295–303.

20. Schannwell CM, Zimmermann T, Schneppenheim M, et al. Left ventricular hypertrophy and diastolic dysfunction in healthy pregnant women. *Cardiology* 2002;97:73–78.

21. De Conti F, Da Corta R, Del Monte D, et al. Left ventricular diastolic function in pregnancy induced hypertension. *Ital Heart J* 2003;4:246–251.

5

Pulmonary Hypertension and Cor Pulmonale

Anita Kedia and Carlos A. Roldan

- Patients with pulmonary hypertension (HTN) and cor pulmonale have high morbidity and mortality (1).
- Cor pulmonale accounts for 20% of hospital admissions for heart failure and for 80,000 deaths/year in the United States.
- Symptoms and physical findings associated with pulmonary HTN and cor pulmonale lack specificity.
- The history and physical examination are limited in defining the etiology, severity, and prognosis of pulmonary HTN and cor pulmonale.

DEFINITION

Right ventricular dilatation, hypertrophy, or diastolic or systolic dysfunction due to pulmonary HTN in the absence of left heart disease.

COMMON ETIOLOGIES OF PULMONARY HYPERTENSION

- Obliterative: Chronic obstructive pulmonary disease characterized by destruction of pulmonary capillary beds.
- Vasoconstrictive: Obstructive sleep apnea and obesity hypoventilation.
- Obstructive: Acute or chronic pulmonary embolism, which accounts for more than 600,000 cases of pulmonary HTN in the United States each year; also includes primary pulmonary HTN (PPH), with an incidence of two cases/million and a female to male ratio of 1.7:1.0 (2).
- Hyperkinetic: Left to right shunting from an atrial or ventricular septal defect, patent ductus arteriosus, or anomalous pulmonary venous drainage leading to right ventricular volume and then to right ventricular pressure overload.

ECHOCARDIOGRAPHY

Class I Indications for Echocardiography

- Transthoracic echocardiography (TTE) can establish the diagnosis, severity, and prognosis of patients with pulmonary HTN with or without cor pulmonale (Table 5-1) (3).

TABLE 5-1. *Class I Indications for Echocardiography in Pulmonary Hypertension and Cor Pulmonale*

Suspected pulmonary hypertension.
For distinguishing cardiac vs. noncardiac etiology of dyspnea in patients in whom clinical and laboratory clues are ambiguous.
Evaluation and follow-up of pulmonary artery pressures in patients with pulmonary hypertension to evaluate response to treatment.
Lung disease with clinical suspicion of cardiac involvement (suspected cor pulmonale).
Edema with clinical signs of elevated central venous pressure when a potential cardiac etiology is suspected or when central venous pressure cannot be estimated with confidence and clinical suspicion of heart disease is high.
Dyspnea with clinical signs of heart disease.
Patient with unexplained hypotension especially in the intensive care unit.
Diagnosis and assessment of hemodynamic severity of right-sided valvular regurgitation.
Assessment of right ventricular size, function, and/or hemodynamics in a patient with right-sided valvular regurgitation.
Pulmonary emboli and suspected clots in the right atrium or ventricle or main pulmonary artery branches.[a]

---

[a]Class IIa indication.
Modified from Cheitlin MD, Armstrong WF, Aurigemma GP, et al. ACC/AHA/ASE guideline update for the clinical application of echocardiography: summary article. *J Am Coll Cardiol* 2003;42:954–970.

- TTE can differentiate acute from chronic cor pulmonale and right heart disease secondary to left heart disease.
- TTE can define the severity of right ventricular dilatation, hypertrophy, and dysfunction.
- Transesophageal echocardiography (TEE) may identify large proximal pulmonary emboli in hemodynamically compromised patients with right ventricular dysfunction by TTE (4).
- TEE is superior to TTE in the detection and characterization of right atrial and right ventricular thrombi or masses and can have complementary diagnostic value to TTE in intracardiac shunts.
- Intravascular ultrasound provides histologic and functional evaluation of the pulmonary vasculature and helps to differentiate PPH from chronic pulmonary thromboembolism (5).

M-Mode and Two-Dimensional Echocardiography: Morphology of the Right Heart

Best Imaging Planes

- TTE parasternal long-axis and short-axis views, and apical and subcostal four-chamber views.
- TEE transgastric long-axis and short-axis views of the right ventricle (RV) and mid-esophageal four-chamber view.

Key Diagnostic Features of Specific Abnormalities

Right Ventricular Dilatation

- A right ventricular end-diastolic diameter >3.5 cm from parasternal and subcostal views and >4 cm from apical four-chamber view indicates right ventricular dilatation.
- With mild right ventricular dilatation, right ventricular area remains less than left ventricular area.
- A right ventricular to left ventricular end-diastolic area ratio <0.6 is normal, 0.6 to 1.0 indicates mild dilatation, and >1.0 indicates severe right ventricular dilatation (Fig. 5-1) (6).
- The right ventricular apex is normally located short of the left ventricular apex by one-third of the distance from the base to the apex. Any alteration from this pattern suggests right ventricular dilatation.

Right Ventricular Hypertrophy

- The normal right ventricular free wall measures 0.2 to 0.5 cm in end-diastole. Right ventricular hypertrophy (RVH) is present if right ventricular free wall measures >0.5 cm.
- RVH is highly predictive of high right ventricular systolic pressure.

Right Ventricular Systolic Dysfunction

- By nuclear techniques, the normal right ventricular ejection fraction is ≥40%.
- Right ventricular systolic function is routinely visually assessed.
- Downward systolic excursion of the tricuspid valve annulus is dependent on right ventricular systolic function.

- Right ventricular function is normal if its excursion toward the apex is >2 cm.
- A right ventricular annular systolic excursion <2 cm, <1 cm, and <0.5 cm indicates mild, moderate, and severe right ventricular dysfunction, respectively.

Right Ventricular Pressure or Volume Overload

- High right ventricular systolic pressure leads to a prolonged right ventricular ejection, and as a result, the right ventricular pressure exceeds the left ventricular pressure during late systole and early diastole.
- Thus, right ventricular pressure overload leads to a flattened or curved septum toward the left ventricle (LV) during late systole and early diastole ("D-shaped LV"), which resumes its usual shape during mid- and late diastole (Fig. 5-1A).
  - ◆ This pattern of septal motion is seen in patients with moderate to severe pulmonary HTN (pressure >45 mm Hg), but it may be absent in those with an elevated left ventricular end-diastolic pressure.
- With right ventricular volume overload, displacement of the septum toward the LV is seen in mid-diastole, as left ventricular diastolic pressure is exceeded during this phase. During systole, the pressure difference reverses, and the septum resumes its normal contour.
  - ◆ This pattern of septal motion is less prominent if pressure and volume overload coexist.
- Paradoxical septal motion is uncommon with mild volume overload and is seen in ≤50% of those with moderate volume overload.
- Chronic pressure overload leads to right ventricular dilatation and dysfunction, with resultant moderate or worse tricuspid regurgitation (TR) and, therefore, a septal motion pattern of pressure and volume overload.
- Chronic pulmonary HTN leads to dilatation of the right ventricular outflow and pulmonary artery (PA) (>3 cm).
- In worse than moderate pulmonary HTN, M-mode of the pulmonic valve shows mid-systolic closure and loss of the normal A wave in 30% to 60% of cases.

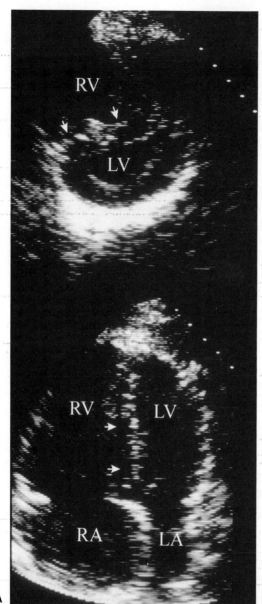

A

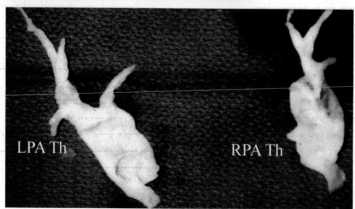

B

FIG. 5-1. Severe cor pulmonale. **A:** Transthoracic echocardiographic short-axis and four-chamber views in a patient with chronic recurrent pulmonary embolism demonstrate severe dilatation of the right heart chambers and abnormal septal motion (*arrows*) consistent with right ventricular pressure overload (estimated pulmonary artery systolic pressure of 75 mm Hg). After pulmonary thromboendarterectomy, pulmonary hypertension and right heart enlargement and dysfunction significantly improved to near normal. **B:** Large, branching, multiple and well-organized thrombi removed from the left (LPA Th) and right (RPA Th) pulmonary arteries. LA, left atrium; LV, left ventricle; RA, right atrium; RV, right ventricle.

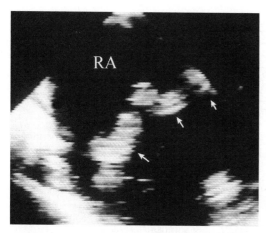

FIG. 5-2. Free-floating right atrial thrombus. Transesophageal echocardiographic four-chamber close-up view of the right atrium (RA) demonstrating multiple and freely mobile thrombi (*arrows*). This patient had severe right ventricular enlargement and dysfunction and multiple lung perfusion defects consistent with pulmonary embolism.

- ◆ In pulmonic valve stenosis, the A wave is increased, and mid-systolic closure of the valve is absent.
- In acute cor pulmonale due to pulmonary embolism, right ventricular size and wall thickness are usually normal, but a global decrease in contractility is seen. In this setting, right ventricular or right atrial thrombi may be seen.

Right Heart Thrombi

- In venous thromboembolism, an in-transit thrombus may be seen in the right atrium, RV, or PAs.
  - ◆ These thrombi are mobile, irregular, and free-floating masses (often prolapsing across the tricuspid valve) (Fig. 5-2).
  - ◆ Thrombi can be attached to a Chiari network or visualized across a patent foramen ovale leading to paradoxical embolism.
- Endocardial damage associated with placement of right heart catheters and pacemakers or automatic implantable cardiac defibrillator electrodes may lead to *in situ* thrombus formation.
  - ◆ These thrombi are nonmobile, have distinct margins and a broad base, and are adhered to the atrial wall or catheter, or both (Figs. 5-3 and 5-4).

Right Atrial Dilatation and Hypertension

- Right atrial enlargement and HTN occur with chronic right ventricular pressure or volume overload.
- Right atrial size or area ≥ the left atrium indicates right atrial enlargement.
- Right atrial pressure is estimated by the diameter and degree of inspiratory collapse of the inferior vena cava (IVC).
  - ◆ Right atrial pressure is <5 mm Hg if IVC is small (<1.0 cm) and collapses with inspiration; 5 to 10 mm Hg if IVC measures 1.0 to 1.5 cm and collapses >50% with inspiration; 10 to 15 mm Hg if IVC is ≥1.5 cm and collapses >50% with inspiration; 15 to 20 mm Hg if IVC is >1.5 cm and collapses <50%; and >20 mm Hg if hepatic veins are dilated and IVC does not collapse with inspiration.
- Failure of the IVC to collapse with a sniff indicates a right atrial pressure >20 mm Hg.
- In severe right atrial HTN, doming of the atrial septum toward the left atrium is seen.
- Dilatation of the hepatic veins and, rarely, the coronary sinus indicates severe right atrial HTN.

Pitfalls

- False positive right ventricular dilatation occurs when the transducer is not located over the left ventricular apex.
- False negative right ventricular dilatation can occur when the LV is concurrently enlarged.
- Assessment of RVH with two-dimensional imaging is less reliable than M-mode because of its slower frame rate and consequent decreased endocardial resolution.
- Because of difficulties in determining the outer edge of the thin right ventricular free wall endocardium, degrees of RVH have not been established.
- The sensitivity of echocardiography (echo) for RVH is also low because the right ventricular response to pressure overload is occasionally dilatation instead of hypertrophy.
- Precise right ventricular ejection fraction is rarely determined by echo, and normal values have not been standardized.

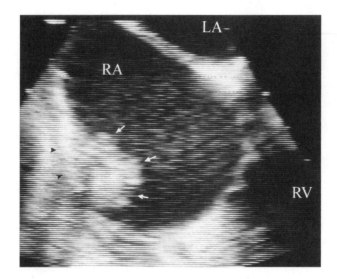

FIG. 5-3. *In situ* right atrial wall thrombi. Transesophageal echocardiographic four-chamber close-up view of the right atrium (RA) demonstrating a large mass (*white arrows*) attached to the right atrial lateral wall (*black arrowheads*). This patient had a right atrial catheter tip extending to the atrial wall and mass. The mass was confirmed to be an organized thrombus. LA, left atrium; RV, right ventricle.

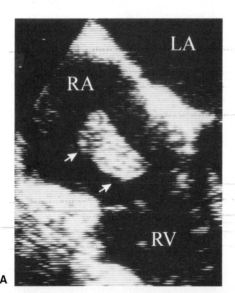

FIG. 5-4. Right atrial thrombi attached to an indwelling catheter. **A:** Transesophageal echocardiographic four-chamber view demonstrating a large and elongated mass (*arrows*) in the right atrium (RA). **B:** A well-organized thrombus (*arrows*) attached and surrounding the catheter is shown (*arrowheads*). LA, left atrium; RV, right ventricle.

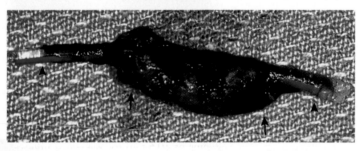

- Difficulties measuring right ventricular volume have made quantification of right ventricular ejection fraction inaccurate.
- Assessment of right atrial pressure by IVC dynamics is not accurate during positive pressure ventilation and in young athletes.

Doppler Echocardiography

Pulmonary Artery Systolic and Diastolic Pressures on Pulsed and Continuous Wave Doppler: Diagnostic Methods and Key Diagnostic Features

- PA systolic pressure is estimated using the simplified Bernoulli equation:

$$\Delta P = 4V^2$$
$$[V = \text{peak TR velocity (TRV)}]$$
$$+ \text{ right atrial pressure}$$

- The time of onset to peak velocity at the pulmonic valve (acceleration time) is an indicator of pulmonary HTN.
  - ◆ An acceleration time <80 msec is highly predictive of pulmonary HTN.
  - ◆ Acceleration time is most useful if normal (>110 msec).
  - ◆ The PA flow velocity curve may also show a mid-systolic reduction in flow, which correlates to the mid-systolic closure of the pulmonic valve seen by M-mode.
- A TRV/TVI ratio of 0.175 correlates with a pulmonary vascular resistance (PVR) of >2 Wood units, and PVR can be estimated as:
  - ◆ PVR = 10 × TRV/TVI$_{RVOT}$, where TRV = peak TR velocity in m/sec and TVI$_{RVOT}$ = time velocity integral at the right ventricular outflow tract (RVOT) by pulsed wave Doppler and from the parasternal short-axis view.
  - ◆ A PVR >2 Wood units indicates pulmonary HTN (7).
- Systolic, diastolic, and atrial reversal flows of the hepatic veins in patients with right atrial HTN show similar changes as those seen in the pulmonary veins of patients with left atrial HTN.
- The majority of patients with pulmonary HTN have pulmonic valve regurgitation.
- PA diastolic pressure, therefore, can be estimated as $4V^2$ + right atrial pressure, where V =

end-diastolic velocity of the pulmonic regurgitant display by continuous wave Doppler.

Right Ventricular Diastolic Dysfunction on Pulsed and Continuous Wave Doppler: Key Diagnostic Features

- Principles used for the evaluation of left ventricular diastolic function can be applied to the RV.
- With pulmonary HTN and RVH, there is a decrease in the E wave and an increase in the A wave of the tricuspid inflow velocity consistent with abnormal right ventricular relaxation.
- With decreased right ventricular compliance, the E wave becomes predominant (pseudonormalization) until a restrictive pattern forms, with an E wave to A wave ratio >2 (8).

Valvular Regurgitation Secondary to Pulmonary Hypertension and Cor Pulmonale

Tricuspid Regurgitation: Diagnostic Methods and Key Diagnostic Features

Pulsed and Continuous Wave Doppler

- The tricuspid valve is structurally normal, and TR is generally mild to moderate.
- An early tricuspid inflow velocity of ≥1 suggests severe TR.
- If moderate TR, the hepatic veins' flow pattern demonstrates a reduction of the normal systolic flow.
- In severe TR, absent or reversed systolic flow can be seen.
- The spectral signal intensity in severe TR is similar to the tricuspid inflow, and often a "V" wave or reduction in velocity during the latter half of systole is seen as right ventricular and right atrial pressures equalize.

Color Doppler

- The following parameters are consistent with severe TR (9–11):
  - ◆ A proximal isovelocity surface area (PISA) radius of 10.6 mm for a Nyquist limit of 28 cm/sec.
  - ◆ A PISA radius of 6.8 mm for a Nyquist limit of 41 cm/sec.

TABLE 5-2. *Stratification of Pulmonary Hypertension and Cor Pulmonale*

Mild	Moderate	Severe
Right atrial hypertension		
Pressure 10–15 mm Hg if IVC ≥1.5 cm and collapses >50%	15–20 mm Hg if IVC >1.5 cm and collapses <50%	>20 mm Hg if IVC is >1.5 and does not collapse; hepatic veins are dilated
Pulmonary hypertension		
Pressure 35–45 mm Hg	46–60 mm Hg	>60 mm Hg
Normal right heart morphology and function	Normal to mildly abnormal right heart morphology and/or function	Always abnormal right heart morphology and/or function
Cor pulmonale		
Usually moderate pulmonary HTN	Unless acute, usually severe pulmonary HTN	Unless acute, always severe pulmonary HTN
Mildly abnormal right heart morphology and function	Moderately abnormal right heart morphology and/or function	Severely abnormal right heart morphology and/or function
Tricuspid valve regurgitation		
Jet area <5 cm²	5–10 cm²	>10 cm², Nyquist at 50–60 cm/sec
Jet/right atrial area <20%	20–40%	>40%
PISA radius ≤5 mm	6–9 mm	≥10 mm, Nyquist limit of 30 cm/sec
		7 mm, Nyquist limit of 40 cm/sec
Vena contracta width <5 mm	<7 mm	≥7 mm
Hepatic vein flow with systolic dominance	Systolic blunting	Systolic reversal
Pulmonic valve regurgitation		
Jet length <10 mm	10–20 mm	>20 mm, Nyquist at 50–60 cm/sec
Pressure half-time >100 msec	Variable but commonly <100 msec	<100 msec

HTN, hypertension; IVC, inferior vena cava; PISA, proximal isovelocity surface area.

- ◆ Jet area of 10.6 cm².
- ◆ Jet length of 5.3 cm.
- ◆ A jet to right atrial area ratio of >40%.
- ◆ A vena contracta width of ≥6.5 mm.
- ■ Accurate assessment of the severity of TR requires integration of Doppler parameters with those of PA pressure, right ventricular size and function, and right atrial size and pressure (Table 5-2).

Pulmonic Regurgitation: Diagnostic Methods and Key Diagnostic Features

Pulsed and Continuous Wave Doppler

- ■ Mild to moderate pulmonic regurgitation (PR) is common in patients with cor pulmonale. If severe PR is seen, associated primary valve disease is likely.
- ■ Although right ventricular total stroke volume subtracted from left ventricular forward stroke volume determines the PR regurgitant volume, cut-off values for grading PR have not been determined.

- ■ The continuous wave signal of PR displays a slow decay in mild to moderate lesions, but it shows a steeper slope and shorter pressure half-time in severe PR (12).
  - ◆ A pressure half-time >100 msec indicates mild PR.
  - ◆ A pressure half-time <100 msec indicates severe PR.
- ■ A deceleration slope greater than 3 m/sec² is associated with significant PR.

Color Doppler

- ■ The severity of PR is related to the ratio of the diameter of the regurgitant jet to the diameter of the RVOT, but specific cut-off values have not been defined.
- ■ The length of the jet is also related to the severity of PR. A jet length of <20 mm is unlikely to be heard on physical examination, but jets >20 mm are associated with significant PR.
- ■ Regurgitant jet area indexed to body surface correlates well with PR regurgitant fraction.

Mild PR is associated with an index of 0.64 ± 0.60 cm/m^2, and severe PR is associated with an index of 2.2 ± 1.67 cm/m^2.

- A jet area >1.5 cm^2 represents significant PR.

Intracardiac Shunts: Key Diagnostic Features

- With significant left to right intracardiac shunting, pulmonary pressures increase, and right heart enlargement or dysfunction may occur. Thus, intracardiac shunts need to be excluded before the diagnosis of cor pulmonale is made.
- Interrogation of the interatrial and interventricular septum and LVOT and RVOT, as well as determination of pulmonary to systemic flow ratio (Qp:Qs), should be performed to exclude intracardiac shunts.
  - The Qp:Qs ratio is approximately 1 in patients with cor pulmonale and >1.5 in those with significant left to right intracardiac shunting.
- By color Doppler, the diameter of the jet through a defect correlates well with the anatomic size of an atrial septal defect (ASD) and can aid in determining which patients are eligible for closure of the defect.
- A saline contrast study increases the sensitivity and specificity for detection of interatrial septal defects in patients with "echo dropout" of the septum on two-dimensional echo images.

Pitfalls

- The modified Bernoulli equation for estimation of PA pressure does not hold true if there is PA or valve stenosis.
- Common underestimation of the PA systolic pressure is due to failure to obtain the true peak TR velocity due to noncoaxial alignment of the Doppler sample and the regurgitant jet.
- The indices used for assessment of mitral or aortic regurgitation severity cannot be applied directly to TR or PR, respectively. Because the RV and PA are low-pressure chambers, regurgitation of a similar volume of blood appears smaller in the right atrium or RV than in the left atrium or LV.
- Conversely, with moderate to severe pulmonary HTN, a jet may appear larger and longer

in relation to the right atrial or right ventricular outflow, despite a smaller volume of regurgitation, and TR or PR are overestimated.

- With right ventricular systolic or diastolic dysfunction and severe right atrial HTN or high right ventricular end-diastolic pressure, the right ventricular to right atrial or PA to right ventricular pressure gradient is decreased. Therefore, color Doppler underestimates the severity of TR or PR.
- Because of difficulties measuring the RVOT diameter, regurgitant volume and fraction are seldom used, and cut-off values for grading severity have not been determined.
- Thus, right ventricular and PA systolic and right atrial pressure, as well as right ventricular systolic function, must be considered when grading the severity of TR or PR.
- False-positive interatrial septal defects may occur with color Doppler because IVC flow is directed along the interatrial septum.
- Although bidirectional flow is the norm with ASDs, a saline contrast study may occasionally show only a "negative" contrast effect (contrast washout), which is sometimes difficult to separate from the effect of IVC flow.
- Unidirectional color flow (right to left) is the norm with a patent foramen ovale. With pulmonary HTN or cor pulmonale, the defect may enlarge, and more saline contrast traverses the defect.

FEATURES OF CHRONIC COR PULMONALE

- Right ventricular dilatation, hypertrophy, and/or dysfunction are hallmark features of chronic pulmonary HTN.
- Right ventricular and tricuspid annular dilatation lead to TR, which causes volume overload and further right ventricular and right atrial enlargement.
- Chronic pressure overload leads to distortion of the intraventricular septum during late systole and early diastole or a D-shaped LV during late systole (Fig. 5-1A).
- Chronic right ventricular volume overload causes the interventricular septum to shift to the left during diastole.

- Chronic right ventricular pressure or volume overload leads to right ventricular diastolic dysfunction. As for the LV, the spectrum of right ventricular diastolic dysfunction includes abnormal relaxation, tricuspid inflow pseudonormalization, and restrictive pattern.
- Ultimately, right ventricular systolic dysfunction of varying degrees occurs.

FEATURES OF ACUTE COR PULMONALE

- Pulmonary embolism and acute respiratory distress syndrome are the most common causes of acute cor pulmonale.
- Right ventricular wall thickness is usually normal, the RV dilates rapidly and right ventricular systolic dysfunction and failure ensue (6).
- Because of the relatively fixed pericardial space, acute right ventricular dilatation occurs with a proportional reduction in left ventricular dimension. Thus, the right ventricular size is often greater than the left ventricular size.
- The right ventricular apex loses its triangular shape and becomes more rounded.
- The right ventricular apex usually has relatively normal contraction despite moderate or severe right ventricular free-wall hypokinesis.
- Acute right ventricular pressure overload causes marked leftward displacement of the interventricular septum during late systole and early diastole.
- The resulting right ventricular dilatation and dysfunction leads to TR and further increase in right atrial pressure.
- A patent foramen ovale (usually maintained closed due to normally higher left atrial pressure) may open when right atrial pressure exceeds left atrial pressure and may lead to right to left shunting, worsening hypoxia, and, potentially, to paradoxic emboli (6).

STRATIFICATION OF PULMONARY HYPERTENSION

Mild Pulmonary Hypertension

- PA systolic pressure between 35 and 45 mm Hg.

- Right ventricular size, wall thickness, function, and septal motion are usually normal.
- Right atrial pressure is generally mildly to moderately elevated.

Moderate Pulmonary Hypertension

- PA systolic pressure is >45 mm Hg but <60 mm Hg.
- When pulmonary HTN is chronic, right ventricular size is normal to mildly dilated, right ventricular wall thickness is normal to mildly increased, but right ventricular systolic function is generally normal.
- Paradoxical septal motion is usually present.
- Right ventricular diastolic dysfunction, usually abnormal right ventricular relaxation, may be present.
- Right atrial HTN is generally present and is mild to moderate.

Severe Pulmonary Hypertension

- PA systolic pressure is >60 mm Hg.
- If chronic, RVH and dilatation vary from mild to severe, and diastolic dysfunction is present.
- Paradoxical septal motion is almost always present.
- Right ventricular systolic dysfunction is a common finding.

STRATIFICATION OF COR PULMONALE

Mild Cor Pulmonale

- Generally associated with moderate or worse pulmonary HTN, unless acute.
- Right ventricular size and wall thickness are usually normal.
- Paradoxical sepal motion is generally absent.
- Right ventricular diastolic and systolic functions are generally normal.
- Right atrial pressure is normal to mildly elevated.

Moderate Cor Pulmonale

- PA pressures are moderate to severely elevated.

- Right ventricular dilatation is moderate to severe, and RVH is generally present (wall thickness 0.6–1.0 cm).
- Paradoxical septal motion is usually present.
- Right ventricular diastolic and systolic functions are at least mildly abnormal.
- Right atrial pressure is moderately or severely elevated.

Severe Cor Pulmonale

- Pulmonary HTN, right ventricular dilatation, and RVH (wall thickness >1 cm) are severe.
- Paradoxical septal motion is always present.
- Right ventricular diastolic and systolic function may be severely compromised.
- Right atrial HTN is severe (usually >20 mm Hg).

DIAGNOSTIC ACCURACY FOR DETECTION OF PULMONARY HYPERTENSION AND COR PULMONALE

- The sensitivity and specificity of right ventricular free-wall thickness >5 mm for detecting pulmonary HTN are 93% and 95%, respectively.
- Assessment of right ventricular systolic function by the degree of downward excursion of the tricuspid annulus correlates highly (0.92) with ejection fraction determined by nuclear methods.
- Pulmonic valve mid-systolic closure and loss of the A wave by M-mode is highly specific (>90%) for pulmonary HTN.
- Paradoxical septal motion is seen in ≥60% of patients with pulmonary HTN (not due to left heart disease) and is present in most patients with moderate to severe pulmonary HTN (2).
- Echo as compared to right heart catheterization has a sensitivity of 78% and a specificity of 75% for detecting pulmonary HTN due to chronic obstructive pulmonary disease.
- Right ventricular free-wall hypokinesis with relatively normal RV apex contraction, known as the *McConnell sign*, has a sensitivity of 77%, a specificity of 94%, and a nega-

tive predictive value of 96% for pulmonary HTN or cor pulmonale, or both, due to pulmonary embolism (13).
- In patients with pulmonary emboli, TTE evidence of acute cor pulmonale is present in 68% of patients; however, in those with lobar or proximal pulmonary emboli, the sensitivity increases to 90% (6).
- The sensitivity of TEE is 60% to 80% in detecting PE. The sensitivity is increased to 84% in detecting proximal pulmonary emboli (4).
- A TRV/TVI_{RVOT} ratio of 0.175 has a 77% sensitivity and 81% specificity for PVR >2 Wood units (7).
- Color Doppler parameters of jet length, jet area, and PISA are ≥80% accurate for the assessment of the severity of TR.
- A TR vena contracta width ≥6.5 mm predicts severe TR with 88% sensitivity and 93% specificity.
- For PR, a pressure half-time <100 msec has a sensitivity of 76% and a specificity of 94% for predicting a significant regurgitant fraction of >20% (12).

USE IN PREGNANT PATIENTS WITH PULMONARY HYPERTENSION AND COR PULMONALE

- Pulmonary HTN is uncommon during pregnancy, but it carries a high risk of maternal and fetal morbidity and mortality.
- Maternal mortality is as high as 50%, and fetal death or prematurity is frequent (13,14).
- Therefore, pregnancy is contraindicated in patients with pulmonary HTN.
- Cardiac catheterization is the gold standard for measurement of PA pressures; it carries a 1% to 5% risk of complications, such as pneumothorax, bleeding, infection, and arrhythmia. In pregnant patients, the technique also adds the risk of fetal radiation exposure.
- In contrast, echo is a noninvasive method of determining PA pressures and may aid in monitoring patients throughout pregnancy.
- During pregnancy, increased blood volume, decreased systemic vascular resistance, and increased cardiac output lead to an increase in

the size of the IVC. Thus, pulmonary HTN may be overestimated.

- In one small study, echo misdiagnosed or overestimated PA pressures compared with cardiac catheterization in 32% of pregnant patients (14,15).
- Therefore, careful and integrated Doppler echo should be used for diagnosis and follow-up of pulmonary HTN during pregnancy.

INDICATORS OF POOR PROGNOSIS IN PULMONARY HYPERTENSION AND COR PULMONALE

- Patients with chronic thromboembolic pulmonary HTN and a mean PA pressure of >40 mm Hg and >50 mm Hg have a 5-year survival of 30% and 10%, respectively (16,17). Their 6-year survival improves to 75% after pulmonary thromboendarterectomy (PTE).
- Right ventricular systolic dysfunction in the setting of pulmonary embolism predicts a six-fold increase in mortality as compared to patients with normal right ventricular function (18).
- Patients with pulmonary embolism with persistent pulmonary HTN and right ventricular dysfunction at 6 weeks have a much higher mortality rate than patients whose pulmonary pressures and right ventricular function normalize.
- In patients with PPH, pericardial effusion, abnormal septal geometry, and right atrial size are independent predictors of increased mortality (19).

PARAMETERS THAT INDICATE THE NEED FOR THERAPEUTIC INTERVENTIONS

Thrombolytic Therapy

- Evidence of right ventricular dysfunction in hemodynamically compromised patients with pulmonary embolism is an indication for thrombolytic therapy.
- Whether patients with pulmonary embolism and right ventricular dilatation or dysfunction who are hemodynamically stable benefit from

thrombolytic therapy remains controversial (18).

- ◆ In a nonrandomized study of 719 hemodynamically stable patients with moderate or severe right ventricular dysfunction, thrombolysis was associated with a 30-day mortality of 4.7% as compared to 11.1% in the anticoagulation alone group.
- ◆ Patients who received thrombolytic therapy, however, tended to be younger and were less likely to have associated cardiac or pulmonary disease than patients treated with heparin.
- ◆ In a retrospective study of 128 patients who were evenly clinically matched, there was 6.25% mortality in the patients treated with thrombolytics versus 0% in those treated with heparin.

Pulmonary Thromboendarterectomy

- PTE is indicated in patients with severe cor pulmonale and chronic pulmonary thromboembolism (Fig. 5-1B).
- PTE is potentially curative and is associated with a relatively low mortality rate of <10% in experienced centers (16,17).
- Patients with severely elevated mean PA pressures (>50 mm Hg) and PVR (>1,100 dynes-sec-cm^{-5}) have a sixfold increase in operative mortality with PTE (16,17).
- Echo can therefore identify candidate patients for PTE and aid in the assessment of right heart pressures, chamber size, and right ventricular systolic and diastolic function after PTE.

Vasodilator Therapy

- Vasodilator therapy is the treatment of choice in patients with PPH.
- Although there are no specific echo criteria for vasodilator therapy in PPH, this technique can assist in identifying candidates for vasodilator therapy and in the assessment of response to therapy.
- Patients with severe cor pulmonale and class III and IV right heart failure from PPH are candidates for vasodilator therapy.

- Beneficial response to intravenous vasodilators is defined as >20% decrease in PA pressure and PVR with an increased or unchanged cardiac output. These patients can then be treated with oral vasodilators.
- "Nonresponder" patients are considered for continuous epoprostenol infusion, oral endothelin receptor antagonists, and/or lung transplantation.
- Administration of bosentan, an orally active endothelin receptor antagonist, significantly improved right ventricular to left ventricular diastolic area ratio, improved right ventricular ejection time and stroke volume, and improved left ventricular diastolic filling (20).
- Moreover, echo can predict vasodilator-induced hypotension. Echo parameters predictive of nifedipine-induced hypotension include leftward ventricular septal bowing, left ventricular transverse diameter in systole <2.7 cm, left ventricular transverse diameter in diastole <4.0 cm, left ventricular area in systole <15.5 cm^2, and left ventricular area in diastole <20.0 cm^2 (21).

Percutaneous or Surgical Closure of Intracardiac Shunts

- TTE, TEE, and intracardiac echo (ICE) can determine the size and location of an ASD. Patients with a secundum ASD with a diameter <38 mm and an adequate circumferential rim are candidates for percutaneous closure (22).
- TEE or ICE can be used during transcatheter repair of ASD by assessing device positioning and adequacy of septal capture, and identifying the presence of significant residual shunts.
- ICE may be as effective or potentially better than TEE in guiding transcatheter device closure of ASDs, and it may eliminate the need for general anesthesia (23).

Heart and Lung Transplantation

Heart and lung transplantation and single-lung or double-lung transplantation are considered in patients with PPH with New York Heart Association class III to IV heart failure who have failed vasodilators or have intolerable side effects.

FOLLOW-UP OF PATIENTS WITH PULMONARY HYPERTENSION AND COR PULMONALE

- Serial postoperative echo studies, initially at 1 month and then every 3 to 6 months, are valuable for follow-up of patients post-PTE to assess reduction in PA pressures.
  - ◆ Improvement in right ventricular size and function, PA pressures, and right ventricular systolic and diastolic function can be seen as early as 5 days after PTE (24).
- Echo every 1 to 3 months is also performed during medical treatment of PPH to evaluate the response to vasodilator therapy and guide decisions regarding alternative therapy.
- Follow-up echo should be performed at approximately 6 weeks after pulmonary embolism with right ventricular dysfunction because persistent pulmonary HTN and right ventricular dysfunction indicate a poor 5-year prognosis (18).

REFERENCES

1. Moraes D, Loscalzo J. Pulmonary hypertension: newer concepts in diagnosis and management. *Clin Cardiol* 1997;20:676–682.
2. Lehrman S, Romano P, Frishman W, et al. Primary pulmonary hypertension and cor pulmonale. *Cardiol Rev* 2002;10:265–278.
3. Cheitlin MD, Armstrong WF, Auriginema GP, et al. ACC/AHA/ASE 2003 guideline update for the clinical application of echocardiography: summary article. *J Am Coll Cardiol* 2003;42:954–970.
4. Vieillard-Baron A, Qanadli SD, Antakly Y, et al. Transesophageal echocardiography for the diagnosis of pulmonary embolism with acute cor pulmonale: a comparison with radiological procedures. *Intensive Care Med* 1998;24:429–433.
5. Rodes-Cabau J, Domingo E, Roman A, et al. Intravascular ultrasound of the elastic pulmonary arteries: a new approach for the evaluation of primary pulmonary hypertension. *Heart* 2003;89:311–315.
6. Jardin F, Dubourg O, Bourdarias JP. Echocardiographic pattern of acute cor pulmonale. *Chest* 1997;111:209–217.
7. Abbas A, Fortuin F, Schiller N, et al. A simple method for noninvasive estimation of pulmonary vascular resistance. *J Am Coll Cardiol* 2003;41:1021–1027.
8. Ozer N, Tokgozoglu L, Coplu L, et al. Echocardiographic evaluation of left and right ventricular diastolic function in patients with chronic obstructive pulmonary disease. *J Am Soc Echocardiogr* 2001;14:557–561.

9. Grossman G, Stein M, Kochs M, et al. Comparison of the proximal flow convergence method for the assessment of the severity of tricuspid regurgitation. *Eur Heart J* 1998;19:652–659.

10. Zoghbi WA, Enriquez-Sarano M, Foster E, et al. Recommendations for evaluation of the severity of native valvular regurgitation with two-dimensional and Doppler echocardiography. *J Am Soc Echocardiogr* 2003; 16:777–802.

11. Tribouiloy CM, Enriquez-Sarano M, Bailey KR, et al. Quantification of tricuspid regurgitation by measuring the width of the vena contracta with Doppler color flow imaging: a clinical study. *J Am Coll Cardiol* 2000;36:472–478.

12. Silversides CK, Veldtman GR, Crossin J, et al. Pressure half time predicts hemodynamically significant pulmonary regurgitation in adult patients with repaired tetralogy of Fallot. *J Am Soc Echocardiogr* 2003;16:1057–1062.

13. Ribeiro A. The role of echocardiography Doppler in pulmonary embolism. *Echocardiography* 1998;15: 769–777.

14. Weiss BM, Zemp L, Seifert B, et al. Outcome of pulmonary vascular disease in pregnancy: a systematic overview from 1978 through 1996. *J Am Coll Cardiol* 1998;31:1650–1657.

15. Penning S, Robinson KD, Major CA, et al. A comparison of echocardiography and pulmonary artery catheterization for evaluation of pulmonary artery pressures in pregnant patients with suspected pulmonary hypertension. *Am J Obstet Gynecol* 2001;184:1568–1570.

16. Fedullo P, Auger W, Kerr K, et al. Chronic thromboembolic pulmonary hypertension. *N Engl J Med* 2001;345:1465–1472.

17. Archibald CJ, Auger WR, Fedullo PF, et al. Long-term outcome after pulmonary thromboendarterectomy. *Am J Respir Crit Care Med* 1999;160:523–528.

18. Dalen JE. The uncertain role of thrombolytic therapy in the treatment of pulmonary embolism. *Arch Intern Med* 2002;162:2521–2523.

19. Raymond R, Hinderliter A, Willis P, et al. Echocardiographic predictors of adverse outcomes in primary pulmonary hypertension. *J Am Coll Cardiol* 2002;39: 1214–1219.

20. Galie N, Hinderliter A, Torbicki A, et al. Effects of the oral endothelin-receptor antagonist bosentan on echocardiographic and Doppler measures in patients with pulmonary arterial hypertension. *J Am Coll Cardiol* 2003;41:1380–1386.

21. Ricciardi M, Bossone E, Bach D, et al. Echocardiographic predictors of an adverse response to a nifedipine trial in primary pulmonary hypertension. *Chest* 1999;116:1218–1223.

22. Du Z, Hijazi Z, Kleinman C, et al. Comparison between transcatheter and surgical closure of secundum atrial septal defect in children and adults. *J Am Coll Cardiol* 2002;39:1836–1844.

23. Hijazi Z, Wang Z, Cao Q, et al. Transcatheter closure of atrial septal defects and patent foramen ovale under intracardiac echocardiographic guidance: feasibility and comparison with transesophageal echocardiography. *Catheter Cardiovasc Interv* 2001;52:194–199.

24. Menzel T, Wagner S, Kramm T, et al. Pathophysiology of impaired right and left ventricular function in chronic embolic pulmonary hypertension: changes after pulmonary thromboendarterectomy. *Chest* 2000;118:897–903.

6

Mitral Regurgitation

Phoebe A. Ashley and Carlos A. Roldan

■ Mitral regurgitation (MR) is the most common acquired valve disease in adults and results from primary disease of the leaflets, chordae tendinea, or papillary muscles (primary MR) or from left ventricular dilatation or systolic global or regional dysfunction (secondary MR).

■ The history and physical examination continue to be the method of choice for the initial assessment of patients with suspected MR.

■ The physical examination, however, has several limitations in the assessment of patients with MR.

◆ Patients with severe MR may develop asymptomatic left ventricular dilatation or systolic dysfunction.

◆ The audibility of mild MR is <20% and that of moderate MR is uncertain; patients with heart failure and severe MR have a soft, even inaudible murmur, and in acute severe MR, the systolic murmur is frequently inaudible.

◆ Eccentric MR jets may produce misleading physical findings. In posterior mitral leaflet prolapse, the mid-systolic to late systolic murmur radiates anteriorly and can be mistaken for aortic stenosis.

◆ Finally, the physical examination is limited in defining the etiology and severity of MR and of associated left ventricular dilatation and dysfunction.

COMMON ETIOLOGIES

Chronic Mitral Regurgitation

■ Mitral valve prolapse (MVP) is the most common cause of MR in the United States.
■ Chordal rupture or flail mitral leaflet.
■ Ischemic heart disease with associated papillary muscle dysfunction.
■ Rheumatic heart disease.

Acute Mitral Regurgitation

■ Primary chordal rupture is the most common cause of severe acute MR.
■ Ischemic papillary muscle dysfunction and partial or complete papillary muscle rupture.
■ Infective endocarditis.
■ Traumatic chordal or papillary muscle rupture.

ECHOCARDIOGRAPHY

Class I Indications for Echocardiography

In patients with MR, transthoracic echocardiography (TTE) and transesophageal echocardiography (TEE) play an essential role in determining the etiology, severity, impact on left ventricular size and function, and timing of valve replacement or repair (Table 6-1) (1,2).

TABLE 6-1. *Class I Indications for Echocardiography in Patients with Mitral Regurgitation (MR)*

Baseline evaluation to quantify severity of MR and left ventricular function in patient with suspected MR.

Delineation of mechanism of MR.

Annual or semiannual surveillance of left ventricular function (estimated by ejection fraction and end-systolic dimension) in asymptomatic severe MR.

To establish cardiac status after a change in symptoms.

Evaluation after mitral valve replacement or repair to establish baseline status.

Intraoperative TEE to establish the anatomic basis for MR and to guide repair.

TEE for evaluation of MR in patients in whom transthoracic echocardiography provides nondiagnostic images regarding severity or mechanism of MR and/or status of LV.

Diagnosis and assessment of hemodynamic severity of MR, leaflet morphology, and ventricular compensation in patients with physical signs of MVP.

To exclude MVP in patients who have been given the diagnosis when there is no clinical evidence to support the diagnosis.

LV, left ventricle; MVP, mitral valve prolapse; TEE, transesophageal echocardiography.
   Adapted from Cheitlin MD, Armstrong WF, Aurigemma GP, et al. ACC/AHA/ASE guideline update for the clinical application of echocardiography: summary article. *J Am Coll Cardiol* 2003;42:954–970; Bonow RO, Carabello B, De Leon, AC, et al. ACC/AHA guidelines for the management of patients with valvular heart disease. *J Am Coll Cardiol* 1998;32:1486–1588.

M-Mode and Two-Dimensional Echocardiography: Mitral Valve Morphology

Best Imaging Planes

■ TTE parasternal long-axis and short-axis and apical four-chamber and two-chamber views.
■ TEE transgastric short-axis and long-axis and mid-esophageal four-chamber, two-chamber, and long-axis views.

Key Diagnostic Features of Specific Morphology Patterns

Myxomatous Mitral Valve Disease

■ MVP is the *sine qua non* of this valve disease.
■ *MVP* is defined as mid-systolic to late systolic or occasionally holosystolic posterior dis-

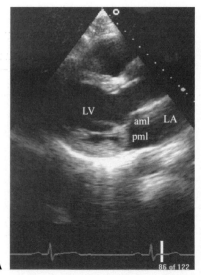
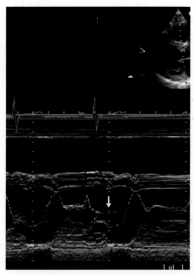

FIG. 6-1. Mitral valve prolapse. **A:** Parasternal long-axis view of the mitral valve demonstrates mid-systolic to late systolic displacement beyond the mitral annulus of the anterior (aml) and predominantly of the posterior mitral leaflet (pml). Diffuse myxomatous thickening of the posterior leaflet is also noted. **B:** The two-dimensional guided M-mode demonstrates mid- to late systolic prolapse predominantly of the posterior leaflet (*arrow*). LA, left atrium; LV, left ventricle.

placement (>2 mm) of the leaflets beyond the annulus plane (Fig. 6-1).
- It is further characterized by leaflet thickening (>5 mm) of soft tissue echoreflectance, redundant chordae, and billowing of the leaflets into the left atrium (LA) during systole.
- Leaflet coaptation of prolapsing leaflets may be symmetric or asymmetric. During symmetric coaptation, the leaflets' tip meet at a common point. During asymmetric coaptation, the tip of one leaflet is displaced toward the LA relative to the other (3).
- The severity of disease varies from mild displacement of the leaflets to complete prolapse or flail of a portion of the leaflet into the LA.

Flail Mitral Leaflet or Chordal Rupture

- During systole, the leaflet tip points and extends freely into the LA (Fig. 6-2).
  - The leaflet tip(s) point(s) toward the left ventricle (LV) in severe MVP without a flail portion (Fig. 6-1).
- There is noncoaptation or separation of the anterior and posterior mitral leaflets.
- There is systolic fluttering of the leaflet in the LA.

- Diastolic chaotic motion of the leaflet is frequently seen.
- Flail mitral leaflet or chordal rupture is always associated with significant and eccentric MR (Fig. 6-3).

Ischemic Mitral Regurgitation

- Ischemic MR occurs post–myocardial infarction (MI) in the absence of primary valve pathology, with an incidence of 20% similar for anterior and inferior MI.
- In inferior MI, akinesis or dyskinesis of the inferior wall associated with thinning, calcification, and/or fibrosis of the ischemic or infarcted posteromedial papillary muscle causes tethering and decreased mobility predominantly of the posterior mitral leaflet, leading to leaflet malcoaptation and relative anterior leaflet prolapse or pseudoprolapse (Fig. 6-4) (4).
  - The anterior mitral leaflet pseudoprolapse explains the characteristic eccentric and posterolaterally directed MR jet.
- In anterior MI, left ventricular dilatation and dysfunction lead to downward and lateral displacement of both papillary muscles, leading

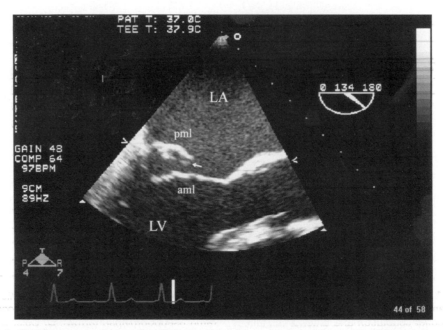

FIG. 6-2. Flail posterior mitral leaflet. This transesophageal echocardiographic (TEE) long-axis view of the mitral valve demonstrates a portion (mid-scallop) of the posterior mitral leaflet (pml) freely prolapsing (flail leaflet) into the left atrium (LA). Myxomatous thickening of the flail leaflet with ruptured chordae is noted (*arrow*). The anterior mitral leaflet (aml) has normal appearance. LV, left ventricle.

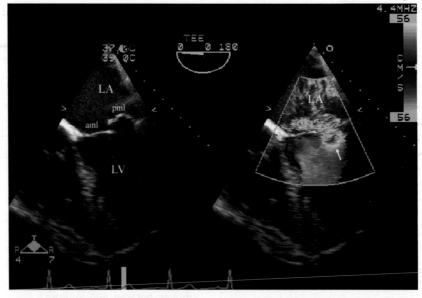

FIG. 6-3. Flail posterior mitral leaflet with severe mitral regurgitation. This mid-esophageal four-chamber transesophageal echocardiographic (TEE) view demonstrates a flail posterior mitral leaflet (pml). The mid-esophageal four-chamber TEE view with color Doppler demonstrates severe eccentric mitral regurgitation as judged by a large (>1 cm) proximal isovelocity surface area (*arrow*) and a large (>10 mm) vena contracta. aml, anterior mitral leaflet; LA, left atrium; LV, left ventricle.

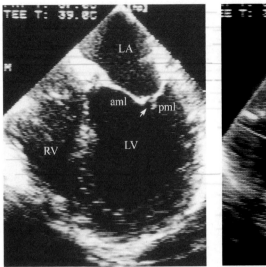
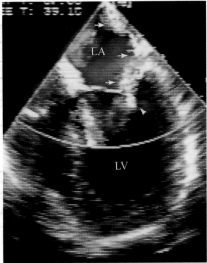

FIG. 6-4. Ischemic mitral valve pseudoprolapse. **A:** This transesophageal echocardiographic (TEE) two-chamber view of a patient with a large inferior myocardial infarction demonstrates incomplete mitral leaflet coaptation and anterior mitral leaflet (aml) pseudoprolapse (*arrow*). **B:** Color Doppler demonstrates a highly eccentric mitral regurgitation jet (*arrows*) with a vena contracta of 4 mm and a proximal isovelocity surface area radius of 7 mm (*arrowhead*). LA, left atrium; LV, left ventricle; pml, posterior mitral leaflet; RV, right ventricle.

to incomplete but symmetric malcoaptation and, therefore, central MR jets.

Papillary Muscle Rupture (Partial or Complete)

■ The detached papillary muscle head is visualized swinging freely from the LV into the LA.
■ The portion of the mitral leaflet attached to the ruptured papillary muscle is flail and associated with severe and eccentric MR.
■ Because of the highly eccentric MR jet, TTE underestimates its severity. Therefore, TEE should be promptly performed in these patients.

Rheumatic Heart Disease

■ Rheumatic heart disease is characterized by thickening and sclerosis, primarily of the leaflet tips.
■ The leaflets have a diastolic "hockey stick" appearance or a 90-degree angulation from the chordae to the leaflet tip due to commissural and chordal fusion.
■ Leaflet retraction with incomplete leaflet coaptation is also common.

■ In acute rheumatic fever, focal nodular thickening or discrete small vegetations may be identified.
  ◆ These nodules measure 1 to 5 mm, have a soft tissue echoreflectance, and are located more commonly at the leaflets' coaptation point.
  ◆ In recurrent rheumatic fever, anterior leaflet prolapse may be seen.
■ Unlike infective endocarditis, rheumatic leaflet nodules do not have independent mobility.

Degenerative Disease

■ Mitral annular calcification (MAC) is the *sine qua non* of degenerative disease.
■ MAC appears as an area of increased echogenicity on the left ventricular side near the insertion of the posterior leaflet, which moves parallel and anterior to the left ventricular posterior wall.
■ MAC may extend to the basal portion of the mitral leaflets, especially the posterior leaflet.
■ MAC may involve a focal area of the annulus or the entire U-shaped posterior annulus.

- MAC increases the rigidity of the annulus and impairs its systolic contraction, which in turn leads to MR.
- The authors define *MAC* as mild when the degree of sclerosis in a cross-sectional view of it is <5 mm, moderate if 5 to 10 mm, and severe if >10 mm.

Infective Endocarditis

- Vegetations are the *sine qua non* of infective endocarditis.
- Recently formed vegetations appear as circumscribed, soft tissue echoreflective masses, generally at the leaflet tips, with irregular borders and variable shape; they are more commonly pedunculated, but they can be sessile.
- Vegetations have a characteristic independent chaotic or rotary motion, involve the anterior or posterior leaflet, and are located on the atrial side of the leaflets' coaptation point.
- Freely mobile vegetations may prolapse into LA during systole and may fall into the LV during diastole. Rarely, large vegetations may cause mild valve obstruction.
- The underlying leaflets are usually structurally abnormal and have a specific underlying morphology (i.e., myxomatous, rheumatic, and so forth).
- Chronic or healed vegetations have homogeneously increased echoreflectance and are less or nonmobile.
- TEE is superior to TTE for the detection of vegetations and associated complications (perforation, abscesses, pseudoaneurysm or fistulas).

Impact of Mitral Regurgitation on the Left Ventricle and Left Atrium

- In acute MR, there is no significant change in left ventricular volume.
- In acute MR, LA is frequently normal in size.
- In acute severe MR, acute pulmonary hypertension leads to right heart chamber dilatation and inferior vena cava plethora.
- In chronic MR, left ventricular volume increases; hence, left ventricular end-diastolic and end-systolic dimensions and left ventricular mass increase.

- Left ventricular shortening fraction is maintained until late in the disease process.
- After mitral valve repair/replacement and elimination of the low-impedance left atrial outflow, ejection fraction decreases by 5% to 10%.
- Despite increases in left ventricular dimensions and left ventricular mass, left ventricular end-systolic wall stress does not change or may decrease. After correction of MR, left ventricular wall stress increases with the removal of the low-impedance left atrial outflow.
- A left atrial diameter of 4.5 cm on M-mode images correlates highly with left atrial hypertension resulting from significant MR and correlates better with natriuretic peptide levels than color Doppler parameters of MR (5).
- Determination of left atrial volumes with two-dimensional echocardiography (echo) is more accurate in assessing left atrial size than the traditional anteroposterior dimension.
- Left atrial dilatation is common in moderate or severe MR, but wide variation exists between MR severity and left atrial size.

Pitfalls

- M-mode is limited in the assessment of valve morphology patterns and in determining the etiology of MR.
- M-mode has limited sensitivity and specificity for detection of flail mitral leaflet or valve vegetation.
- M-mode has low sensitivity but high specificity for diagnosis of MVP.

Doppler Echocardiography for Assessment of the Severity of Mitral Regurgitation

Pulsed Wave Doppler

Best Imaging Planes

TTE apical and TEE mid esophageal two-chamber and four-chamber views.

Diagnostic Methods and Formulas

Regurgitant Flow and Regurgitant Fraction

- Total flow (TF) = mitral valve orifice area × time velocity integral across mitral valve.

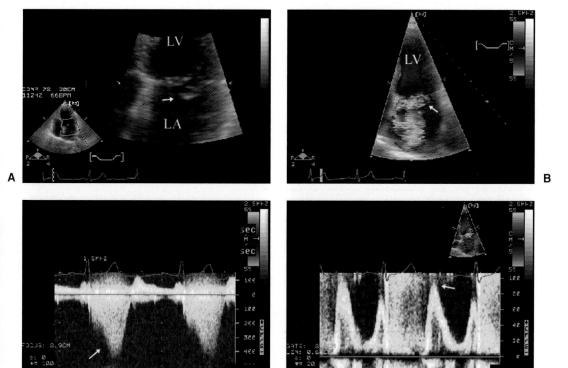

FIG. 6-5. Flail posterior mitral leaflet with severe mitral regurgitation. **A:** The two-dimensional close-up four-chamber view of the mitral valve demonstrates a flail posterior mitral leaflet (*arrow*). **B:** The corresponding color Doppler image demonstrates severe and highly eccentric (anteromedially directed) mitral regurgitation jet (*arrow*). **C:** The continuous wave spectral Doppler demonstrates late blunting of the regurgitant jet or V wave (*arrow*), as well a signal intensity similar to the mitral inflow. **D:** Finally, pulsed Doppler of the mitral inflow demonstrates an early diastolic transmitral velocity (E wave)/atrial filling transmitral velocity (A wave) ratio >1.5, a high E velocity (up to 1 m/sec) (*arrow*), and a rapid E wave deceleration slope. LA, left atrium; LV, left ventricle.

- Mitral valve orifice area = πr^2 (r = radius of mitral annulus from four-chamber view).
- Forward flow = left ventricular outflow tract area × time velocity integral across left ventricular outflow tract.
- Regurgitating flow = TF – forward flow.
- Regurgitant fraction (RFx) = regurgitating flow/TF.
- These methods are valid with eccentric and multiple MR jets.
- A regurgitant volume of ≥50 mL/beat and a RFx ≥60% indicate severe MR (6,7).

Mitral and Pulmonary Veins' Inflow Patterns

- Mitral and pulmonary veins' inflow patterns provide information regarding the hemody-

namic impact of MR on left ventricular and left atrial pressure (8).
- Mitral and pulmonary veins' Doppler patterns do not quantify MR severity.
- An increased early diastolic transmitral velocity (E wave) and E wave/atrial filling transmitral velocity (A wave) (E/A) ratio and a shortening of the isovolumic relaxation time and E wave deceleration time correlate with a high left atrial pressure, which is usually associated with significant MR (Fig. 6-5) (9).
- In severe MR, mitral E velocity is higher than A velocity, and it is usually >1.2 m/sec.
- As MR increases in severity, left atrial pressure increases, and in turn, the antegrade systolic flow in the pulmonary veins diminishes.

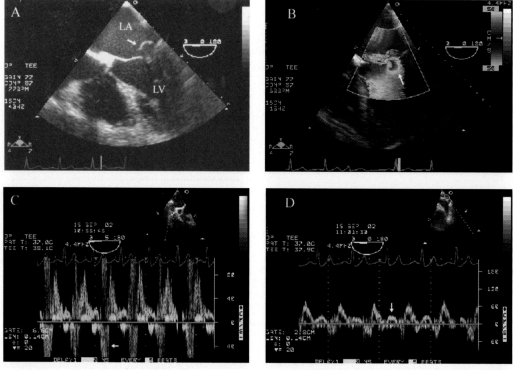

FIG. 6-6. Flail posterior mitral leaflet with severe mitral regurgitation. **A:** This mid-esophageal four-chamber transesophageal echocardiographic (TEE) view demonstrates a flail posterior mitral leaflet (*arrow*). **B:** This mid-esophageal four-chamber TEE view with color Doppler demonstrates severe mitral regurgitation as judged by a vena contracta width and proximal isovelocity surface area radius of >10 mm (*arrow*). The highly eccentric and anteromedially directed regurgitant jet extends into the right upper pulmonary vein. **C:** Pulsed Doppler interrogation of the right upper pulmonary vein demonstrates systolic reversal (*arrow*). **D:** Pulsed Doppler interrogation of the left upper pulmonary vein demonstrates blunting (*arrow*) followed by minimal systolic reversal. LA, left atrium; LV, left ventricle.

■ Systolic flow reversal in the pulmonary veins, especially identified in pulmonary veins not in the direction of the regurgitant jet, is very specific for severe MR and correlates well with high pulmonary wedge pressure (Fig. 6-6).

Continuous Wave Doppler

Best Imaging Planes

Same as listed in Pulsed Wave Doppler.

Key Diagnostic Features

■ The density of the continuous wave (CW) Doppler spectral of the MR jet is proportional to the number of red blood cells within the range of the ultrasound beam, and therefore, it provides an estimate of the severity of MR.
  ◆ If spectral signal is as intense as mitral inflow, MR is likely moderate or worse (Fig. 6-5).
■ The CW spectral recording of MR demonstrates a smooth curve throughout the regurgitant cycle. In acute MR, a notch (V wave) is noted along the velocity curve as left atrial pressure rises, left ventricular to left atrial pressures equalize, and the transmitral systolic pressure gradient falls abruptly (Fig. 6-5C).
■ The presence of pulmonary hypertension also provides an indirect clue to the severity of MR.

Color Doppler

Best Imaging Planes

- TTE parasternal long-axis and apical four-chamber and two-chamber views.
- TTE parasternal long-axis and short-axis views for assessment of the jet's vena contracta when the ultrasound beam is perpendicular to mitral orifice.
- TEE mid-esophageal four-chamber, two-chamber, and long-axis views (110–130 degrees).

Diagnostic Methods, Formulas, and Key Diagnostic Features

Jet Length or Depth

- MR is mild when the jet length is limited to the space immediately behind the leaflet coaptation point.
- Severe MR is suggested by a jet length that occupies more than one-half the length of LA.

Jet Area and Jet Area to Left Atrial Area Ratio

- A jet area <4 cm² and >10 cm² separates mild from severe MR (10,11).
- Jet to left atrial area ratios <20% and >40% correspond to mild and severe MR, respectively.
- The jet area method is simple and quick; however, it is subject to technical and hemodynamic variation.

Jet Width or Vena Contracta

- Vena contracta is the narrowest portion of the regurgitant jet, relates well to the regurgitant orifice area (ROA), and is a reliable indicator of the severity of MR.
- This method is particularly useful with eccentric MR jets.
  - ◆ Vena contracta <3 mm indicates mild MR, and vena contracta >7 mm indicates severe MR (Figs. 6-3 and 6-6) (12–15).

Flow Convergence or Proximal Isovelocity Surface Area

- Flow proximal to the regurgitant orifice or on the ventricular side of the orifice is equal to flow that passes through the regurgitant orifice into the LA.
- The proximal isovelocity surface area (PISA) is a semiquantitative method for evaluation of MR severity. It is simple, fast, reproducible, and reliable.
- The presence of PISA at a Nyquist limit of 50 to 60 m/sec should alert the examiner to the presence of significant MR.
- PISA should be assessed from TTE apical views, usually the four-chamber view, and from mid-esophageal four-chamber and two-chamber and longitudinal views (110–120 degrees).
- Using the concept of the continuity equation, PISA allows assessment of regurgitant volume and effective ROA as follows:

  Regurgitant flow = PISA area × Nyquist jet velocity
  PISA area = $2\pi r^2$ (r = radius of PISA)
  ROA = PISA area × Nyquist velocity/peak MR velocity by CW

- By adjusting down the Nyquist limit (the color Doppler velocity scale) to 30 to 40 cm/sec, a measurable radius at the point of aliasing can be more easily achieved.
- A PISA radius >8 mm and derived ROA >0.4 cm² using the PISA indicates severe MR (Figs. 6-3, 6-5, and 6-6) (16,17).
- A simplified PISA method allows the ROA to be estimated as ROA = r/2 (18).
  - ◆ This method assumes a driving pressure between the LV and LA of 100 mm Hg (MR jet = 5 m/sec).
  - ◆ The aliasing velocity is set at approximately 40 cm/sec.
  - ◆ The radius of the first aliasing contour is obtained.

Mitral Regurgitation Index

- The most accurate method for assessment of the severity of MR should include the integration of Doppler parameters with those of left ventricular and left atrial size, function, and pressure, as well as pulmonary artery pressure (Table 6-2) (18,19).
- This index includes six parameters: jet penetration or length, PISA, CW Doppler jet density, pulmonary vein inflow pattern, and left atrial size.

TABLE 6-2. *Summary of the Assessment of the Severity of Mitral Regurgitation (MR)*

Method	Mild	Moderate/ moderate to severe	Severe
Mitral inflow in patients >50 yr old	Dominant A wave	Variable	Dominant E wave (≥1.2 m/ sec)
Pulmonary vein inflow	Systolic filling predominates	Systolic blunting/systolic blunting or absence	Systolic flow absence or reversal and diastolic pre- dominance
CW jet density	Faint or incom- plete	Less dense than inflow/ as dense as inflow	As dense as inflow
CW jet contour	Parabolic	Usually parabolic	Blunted peak (V-notch wave)
Jet length (cm)	<1.5	1.5–2.9/3.0–4.4	>4.4
Jet area (cm²)	≤4	4–10	>10
Jet area/ left atrial area ratio (%)	<20	20–40	≥40
Vena contracta width (cm)	0.3	0.3–0.69	0.6–0.8
Regurgitant volume (mL/beat)	<30	30–39/40–49	≥50
Regurgitant fraction	<30	30–44/45–59	≥60
ROA (cm²)	≤0.2	>0.2–0.29/0.3–0.39	≥0.4
MR index (mean ± SD)	1.2 ± 0.4	1.7 ± 0.4	2.4 ± 0.3
Left atrial size	Normal	Normal or dilated	Usually dilated
Left ventricular size	Normal	Normal or dilated	Usually dilated

CW, continuous wave; ROA, regurgitant orifice area.

Adapted from Bonow RO, Carabello B, De Leon AC, et al. ACC/AHA guidelines for the management of patients with valvular heart disease. *J Am Coll Cardiol* 1998;32:1486–1588; Quinones MA, Otto CM, Stoddard M, et al. Recommendations for quantification of Doppler echocardiography: a report from the Doppler Quantification Task Force of the Nomenclature and Standards Committee of the American Society of Echocardiography. *J Am Soc Echocardiogr* 2002;15:167–184; Zoghbi WA, et al. Recommendations for evaluation of the severity of native valvular regurgitation with two-dimensional and Doppler echocardiography. *J Am Soc Echocardiogr* 2003;16:777–802; Irvine T. Assessment of mitral regurgitation. *Heart* 2002;88[Suppl IV]:iv11–iv19; Zhou X, Jones M, et al. Vena contracta imaged by Doppler color flow mapping predicts the severity of eccentric mitral regurgitation better than color jet area: a chronic animal study. *J Am Coll Cardiol* 1997;30:1393–1398; Heinle SK, Hall SA, Brickner ME, et al. Comparison of vena contracta width by multiplane transesophageal echocardiog- raphy with quantitative Doppler assessment of mitral regurgitation. *Am J Cardiol* 1998;81:175–179; Mele D, Schwammenthal E, Torp H, et al. A semiautomated objective technique for applying the proximal isovelocity sur- face area method to quantitate mitral regurgitation: clinical studies with the digital flow map. *Am Heart J* 2001;141:653–660; and Thomas L, Foster E, Schiller NB. Mitral regurgitation index: a new semiquantitative guide to evaluate severity. *Circulation* 1997;96:Suppl I-541.

- Each variable is scored 0 to 3, and an aver- aged global score is obtained.
- An MR index <1.7 or >2.0 indicates mild or severe MR, respectively.

Diastolic Mitral Regurgitation

- Diastolic MR is uncommon and is seen in patients with atrioventricular dissociation (high degree atrioventricular block or in patients with atrial tachycardia or flutter) who have high left ventricular end-diastolic pres- sure for any reason.
- It is generally trivial to mild and occurs dur- ing mid-diastole to late diastole. At this point, left ventricular end-diastolic pressure is high or highest, and mitral valve opening during

this time due to atrioventricular dissociation leads to diastolic MR (Fig. 6-7).

Pitfalls

- Determining regurgitant volume and fraction by pulsed Doppler is time-consuming, requires multiple measurements (from a variety of views) and calculations, and is, therefore, sensitive to errors (Table 6-3) (2,6,7).
- Left atrial pressure, left ventricular relax- ation, mitral valve area, and atrial fibrillation influence mitral and pulmonary vein inflow patterns.
- Assessment of flow at the mitral valve annu- lus is less reliable if valve and/or annulus are calcified.

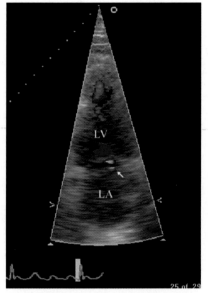
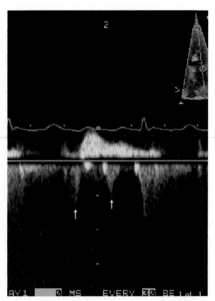

FIG. 6-7. Diastolic mitral regurgitation. **A:** Two-dimensional two-chamber view with color Doppler in a patient with atrial flutter and severe left ventricular diastolic dysfunction demonstrates trivial diastolic mitral regurgitation (*arrow*). **B:** The corresponding continuous wave Doppler demonstrates short-lasting and low peak velocity diastolic regurgitant jets (*arrows*). LA, left atrium; LV, left ventricle.

- Pulsed wave flow quantitation is not valid when concomitant significant AR is present, unless the pulmonic valve site is used.
- Left atrial hypertension is not specific for significant MR. Other causes of left ventricular diastolic dysfunction need to be considered or excluded.
- Reduced preload or afterload (i.e., hypovolemia or hypotension) leads to a decrease in left ventricular pressure and underestimation of the severity of MR.
- CW Doppler is sensitive for the detection of MR but nonspecific for assessment of its severity.
- With CW Doppler, it may be difficult to record the full envelope of an eccentric MR jet.
- Factors such as instrument settings (color gain, wall filter, transducer frequency, pulsed repetition frequency), transducer position, left atrial compliance and pressure, left ventricular pressure, and systolic function can affect the size of a regurgitant jet by color Doppler.
- Unlike the jet area and jet/left atrial area ratio, jet length and height correlate poorly with angiography.

- MR jet area and severity are underestimated in eccentric jets.
  - ◆ Eccentric MR jets hug the left atrial wall and appear smaller, and therefore, MR severity is underestimated (the Coanda effect).
  - ◆ In an eccentric MR jet, the jet area method should not be used.
- Central MR jets appear larger due to entrainment of red blood cells on the side of the jet when the Nyquist limit is set up at <50 cm/sec.
- Assessment of vena contracta from the two-chamber view should be avoided. As the ultrasound beam is parallel to the coaptation line, a wide vena contracta even in mild MR can be seen.
- The vena contracta may appear smaller with decreased left ventricular afterload, eccentric jets, multiple jets, and a nonspherical orifice.
- Assessment of the vena contracta is also limited by the decreased lateral resolution of color Doppler. Small errors in defining its

width lead to significant underestimation or overestimation of MR severity.

- Analysis of PISA may be limited in some cases if the hemisphere is difficult to define or the radius is difficult to measure.
- The time necessary to perform PISA measurements limits its routine applicability.
- Other limitations of the PISA method include (a) flattening of the contours near the orifice (underestimates flow across the valve), (b) constraint of flow by proximal structures, (c) uncertainty in localizing the regurgitant orifice in eccentric or multiple jets, and (d) variability in regurgitant orifice throughout the cardiac cycle.

Diagnostic Accuracy for Assessment of Mitral Regurgitation

- TTE and TEE are accurate for assessment of the etiology and severity of MR.
- Pulsed wave Doppler has a sensitivity of ≥90% and a specificity of ≥95% for detection of MR.
- Color Doppler jet area and jet/left atrial area ratio for assessing the severity of MR have high sensitivity and specificity and correlate highly with angiography (r = 0.78) (11).
- The vena contracta width correlates well with mitral regurgitant volume [r = 0.85; standard error of estimate = 10–20 mL] and ROA (r = 0.88, standard error of estimate = 0.15 cm^2) (7,12–15).
- In the setting of eccentric MR, vena contracta width correlates well with regurgitation severity as determined by electromagnetic flowmeters (r = 0.95 for peak flow rate, r = 0.85 for regurgitant stroke volume, and r = 0.90 for RFx) (12–15).
- A high correlation exists between the MR regurgitant volume and fraction assessed by the PISA method and angiography (r = 0.77 – 0.88 for regurgitant volume and 0.82 – 0.85 for RFx) (16,17).
- An MR index ≥2 has a sensitivity of 100%, specificity of 95%, and a positive predictive value of 91% for mitral RFx >40% (18).
- TEE has a sensitivity and specificity of 100% for the detection of ruptured chordae, compared to a sensitivity of 35% and a specificity of 100% using TTE.

TABLE 6-3. *Pitfalls of Color Doppler for Assessment of Mitral Regurgitation*

Pitfalls	Effect on color jet size
Hemodynamic effects	
Increased left atrial compliance	Increases
Increased left atrial pressure	Decreases
Decreased left ventricular systolic function	Decreases
Increased left ventricular pressure	Increases
Instrument settings	
Increased color gain	Increases
Wall filter	Decreases
Increased transducer frequency	Increases
Pulsed repetition frequency	Decreases
Transducer position	
Flow directed	Doppler angle effects
Inadequate alignment	Underestimates jet size
Jet eccentricity	
Coanda effect	Underestimates jet size

Adapted from Bonow RO, Carabello B, De Leon AC, et al. ACC/AHA guidelines for the management of patients with valvular heart disease. *J Am Coll Cardiol* 1998;32:1486–1588; Quinones MA, Otto CM, Stoddard M, et al. Recommendations for quantification of Doppler echocardiography: a report from the Doppler Quantification Task Force of the Nomenclature and Standards Committee of the American Society of Echocardiography. *J Am Soc Echocardiogr* 2002;15: 167–184; and Zoghbi WA, et al. Recommendations for evaluation of the severity of native valvular regurgitation with two-dimensional and Doppler echocardiography. *J Am Soc Echocardiogr* 2003;16:777–802.

Use in the Pregnant Patient with Mitral Regurgitation

- Unless severe, MR is generally well tolerated in pregnancy. The volume overload could increase, but the decrease associated with low systemic vascular resistance results in no change in the severity of MR.
- Women with more than mild MR should undergo echo if the intensity of the MR murmur increases or if symptoms develop during pregnancy.
- Women with known or suspected moderate or severe MR should have an echo performed in the first trimester, second to third trimester, 1

TABLE 6-4. *Echocardiography Follow-Up of Asymptomatic Patients with Mitral Regurgitation (MR)*

Severity of MR	Left ventricular size and EF	Echo follow-up
Mild	Normal ESD and EF	Every 5 yr
Moderate	Normal ESD and EF	Every 1–2 yr
Moderate	ESD >40 mm or EF <65%	Annually
Severe	Normal ESD and EF	Annually
Severe	ESD >40 mm or EF <65%	Every 6 mo

EF, ejection fraction; ESD, end-systolic diameter.
Adapted from Irvine T. Assessment of mitral regurgitation. *Heart* 2002;88[Suppl IV];iv11–iv19; and Otto CM. Evaluation and management of chronic asymptomatic mitral regurgitation. *N Engl J Med* 2001;345:740–746.

TABLE 6-5. *Echocardiography Parameters That Indicate Need for Mitral Valve Replacement or Repair*

Acute symptomatic MR in which repair is likely.
Symptomatic patients with EF >60% and left ventricular end-systolic diameter <45 mm
Symptomatic or asymptomatic patients with severe MR and EF 50–60% and left ventricular end-systolic dimension of 45–50 mm
Patients with severe MR and left ventricular end-systolic dimension of 50–55 mm
Patients with severe MR and moderate left ventricular dysfunction (EF 30–50%)
Asymptomatic patients with normal EF and atrial fibrillation or pulmonary hypertension (>50 mm Hg at rest or >60 mm Hg with exercise)[a]

EF, ejection fraction; MR, mitral regurgitation.
[a]Class IIa indication.
Adapted from Cheitlin MD, Armstrong WF, Aurigemma GP, et al. ACC/AHA/ASE guideline update for the clinical application of echocardiography: summary article. *J Am Coll Cardiol* 2003;42:954–970; and Bonow RO, Carabello B, De Leon AC, et al. ACC/AHA guidelines for the management of patients with valvular heart disease. *J Am Coll Cardiol* 1998;32:1486–1588.

to 2 months after delivery, and at any time if symptoms develop.

Follow-Up of Asymptomatic Patients with Severe Mitral Regurgitation

Regular echo follow-up is necessary in asymptomatic patients with moderate to severe MR to detect left ventricular dilatation and dysfunction (Table 6-4) (1,2,20).

Indicators of Poor Prognosis in Mitral Regurgitation

- Preoperative left ventricular end-systolic dimension >50 mm and left ventricular end-diastolic dimension >70 mm are predictive of postoperative left ventricular dysfunction and heart failure.
- A left ventricular end-systolic diameter index >2.6 cm/m^2, an end-systolic volume index >50 mL/m^2, a fractional shortening <31%, and a high wall stress index are predictors of postoperative left ventricular dysfunction, lack of regression of left ventricular dilation, and persistent symptoms.
- An effective ROA ≥0.4 cm^2 indicates severe primary MR, but in ischemic MR, an effective ROA ≥0.2 cm^2 predicts excess mortality.
- Atrial fibrillation and pulmonary hypertension are poor prognostic indicators in asymptomatic patients with severe MR and normal left ventricular ejection fraction.

Parameters That Indicate Need for Mitral Valve Replacement or Repair

- Echo is currently the diagnostic method of choice to determine when an asymptomatic patient with severe MR should undergo valve replacement or valve repair (Table 6-5) (1,2).
- In asymptomatic patients with severe MR, echo accurately separates patients who need valve replacement from those who need valve repair.
- Atrial fibrillation or pulmonary hypertension in asymptomatic patients may be indicators of left ventricular decompensation. There is a higher likelihood of conversion to normal sinus rhythm if surgery is performed within 6 months of the onset of atrial fibrillation.

Intraoperative Use in Patients Undergoing Mitral Valve Replacement or Repair

- TEE is invaluable intraoperatively before and after mitral valve repair or replacement.
- Intraoperative presurgical assessment of the mitral valve is important to define the valve pathology, determine the mechanism of MR,

and better define the type of valve surgery needed.

■ Intraoperative echo should not be used to assess the severity of MR, because a decrease in preload and especially afterload during anesthesia leads to underestimation of the true severity of MR.

■ In the immediate postoperative TEE, the following four parameters need to be assessed after valve repair.
  ◆ Severity of residual MR
  ◆ Absence of inflow obstruction or mitral stenosis
  ◆ Systolic anterior motion of the anterior mitral leaflet
  ◆ Left ventricular outflow obstruction

■ Preservation of the subvalvular structures is critical during mitral valve replacement to prevent left ventricular dilatation and dysfunction.
  ◆ Rarely, a retained chordae becomes entrapped in the prosthetic leaflets, leading to MR.

■ Carefully search for the presence and severity of paraprosthetic regurgitation after valve replacement.

■ Recognition of intracardiac air bubbles must be relayed to the surgical and anesthesia teams. Air emboli, more frequently to the right coronary artery, may result in hypotension due to ischemic right and left ventricular systolic dysfunction.

Use after Mitral Valve Repair or Replacement

■ Post–mitral valve repair:
  ◆ Baseline TTE at 1 to 3 months after surgery.
  ◆ Follow-up studies as clinically indicated.

■ Clinically normally functioning bioprosthetic valves:
  ◆ Baseline TTE at 1 to 2 months post surgery. At this point, the heart is healed, anemia is corrected, and serum catecholamine levels are reduced.
  ◆ Follow-up studies at 2 to 3 and 5 years postoperatively.
  ◆ After the fifth year, echo should be performed every 2 years and after 10 years, every year.

■ Clinically normally functioning mechanical prosthetic valves:

◆ A baseline echo should be obtained at 1 to 2 months.

◆ Follow-up echoes are recommended at 5 years, 10 years, then every 2 years until 15 years, after which echoes are recommended yearly.

REFERENCES

1. Cheitlin MD, Armstrong WF, Aurigemma GP, et al. ACC/AHA/ASE guideline update for the clinical application of echocardiography: summary article. *J Am Coll Cardiol* 2003;42:954–970.
2. Bonow RO, Carabello B, De Leon AC, et al. ACC/AHA guidelines for the management of patients with valvular heart disease. *J Am Coll Cardiol* 1998;32:1486–1588.
3. Playford D, Weyman AE. Mitral valve prolapse: time for a fresh look. *Rev Cardiovasc Med* 2001;2:73–81.
4. Roldan CA, Chai A, Coughlin C, et al. Mechanisms of mitral regurgitation post myocardial infarction. *J Am Coll Cardiol* 1998;31:255C.
5. Sutton TM, Stewart RAH, Gerber IL, et al. Plasma natriuretic peptide levels increase with symptoms and severity of mitral regurgitation. *J Am Coll Cardiol* 2003;41:2280–2287.
6. Quinones MA, Otto CM, Stoddard M, et al. Recommendations for quantification of Doppler echocardiography: a report from the Doppler Quantification Task Force of the Nomenclature and Standards Committee of the American Society of Echocardiography. *J Am Soc Echocardiogr* 2002;15:167–184.
7. Zoghbi WA, et al. Recommendations for evaluation of the severity of native valvular regurgitation with two-dimensional and Doppler echocardiography. *J Am Soc Echocardiogr* 2003;16:777–802.
8. Pu M, Griffin BP, Vandervoort PM, et al. The value of assessing pulmonary venous flow velocity for predicting severity of mitral regurgitation: a quantitative assessment integrating left ventricular function. *J Am Soc Echocardiogr* 1999;12:736–743.
9. Thomas L, Foster E, Schiller NB. Peak mitral inflow velocity predicts mitral regurgitation severity. *J Am Coll Cardiol* 1998;31:174–179.
10. The patient with mitral regurgitation. In: Roldan CA, Abrams J, eds. *Evaluation of the patient with heart disease: integrating the physical exam and echocardiography*. Philadelphia: Lippincott Williams & Wilkins, 2002.
11. Irvine T. Assessment of mitral regurgitation. *Heart* 2002;88[Suppl IV]:iv11–iv19.
12. Zhou X, Jones M, et al. Vena contracta imaged by Doppler color flow mapping predicts the severity of eccentric mitral regurgitation better than color jet area: a chronic animal study. *J Am Coll Cardiol* 1997;30:1393–1398.
13. Heinle SK, Hall SA, Brickner ME, et al. Comparison of vena contracta width by multiplane transesophageal

echocardiography with quantitative Doppler assessment of mitral regurgitation. *Am J Cardiol* 1998;81: 175–179.

14. Kizilbash AM, Willet DL, Brickner ME, et al. Effects of afterload reduction on vena contracta width in mitral regurgitation. *J Am Coll Cardiol* 1998;32:427–431.

15. Hall SA, Brickner ME, et al. Assessment of mitral regurgitation severity by Doppler color flow mapping of the vena contracta. *Circulation* 1997;95: 636–642.

16. Mele D, Schwammenthal E, Torp H, et al. A semiautomated objective technique for applying the proximal isovelocity surface area method to quantitate mitral

regurgitation: clinical studies with the digital flow map. *Am Heart J* 2001;141:653–660.

17. Pu M, Prior DL, Fan X, et al. Calculation of mitral regurgitant orifice area with the use of a simplified proximal convergence method: initial clinical application. *J Am Soc Echocardiogr* 2001;14:180–185.

18. Thomas JD. Doppler echocardiographic assessment of valvular regurgitation. *Heart* 2002;88:651–657.

19. Thomas L, Foster E, Schiller NB. Mitral regurgitation index: a new semiquantitative guide to evaluate severity. *Circulation* 1997;96:Suppl I-541.

20. Otto CM. Evaluation and management of chronic asymptomatic mitral regurgitation. *N Engl J Med* 2001;345:740–747.

7

Mitral Stenosis

Carlos A. Roldan

The history and physical examination are essential in the assessment of mitral stenosis, but they are especially limited in establishing the severity of the disease and in defining the suitability of the valve for percutaneous valvuloplasty or valve surgery.

DEFINITION

- Mitral stenosis results from chronic or recurrent rheumatic valvulitis leading to commissural fusion; thickening, calcification, and retraction of the anterior and posterior leaflets; and thickening, calcification, retraction, and fusion of the chordae tendinea.

- The mitral valve apparatus becomes a funnel-like sleeve and when severe, the mitral valve looks like a "fish mouth" and loses the ability to open during diastole.

COMMON ETIOLOGIES

- Rheumatic fever is the most common cause of mitral stenosis.

- Systemic lupus erythematosus and congenital mitral stenosis are rare causes.
- Degenerative severe mitral annular calcification rarely results in mild mitral stenosis.
- Pure mitral stenosis occurs in 25% of patients, combined mitral stenosis and mitral regurgitation (MR) occurs in 40%, and MR only occurs in 35% of patients.

ECHOCARDIOGRAPHY

Class I Indications for Echocardiography in Mitral Stenosis

- Transthoracic echocardiography (TTE) and transesophageal echocardiography (TEE) M-mode; two-dimensional (2D); pulsed, continuous wave, and color Doppler echocardiography (echo) are essential in the diagnosis, assessment of severity, and management of mitral stenosis (Table 7-1) (1,2).
- TTE or TEE M-mode or 2D and recently three-dimensional and intracardiac echo accurately characterize the morphology of the mitral valve and subvalvular apparatus and identify patients for valvuloplasty or valve replacement.
- TEE can detect atrial thrombi, guide a balloon valvuloplasty, and determine postprocedure mitral valve area, gradient, and degree of MR (3).

M-Mode and Two-Dimensional Echocardiography

Mitral Valve and Subvalvular Apparatus Morphology

Best Imaging Planes

- TTE parasternal long-axis and short-axis views and apical four-chamber and two-chamber views.
- TEE transgastric short-axis and long-axis views and mid-esophageal four-chamber and two-chamber views.

Key Diagnostic Features

M-Mode

- Mitral leaflets' tips thickening with markedly decreased mobility.

TABLE 7-1. *Indications for Echocardiography in Patients with Mitral Stenosis*

Diagnosis of mitral stenosis, assessment of hemodynamic severity (mean gradient, mitral valve area, pulmonary artery pressure), and assessment of right ventricular size and function

Assessment of valve morphology to determine suitability for percutaneous mitral balloon valvotomy

Diagnosis and assessment of concomitant valvular lesions

Reevaluation of patients with known mitral stenosis with changing symptoms or signs

Assessment of changes in hemodynamic severity and ventricular compensation in patients with known mitral stenosis during pregnancy

Postintervention (percutaneous valvotomy) baseline studies for valve function (early) and ventricular remodeling (late)

Use of TEE for performing percutaneous balloon valvotomy

Assessment of mean gradient and pulmonary artery pressure by exercise Doppler echocardiography in patients with discrepant resting hemodynamics and clinical findings[a]

TEE for assessment of atrial thrombus before mitral balloon valvotomy or cardioversion[a]

TEE to evaluate mitral valve morphology and hemodynamics when TTE is suboptimal[a]

TEE, transesophageal echocardiography; TTE, transthoracic echocardiography.
[a]Class IIa indication.

- Blunting to disappearance of the E to F slope.
- Parallel anterior motion of leaflets due to commissural fusion and chordal thickening and fusion (Fig. 7-1A).

Two-Dimensional
Transthoracic echocardiography

- Thickening with restricted mobility, predominantly of the leaflets' tips, leads to a characteristic diastolic doming mobility pattern, especially of the anterior leaflet known as the *hockey stick* (Fig. 7-1B).
- The diastolic doming mobility of the mitral leaflets is due to tethering of the leaflets by retracted and fused chordae tendinea and commissural fusion.
- The thickening, mobility, and calcification of the mitral leaflets as well as of the chordae tendinea can be assessed and scored from 1 (mild) to 4 (severe involve-

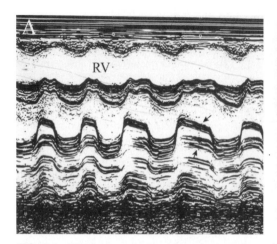
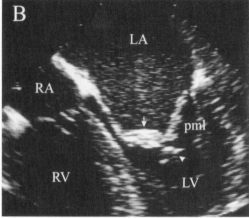

FIG. 7-1. Mitral stenosis by M-mode transthoracic echocardiography (TTE) and two-dimensional transesophageal echocardiography (TEE). **A:** By TTE M-mode, note the marked thickening, decreased mobility, and parallel anterior motion of both anterior and posterior mitral leaflets (*arrows*). **B:** By TEE two-dimensional imaging, note the severe thickening predominantly of the anterior mitral leaflet tip (*arrow*). Tethering of the anterior mitral leaflet results in doming mobility of the leaflet and its character-istic "hockey stick" appearance (*arrow*). The posterior leaflet (pml) appears diffusely thickened and is fixed. Also, note the involvement of the subvalvular apparatus (*arrowhead*). Mild left atrial spontaneous echo contrast is noted. LA, left atrium; LV, left ventricle; RA, right atrium; RV, right ventricle.

ment) (Table 7-2). The lowest score is 4, and the highest is 16.

♦ A score <8 predicts feasibility and short- and long-term success of balloon valvulo-plasty, defined as an increase in valve area

of >50%, valve area >1.5 cm², and ≤2+ MR (4).

♦ The degree of increase in mitral valve area is related to a complete or partial splitting of the commissural fusion.

TABLE 7-2. *Echocardiography Characterization of Mitral Valve and Subvalvular Apparatus*

Grade	Mobility[a]	Subvalvular thickening	Valve thickening[b]	Calcification[c]
1	Highly mobile valve with only leaflet tip restricted	Minimal thickening just below the mitral leaflets	Leaflets near normal in thickness (4–5 mm)	A single area of increased bright-ness
2	Leaflet middle and base portions have normal mobility	Thickening of chordal struc-tures extending up to one-third of the chordal length	Mid-leaflets normal, considerable thicken-ing of margins (5–8 mm)	Scattered areas of brightness con-fined to leaflet margins
3	Valve continues to move forward in diastole, mainly from the base	Thickening extending to the distal third of the chordal length	Thickening extending through the entire leaflet (5–8 mm)	Brightness extend-ing into the mid-portion of the leaflets
4	No or minimal for-ward movement of the leaflets in diastole	Extensive thickening and shortening of all chordal structures extending down to the papillary muscles	Considerable thicken-ing of all leaflet tis-sue (>8–10 mm)	Extensive bright-ness throughout much of the leaf-let tissue

[a]A ratio of the height vs. length of the doming of the mitral valve of ≥0.45 is predictive of optimal results in con-trast to a ratio of ≤0.25.
[b]Leaflet thickness <4–5 mm or a ratio of the mitral valve thickness vs. the thickness of the aortic root posterior wall of 1.5–2.9 is predictive of optimal results in contrast to leaflet thickness >8.0 mm or a valve to root wall thick-ness ratio of ≥5.
[c]Heavy calcification of both commissures is also associated with suboptimal results.

♦ Balloon dilatation does not split chordal fusion.

♦ Thus, severe subvalvular fibrosis and calcification predicts suboptimal results.

♦ Moderate MR is caused by excessive commissural tear (60–65%) and either leaflet or chordal rupture or perforation (35–40%).

♦ Severe MR is caused by leaflet rupture (73%), chordal rupture (18%), or excessive commissural tear (9%) (5).

■ Left atrial thrombi occur in 7% to 15% of patients with mitral stenosis, even in those in normal sinus rhythm (6).

■ With harmonic imaging, TTE can detect left atrial thrombi in patients with spontaneous contrast on TEE (7).

■ Systemic embolism during mitral valvuloplasty occurs in up to 4% of patients and is most commonly due to left atrial thrombi, then aortic atheromatous disease, and finally, catheter thrombi.

■ During balloon valvuloplasty, a left atrial size >6 cm poses difficulties for transseptal puncture and predicts a suboptimal increase in valve area.

■ With TTE 2D images, the mitral valve orifice area can be planimetered (8).

Transesophageal echocardiography

■ From the TEE mid-esophageal four-chamber and two-chamber views and using M-mode or 2D images, thickness of the mitral leaflets can be quantitatively assessed (9).

■ TEE can accurately assess the extent of leaflets' calcification and decreased mobility, as well as the extent of subvalvular apparatus involvement.

■ TEE can define the extent of commissural fusion, which predicts feasibility and outcome of percutaneous mitral valvuloplasty.

■ The prevalence of left atrial thrombi (more common in the appendage and left atrial posterior wall) in patients with mitral stenosis is 7% to 15%.

■ Left atrial thrombi and pseudocontrast are related to the severity of mitral stenosis, left atrial size, and atrial fibrillation (10). Pseudocontrast can be detected by TEE in approximately 25% of patients in normal sinus rhythm and in >60% of patients in atrial fibrillation (6).

■ The prevalence of left atrial thrombi and pseudocontrast is lower in patients with moderate or worse MR (17%), as compared to those without significant MR (94%) (11).

■ The presence of left atrial thrombus is a contraindication to balloon valvuloplasty.

Pitfalls

■ A reduced E to F slope on M-mode is nonspecific for mitral stenosis.

■ A reduced E to F slope can be seen in patients with left ventricular systolic dysfunction, elevated left ventricular end-diastolic pressure, and in those with aortic regurgitation (regurgitant jet does not allow normal opening of the anterior leaflet).

■ Definition of the mitral valve orifice by planimetry is difficult when the mitral valve and subvalvular apparatus are heavily calcified.

■ The mitral valve orifice is more irregular and more difficult to define after balloon valvuloplasty.

■ The true valve orifice may be overestimated if the imaging plane is above the leaflets' tip. Use of the long-axis view for orientation to the true orifice may prevent this pitfall.

■ By TEE and from the mid-esophageal four-chamber and two-chamber views, the extent of involvement of the subvalvular apparatus can be underestimated due to overshadowing by severely thickened and calcified mitral leaflets. This pitfall can be avoided by imaging the subvalvular apparatus from the transgastric short- and long-axis views of the mitral valve.

Three-Dimensional Echocardiography

Indications for Use

■ Three-dimensional TTE or TEE is feasible in 80% to 95% of patients and provides additional information to conventional echo regarding mitral valve morphology, especially of the valve commissures (12).

■ Three-dimensional echo is most valuable for evaluation of commissural fusion, an important predictor of outcome after percutaneous mitral valvuloplasty (Fig. 7-2) (13). Complete and partial commissural split are the main determinants of postprocedure valve area.

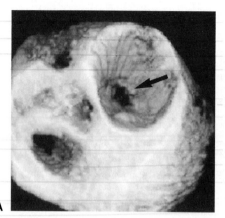 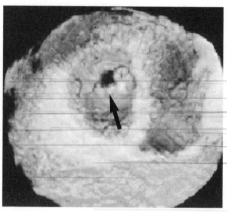

A   **B**

FIG. 7-2. Mitral stenosis by three-dimensional echocardiography. This three-dimensional echocardiogram shows a severely stenotic mitral valve viewed from above (**A**, *arrow*) and below (**B**, *arrow*) the valve. (Courtesy of Edward A. Gill, M.D.)

■ Three-dimensional echo accurately detects tears within the mitral leaflets leading to postprocedural MR.

Pitfalls

Prolonged acquisition time (>20 minutes), limited availability, and requirement of additional training and expertise.

Doppler Echocardiography for Assessment of the Severity of Mitral Stenosis

Pulsed and Continuous Wave Doppler Echocardiography

Best Imaging Planes

■ TTE parasternal long-axis or TEE mid-esophageal longitudinal view to assess left ventricular outflow tract diameter.
■ TTE and TEE four-chamber and two-chamber views for assessment of mitral valve peak and mean gradients, pressure half-time ($P_{1/2}$), velocity time integrals (VTIs), proximal isovelocity surface area (PISA), and vena contracta.

Diagnostic Methods and Key Diagnostic Features

Valve Gradients

■ Continuous wave VTI across the mitral valve orifice defines the peak and mean gradients.

Stenosis is mild if mean gradient <5 mm Hg, moderate if 5 to 10 mm Hg, and severe if >10 mm Hg (Table 7-3) (Fig. 7-3C).

Valve Area
Continuity equation

■ The principle of the continuity equation is that flow rate through a stenotic valve is the same as that of a nonstenotic valve (12).

Mitral valve area in cm^2 =
left ventricular outflow tract area [$\Pi(r)^2$ in cm^2] ×
pulsed Doppler VTI of left ventricular outflow tract (cm/sec) ÷
continuous wave Doppler VTI across the mitral valve (cm/sec)

■ Mitral stenosis is mild if valve area is >1.5 cm^2, moderate if 1.0 to 1.5 cm^2, and severe if <1 cm^2.

Pressure half-time

■ By continuous wave Doppler, $P_{1/2}$ measures the time (msec) it takes for the peak

TABLE 7-3. *Severity of Mitral Stenosis*

Severity	Valve area (cm^2)	Mean gradient (mm Hg)	Pressure half-time (msec)
Mild	1.6–2.0	<5	≤130
Moderate	1.1–1.5	6–10	130–220
Severe	≤1.0	>10	>220

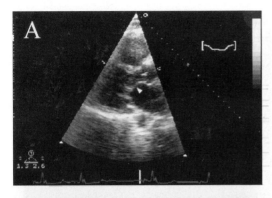

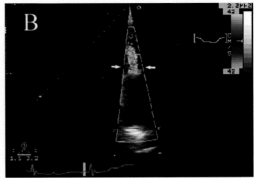

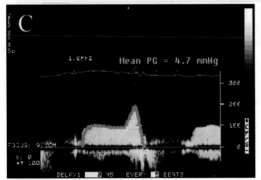

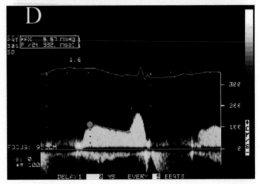

FIG. 7-3. Mitral stenosis by two-dimensional and color Doppler transthoracic echocardiography (TTE). **A:** Two-dimensional TTE parasternal long-axis view of the mitral valve showing thickening of the mitral leaflets' tip and diastolic doming mobility of the anterior mitral leaflet (*arrowhead*). **B:** Narrow sector scan TTE apical four-chamber view of the mitral valve with color Doppler illustrating the vena contracta (*arrows*) of the mitral valve to orient the most appropriate sampling site by continuous wave Doppler. **C:** Mitral valve mean gradient of 4.7 mm Hg is suggestive of mild to moderate mitral stenosis, but patient's volume depletion led to underestimation of valve gradient. **D:** By pressure half-time (332 msec), mitral stenosis was severe, with a valve area of 0.7 cm².

mitral valve gradient to decrease by 50%. The longer the $P_{1/2}$, the worse is the mitral stenosis.

- ◆ *Stenosis is mild if $P_{1/2}$ is <130 msec, moderate if 130 to 220 msec, and severe if >220 msec* (Fig. 7-3D).
- ◆ *Mitral valve area is calculated as the constant 220 ÷ $P_{1/2}$.*

Other Doppler parameters

- By pulsed Doppler, pulmonary veins' inflow demonstrates a decrease in systolic, diastolic, and atrial reversal velocities (14). These velocities increase significantly post–mitral valvuloplasty.
- The severity of pulmonary hypertension correlates with the severity of mitral stenosis.

- Pulmonary hypertension, and right ventricular dilatation and hypertrophy result from chronically elevated left atrial and pulmonary capillary wedge pressures.

Pitfalls

- Pressure gradients are flow-rate dependent. Therefore, volume overload or dehydration can lead to overestimation or underestimation of pressure gradients, respectively (Fig. 7-3C).
- The continuity equation is less accurate in patients with more than mild aortic regurgitation or MR.
- If alignment of Doppler beam is not parallel to the direction of blood flow or within the center of the mitral stenotic jet, $P_{1/2}$ can be overestimated (longer in duration), and valve area can

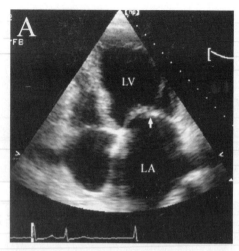
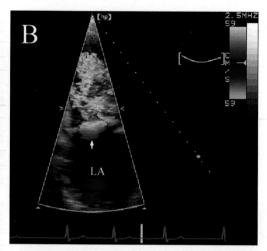

FIG. 7-4. Mitral stenosis by two-dimensional and color Doppler transthoracic echocardiography (TTE). **A:** This four-chamber TTE shows marked thickening and decreased doming mobility of anterior and posterior mitral leaflets (*arrow*). **B:** A large flow convergence zone (*arrow*) is noted proximal to the mitral orifice. The mitral valve area was 0.9 cm² as calculated with the proximal isovelocity surface area. LA, left atrium; LV, left ventricle.

be underestimated. Orientation of beam with the color Doppler vena contracta may help to prevent this pitfall (Fig. 7-3B).

- Moderate or worse aortic regurgitation and other conditions associated with high left ventricular end-diastolic pressure lead to shortening of the $P_{1/2}$ and overestimation of the mitral valve area.
- Decreased left ventricular relaxation (especially in the elderly) can result in prolongation of the $P_{1/2}$ and underestimation of the mitral valve area.
- During tachycardia, fusion of initial and late velocities of the mitral inflow preclude assessment of $P_{1/2}$.
- Finally, $P_{1/2}$ is unreliable for assessment of stenosis severity immediately after valvuloplasty because of worsening of left atrial compliance.

Color Doppler Echocardiography

Best Imaging Planes

- TTE apical and TEE mid-esophageal four-chamber and two-chamber views.

Diagnostic Methods and Key Diagnostic Features

- With color Doppler, high-velocity flow can be demonstrated at the valve orifice (vena contracta).
- Proximal to the stenotic orifice (atrial side), the flow convergence zone or PISA is seen by adjust-

ing the color Doppler settings to define a hemispheric aliasing surface area (Figs. 7-4 and 7-5).

- The PISA can be used to calculate flow rate and the mitral valve area (13).
  - ◆ The velocity at the outer shells of the PISA equals that of the Nyquist limit.
  - ◆ The PISA length allows for calculation of flow rate proximal to the stenotic valve orifice, which equals flow rate across the stenotic orifice (principle of the continuity equation).
    - • Proximal flow rate (cm³/sec) using the formula for a hemielliptic model:

$$2 \times \pi \times r^2 \times Vr$$

    - • Where r = radius or length of the PISA and Vr = color Doppler aliasing velocity (cm/sec). This value can be multiplied by a factor that corrects for the inflow angle (∅/180).
  - ◆ Valve area = proximal flow rate ÷ continuous wave early peak velocity across the mitral valve (Fig. 7-5B,D).
- The vena contracta also can be used for calculation of mitral valve area (15).
  - ◆ By TTE or TEE, using the four-chamber and two-chamber views, mitral valve area is calculated using the color Doppler inflow jet widths within 1 cm below the leaflets' coaptation point as follows:

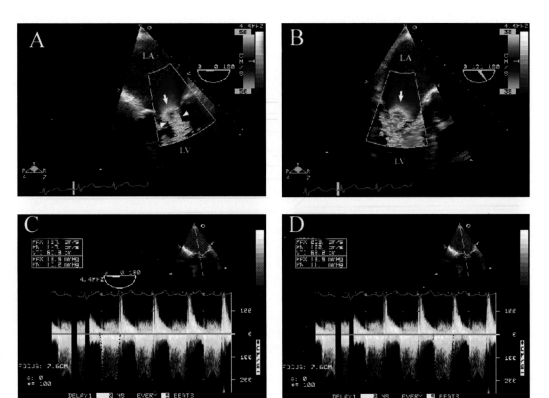

FIG. 7-5. Mitral stenosis by color and continuous wave Doppler transesophageal echocardiography (TEE). **A:** Close-up four-chamber TEE view of the mitral valve with color Doppler illustrating a well-defined proximal isovelocity surface area (PISA) (*arrow*) (at a Nyquist limit of 56 cm/sec) and a vena contracta width of 1 cm (*arrowheads*). By the vena contracta method, mitral stenosis was defined as severe, with a valve area of 0.7–0.8 cm². **B:** Close-up four-chamber TEE view of the mitral valve with color Doppler illustrating a well-defined PISA of 1.4 cm (*arrow*) (at a Nyquist limit of 38 cm/sec). By the PISA method, mitral stenosis was defined as severe, with a valve area of 0.6–0.7 cm². **C,D:** By continuous wave Doppler, mitral valve mean gradients were 11–12 mm Hg, consistent with severe mitral stenosis.

π(jet width by horizontal plane ÷ 2 × jet width by vertical plane ÷ 2) (Figs 7-3B and 7-5A)

◆ The accuracy of this method is similar to that of other echo methods for assessment of mitral valve area.

■ Color Doppler allows assessment of the presence and severity of MR.

◆ The presence of 2+ MR is considered a contraindication to mitral balloon valvuloplasty.

Diagnostic Accuracy in the Assessment of Mitral Stenosis

■ Three-dimensional planimetry of the mitral valve area prevalvuloplasty and postvalvuloplasty correlates highly with valve areas measured by 2D planimetry, $P_{1/2}$, and continuity equation, with less intraobserver and interobserver variability than 2D echo and $P_{1/2}$.

■ Pressure gradients and valve area by the different echo methods have shown high correlation when compared among themselves and against catheter-derived gradients and area and anatomic orifice measurements (Table 7-4).

◆ Planimetry of the mitral valve orifice by 2D TTE correlates well with other echo methods, correlates moderately against the Gorlin formula, and has up to a 0.95 correlation when compared with a true anatomic orifice (8).

◆ Calculation of mitral valve area using the $P_{1/2}$ method has demonstrated a correlation coeffi-

TABLE 7-4. *Diagnostic Accuracy of Echocardiography for Assessment of Mitral Stenosis*

Diagnostic methods	Correlation coefficient	Standard error
2D planimetry vs. cardiac catheterization (valve area)	0.71–0.81[a]	0.17 cm^2
Pressure gradients vs. cardiac catheterization	0.70–0.89	
P$_{1/2}$ vs. cardiac catheterization (valve area)	0.71–0.81[a]	0.11–0.15 cm^2
Continuity equation vs. cardiac catheterization (valve area)	0.71–0.84	0.22 cm^2
PISA method by TTE or TEE vs. cardiac catheterization or P$_{1/2}$ (valve area)	0.87–0.90	0.13 cm^2
Color Doppler jet widths vs. cardiac catheterization, 2D planimetry, or Doppler P$_{1/2}$ (valve area)	0.83–0.94	0.13–0.24 cm^2
3D echo planimetry vs. 2D echo and P$_{1/2}$ (valve area)	0.93 and 0.87, respectively	0.09 ± 0.14 cm^2 and 0.16 ± 0.19 cm^2, respectively

2D, two-dimensional; 3D, three-dimensional; P$_{1/2}$, pressure half-time; PISA, proximal isovelocity surface area; TEE, transesophageal echocardiography; TTE, transthoracic echocardiography.
[a]Lowest values of 0.51–0.71 in patients post–balloon valvuloplasty are due to technical difficulties, rapidly changing hemodynamics, or development of atrial septal defect.

cient of ≥0.80 compared with direct measurement of an anatomic valve orifice.

◆ Calculation of mitral valve area using the color Doppler PISA method has demonstrated a correlation coefficient of 0.87 when compared with measurement of an anatomic valve orifice (16).

■ In patients with mitral stenosis, TTE has a sensitivity of 32% and a specificity of 94% for detecting left atrial thrombi.

■ In patients with mitral stenosis, TEE has a sensitivity of 98% and a specificity of 98% for detecting left atrial appendage thrombi. TEE has a sensitivity of 81% and specificity of 99% for detecting thrombi in the main left atrial cavity (10).

Prognostic Value in Mitral Stenosis

■ A mitral valve morphology score ≤8 predicts feasibility and short-term and long-term success of mitral balloon valvuloplasty (4).

■ Patients with a successful valvuloplasty have an event-free survival (death, repeat valvuloplasty, or valve replacement) of 80% to 96% at 1 year, >60% at 4 years, and >55% at 6 years (17,18).

◆ A mitral valve morphology score >10 and commissural calcification have been associated with a 9% to 13% incidence of moderate to severe MR after balloon valvuloplasty.

■ The severity of tricuspid regurgitation is related to the severity of mitral stenosis. Therefore, the presence of severe tricuspid regurgitation predicts a lower event-free survival after mitral balloon valvuloplasty than does mild or moderate tricuspid regurgitation.

■ A left atrial diameter of >6 cm is associated with more severe mitral stenosis and lower success and higher complication rates during mitral balloon valvuloplasty.

■ Patients with mitral stenosis and severe pulmonary hypertension have a <3-year survival rate (19).

Indicators for Mitral Valvuloplasty, Valve Repair, or Valve Replacement

■ The ideal candidate for balloon valvuloplasty is a patient with highly mobile and noncalcified mitral leaflets and subvalvular apparatus or a valve morphology score <8 and none or mild MR (Table 7-5).

■ In patients with bilateral commissural calcification or in those with moderately thickened leaflets but severe subvalvular thickening and fusion and a valve score >8 and valve area <0.8 cm^2, open mitral commissurotomy is the therapy of choice.

■ In patients with a mitral valve morphology score >10, severe bilateral commissural, or subvalvular calcification, valve replacement is probably the best therapeutic alternative.

■ Patients with 2+ MR or left atrial thrombi should undergo mitral valve replacement.

TABLE 7-5. *Value of Echocardiography in Determining Class I Indications for Mitral Valvuloplasty, Valve Repair, or Valve Replacement in Patients with Mitral Stenosis*

Balloon valvuloplasty for symptomatic patients (NYHA functional class II–IV), moderate or severe stenosis (valve area ≤1.5 cm^2), and valve morphology favorable for valvuloplasty in the absence of left atrial thrombus or moderate or severe MR.

Valve repair for symptomatic patients (functional class III–IV), valve area ≤1.5 cm^2, valve morphology favorable for repair, and balloon valvuloplasty is not available.

Valve repair for symptomatic patients (class III–IV), valve area ≤1.5 cm^2, valve morphology favorable for repair, and left atrial thrombus present despite anticoagulation.

Valve repair for symptomatic patients (class III–IV), valve area ≤1.5 cm^2, and nonpliable or calcified valve with the decision to proceed with repair or replacement made at the time of the operation.

Valve replacement for symptomatic patients (class III–IV) with a valve area ≤1.5 cm^2 who are not considered candidates for percutaneous balloon valvuloplasty or valve repair.

MR, mitral regurgitation; NYHA, New York Heart Association.

- Patients with unsuccessful (valve area <1.5 cm^2) or complicated mitral balloon valvuloplasty with cardiac perforation or acute severe MR require emergent valve replacement.
- Patients with mitral restenosis or a large left to right shunt post–mitral valvuloplasty require valve replacement.

Use in the Pregnant Patient with Mitral Stenosis

- The diagnostic accuracy of echo for detection and assessment of the severity of mitral stenosis is similar in pregnant and nonpregnant patients.
- Mitral stenosis is the most common clinically relevant valve disease associated with pregnancy.
- Maternal and fetal morbidity and mortality are highest among patients with valve area <1.5 cm^2 and New York Heart Association functional class III to IV.
- The physiologic volume overload and increase in heart rate associated with pregnancy lead to an increase in transmitral flow rate, decreased diastolic filling time, and increases in left atrial

and pulmonary capillary wedge pressure and left heart failure.

- Therefore, pregnant, asymptomatic patients with moderate to severe mitral stenosis need clinical and echo surveillance during the second to third trimesters and during labor.
- Balloon valvuloplasty is the therapy of choice in symptomatic pregnant patients (class III–IV) with severe mitral stenosis (valve area <1 cm^2).
  - ◆ With echo guidance (TEE or intracardiac echo), balloon valvuloplasty can be successfully performed in 94% to 98% of pregnant patients with none or minimal (<10 minutes) radiation exposure of the mother and fetus (20).
  - ◆ This technique performed early during the third trimester allows term pregnancies and vaginal deliveries, and it reduces the morbidity and mortality of patients and offspring.
- The immediate and long-term results of balloon valvuloplasty (increase in mitral valve area, reduction in valve gradients and pulmonary artery pressure) under echo guidance are similar to those achieved with fluoroscopic guidance in nonpregnant patients.

Stress Echocardiography in Patients with Mitral Stenosis

In patients in whom valve area, peak and mean gradients, or pulmonary artery pressure are disproportional to symptoms, an increase in mean gradient (>15 mm Hg) and pulmonary artery systolic pressure (>60 mm Hg) during stress echo indicate severe stenosis and need for valvuloplasty or valve replacement (21–23).

Intraoperative or Periprocedural Use in Patients with Mitral Stenosis

- On-line TEE is a feasible, safe, and well-tolerated alternative to fluoroscopy for guiding percutaneous balloon valvuloplasty (3).
- Intraoperative or periprocedural echo, especially TEE, is indicated in patients undergoing balloon mitral valvuloplasty or open (surgical) mitral commissurotomy.
- During mitral balloon valvuloplasty, echo assists in transseptal catheterization by

- ◆ Noting tenting of atrial septum or by saline-contrast injection.
- ◆ Positioning balloon in the mitral valve.
- ◆ Avoiding placement and inflation of balloon close to the interatrial septum, which can lead to atrial septal defect.
- ◆ Preventing inflation of the catheter in the left atrial appendage.
- ◆ Detecting left atrial thrombi.
- As for mitral balloon valvuloplasty, TEE can also assist, define the success, and detect complications associated with open-heart valvuloplasty.
  - ◆ TEE also helps select balloon size (ratio of mitral annulus to balloon diameters >1) and immediately assess the effects of balloon dilations on valve area, gradient, and degree of MR.
  - ◆ Using TEE, fluoroscopy time can be reduced to <10 minutes.
  - ◆ TEE also assists in defining the success of the procedure (increase in mitral valve area >2 cm^2, <2+ MR, and >60% decrease in peak and mean gradients).
- Echo detects and guides immediate therapy of procedure-related complications [severe MR (3%), atrial septal defect (10%), and atrial or ventricular rupture with cardiac tamponade (0.2–4.0%)].
- New or worsening MR (generally of one degree) occurs in 19% to 85% of patients undergoing mitral balloon valvuloplasty.
  - ◆ An increase of two or more degrees occurs in 3% to 10%, and the need for emergent surgery due to severe MR occurs in 1.1% to 2.0% of cases.
- Atrial septal defects as a result of transseptal catheterization range from 0.3 to 1.5 cm in diameter and are detected in 7% to 33% of cases by oximetry (this technique does not detect defects <0.5 cm); in approximately 50% of cases by TTE; and in up to 87% by TEE.
  - ◆ Defects of >1 cm are of hemodynamic importance, and those of <0.7 cm generally close within 6 months.
  - ◆ Atrial perforation during transseptal catheterization can be treated with pericardiocentesis, close observation, or surgery.

- Perforation of the left ventricle during balloon inflation is the most common indication for emergent surgery and the most common cause of death.
- Intracardiac echo may become the procedure of choice to guide and assess the results of percutaneous and surgical valvuloplasty in patients with mitral stenosis (24).

Follow-Up of Patients with Mitral Stenosis Pre– and Post–Mitral Valvuloplasty, Open Commissurotomy, or Valve Replacement

- Reevaluation of patients with known mitral stenosis with changing symptoms or signs (1,2).
- In patients post–percutaneous valvuloplasty or open commissurotomy, baseline echo for valve function and hemodynamics should be performed.
- In patients with a successful balloon valvuloplasty (mitral valve area >2 cm^2 and <2+ MR), valve restenosis (loss of 50% of post-procedure valve area or a valve area <1.5 cm^2) occurs in 6% to 21% of patients at 19 to 22 months.
  - ◆ Therefore, patients post–successful balloon valvuloplasty should have follow-up echo at 18 to 24 months. Those with less optimal results should have follow-up echo at least at 12 months.
- Patients with MR before or after balloon valvuloplasty have a lower event-free survival and probably should have echo follow-up at 6 to 12 months.
- Approximately two-thirds of atrial septal defects post–balloon valvuloplasty close during follow-up, and persistent small defects are well tolerated. These patients should have follow-up echo at least once a year to assess development of right ventricular volume overload and pulmonary hypertension.
- Exercise Doppler echo should be performed for assessment of mean gradient and pulmonary artery pressure in patients with discrepant resting hemodynamics and clinical findings.
- Patients who have undergone bioprosthetic or mechanical valve replacement should

undergo follow-up echo studies as delineated in Chapter 10.

REFERENCES

1. Cheitlin MD, Armstrong WF, Aurigemma GP, et al. ACC/AHA/ASE guideline update for the clinical application of echocardiography: summary article. *J Am Coll Cardiol* 2003;42:954–970.
2. Bonow RO, Carabello B, De Leon AC, et al. ACC/AHA guidelines for the management of patients with valvular heart disease. *J Am Coll Cardiol* 1998;32: 1486–1588.
3. Park SH, Kim MA, Hyon MS. The advantages of on-line transesophageal echocardiography guide during percutaneous balloon mitral valvuloplasty. *J Am Soc Echocardiogr* 2000;13:26–34.
4. Hildick-Smith DJ, Taylor GJ, Shapiro LM. Inoue balloon mitral valvuloplasty: long-term clinical and echocardiography follow-up of a predominantly unfavorable population. *Eur Heart J* 2000;21:1690–1697.
5. Kaul UA, Singh S, Kalra GS, et al. Mitral regurgitation following percutaneous mitral commissurotomy: a single center experience. *J Heart Valve Dis* 2000;9: 262–266.
6. Agarwal AK, Venugopalan P. Left atrial spontaneous echo contrast in patients with rheumatic mitral valve stenosis in normal sinus rhythm: relationship to mitral valve and left atrial measurements. *Int J Cardiol* 2001;77:63–68.
7. Ha JW, Chung N, Kang SM, et al. Enhanced detection of left atrial spontaneous echo contrast by transthoracic harmonic imaging in mitral stenosis. *J Am Soc Echocardiogr* 2000;13:849–854.
8. Shiran A, Goldstein SA, Ellahham S, et al. Accuracy of two-dimensional echocardiographic planimetry of the mitral valve area before and after balloon valvuloplasty. *Cardiology* 1998;90:227–230.
9. Crawford MH, Roldan CA. Quantitative assessment of valve thickness in normal subjects by transesophageal echocardiography. *Am J Cardiol* 2001;87:1419–1423.
10. Koca V, Bozat T, Akkaya V, et al. Left atrial thrombus detection with multiplane transesophageal echocardiography: an echocardiographic study with surgical verification. *J Heart Valve Dis* 1999;8:63–66.
11. Kranidis A, Koulouris S, Filippatos G. Mitral regurgitation protects from left atrial thrombogenesis in patients with mitral valve disease and atrial fibrillation. *Pacing Clin Electrophysiol* 2000;23:1863–1866.
12. Applebaum RM, Kasliwal RR, Kanojia A, et al. Utility of three-dimensional echocardiography during balloon mitral valvuloplasty. *J Am Coll Cardiol* 1998;32:1405–1409.
13. Binder TM, Rosenhek R, Prenta G, et al. Improved assessment of mitral valve stenosis by volumetric real-time three-dimensional echocardiography. *J Am Coll Cardiol* 2000;36:1355–1361.
14. Srinivasa KH, Manjunath CN, Dhanalakshmi C, et al. Transesophageal Doppler echocardiographic study of pulmonary venous flow pattern in severe mitral stenosis and the changes following balloon mitral valvuloplasty. *Echocardiography* 2000;17:151–157.
15. Abaci A, Oguzhan A, Unal S, et al. Application of the vena contracta method for the calculation of the mitral valve area in mitral stenosis. *Cardiology* 2002;98:50–59.
16. Bennis A, Drighil A, Tribouilloy C, et al. Clinical application in routine practice of the proximal flow convergence method to calculate the mitral surface area in mitral valve stenosis. *Int J Cardiovasc Imaging* 2002;18:443–451.
17. Arora R, Kalra GS, Singh S, et al. Percutaneous transvenous mitral commissurotomy: immediate and long-term follow-up results. *Catheter Cardiovasc Interv* 2002;55:450–456.
18. Ben-Farhat M, Betbout F, Gamra H, et al. Predictors of long-term event-free survival and of freedom from restenosis after percutaneous balloon mitral commissurotomy. *Am Heart J* 2001;142:1072–1079.
19. Sajja LR, Mannam GC. Role of close mitral commissurotomy in mitral stenosis with severe pulmonary hypertension. *J Heart Valve Dis* 2001;10:288–293.
20. de Souza JA, Martinez EE Jr, Ambrose JA, et al. Percutaneous balloon mitral valvuloplasty in comparison with open mitral valve commissurotomy for mitral stenosis during pregnancy. *J Am Coll Cardiol* 2001; 37:900–903.
21. Aviles RJ, Nishimura RA, Pellika PA, et al. Utility of stress Doppler echocardiography in patients undergoing percutaneous mitral valvotomy. *J Am Soc Echocardiogr* 2001;14:676–681.
22. Eren M, Arikan E, Gorgulu S, et al. Relationship between resting parameters of the mitral valve and exercise capacity in patients with mitral stenosis: Can the diastolic filling period predict exercise capacity? *J Heart Valve Dis* 2002;11:191–198.
23. Mohan JC, Patel AR, Passey R, et al. Is the mitral valve area flow-dependent in mitral stenosis? A dobutamine stress echocardiographic study. *J Am Coll Cardiol* 2002;40:1809–1815.
24. Salem MI, Makaryus AN, Kort S, et al. Intracardiac echocardiography using the AcuNav ultrasound catheter during percutaneous balloon mitral valvuloplasty. *J Am Soc Echocardiogr* 2002;15:1533–1537.

8

Aortic Regurgitation

Carlos A. Roldan

■ The physical examination is inaccurate for determining the etiology and severity of chronic and acute aortic regurgitation (AR). Acute severe AR manifests mainly by heart failure or pulmonary edema, and physical findings of AR in these patients are frequently absent.

■ Aortic root disease is a common cause of severe isolated AR, and the physical examination is limited in assessing its presence and severity. Approximately 25% of patients with moderate to severe AR develop asymptomatic left ventricular dilatation or systolic dysfunction. The physical examination is also limited in defining the severity of left ventricular dilatation and dysfunction.

COMMON ETIOLOGIES

■ Chronic AR: degenerative valve disease, bicuspid valve, rheumatic heart disease, healed infective endocarditis, idiopathic aortic root dilatation, and aortic annuloectasia.

■ Acute AR: infective endocarditis, aortic dissection, and aortic trauma.

ECHOCARDIOGRAPHY

Indications for Echocardiography

■ Transthoracic echocardiography (TTE) is indicated to define the presence, etiology, severity, and follow-up of patients with AR (Table 8-1) (1,2).

TABLE 8-1. *Class I Indications for Echocardiography in Aortic Regurgitation (AR)*

Confirm the presence and severity of acute AR.
Assessment of the etiology of AR.
Semiquantitative estimate of the severity of AR.
Diagnosis of chronic AR in patients with equivocal physical findings.
Assessment of left ventricular hypertrophy, dimensions, volumes, and systolic function.
Reevaluation of patients with mild, moderate, or severe AR with new or changing symptoms.
Reevaluation of left ventricular size and function in asymptomatic patients with severe AR.
Reevaluation of asymptomatic patients with mild, moderate, or severe AR and dilated root.

- Transesophageal echocardiography (TEE) is indicated for diagnosis and determination of the need and type of surgery in AR due to aortic dissection, aortic aneurysm, or infective endocarditis.

M-Mode and Two-Dimensional Transthoracic Echocardiography or Transesophageal Echocardiography

Aortic Valve and Root Morphology

Best Imaging Planes

- M-mode echocardiography (echo): TTE parasternal long-axis and short-axis and TEE basal long-axis and short-axis views.
- Two-dimensional (2D) echo: TTE parasternal long-axis and short-axis and apical five-chamber and three-chamber views; TEE basal long-axis and short-axis views.

Key Diagnostic Features

- *Aortic valve mobility:* Subjectively assessed by TTE and TEE. No specific parameters have been defined for assessing the severity of decreased cusps' mobility.
- *Aortic valve sclerosis:* Occurs when any cusp has increased reflectance and thickness >2 mm (3). In the author's laboratory, *mild sclerosis* is defined as any cusp with sclerosis with normal mobility; *moderate sclerosis* if decreased cusp mobility; and *severe sclerosis* if associated with decreased mobility and increased, but <2 m/sec, valve peak velocity.

- *Aortic valve regurgitant orifice area:* Central gap bordered by the cusps' commissural edges during end-diastole using 2D TEE basal short-axis view (4). An orifice area of <0.2 cm², >0.2 and ≤0.4 cm², and >0.4 cm² predicts mild, moderate, and severe AR, respectively.
- *Degenerative aortic valve disease:* Sclerosis of one or more cusps predominantly at the margins and basal portions with decreased mobility. Sclerosis can be localized, nodular, or diffuse, but a mixed pattern is most common (5).
- *Bicuspid aortic valve:* Has two cusps of unequal size, single linear commissure, sclerosed raphe, systolic doming of pliable cusps, and eccentric closure in relation to root walls.
- *Rheumatic valve disease:* There is commissural fusion (best seen from short-axis view), thickening of the tip portions, and retraction of the cusps. Often, all commissures are affected.
- *Infective endocarditis:* Characterized by leaflet vegetations, perforation, and/or prolapse; leaflet, annulus, or root abscesses; and leaflet or root aneurysm or pseudoaneurysms.
- *Aortic root dilatation:* Categorized as *mild* if the tubular portion measures 3.7 to 4.5 cm, *moderate* if it measures 4.6 to 5.0 cm, and *severe* if it measures >5 cm.
- *Aortic root sclerosis:* Anterior or posterior root wall has increased reflectance, and thickness is >2.2 mm (6). The author defines it as *mild* when a sclerotic wall measures 2.3 to 3.0 mm; *moderate* if it measures 3.1 to 4.0 mm; and *severe* if it measures >4 mm.
- *Diastolic fluttering of the anterior mitral leaflet:* By M-mode, it is specific but not sensitive, and its presence is not related to the severity of AR (Fig. 8-1A).
- *Premature closure of the mitral valve (before onset of left ventricular isovolumic contraction or onset of QRS):* By M-mode, it indicates severe, especially acute AR (Fig. 8-1B).

Hemodynamic Impact of Aortic Regurgitation on the Left Ventricle and Left Atrium

Best Imaging Planes

- TTE parasternal long-axis and short-axis and apical views.

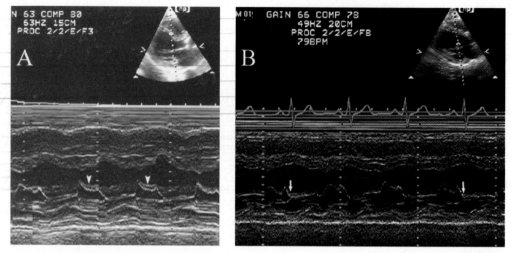

FIG. 8-1. M-mode images of **(A)** diastolic fluttering of the anterior mitral leaflet (*arrowheads*) and **(B)** premature closure of the mitral valve (*arrows*).

■ TEE transgastric short-axis and long-axis and basal four-chamber and two-chamber views.

Diagnostic Methods

■ By M-mode, left ventricular end-diastolic and end-systolic diameters and respective indexes, and left ventricular shortening fraction provide key information concerning the severity and prognosis of AR and indicate whether valve replacement or repair is needed.

■ By 2D echo using the modified Simpson's rule, left ventricular end-diastolic and end-systolic volumes, total stroke volume, and ejection fraction (EF) can be accurately quantified.

■ Left ventricular radius to wall thickness ratio and end-systolic wall stress also assess AR severity.

Key Diagnostic Features

■ Left ventricular and left atrial size and volumes are normal in mild AR.

■ Left ventricular and left atrial size and volumes are frequently normal in mild to moderate or moderate AR.

■ Left ventricular and left atrial size and volumes are generally increased with moderate to severe or severe AR.

Pitfalls

■ Etiology of AR cannot be defined, and localized valve sclerosis can be missed by M-mode.

■ Diastolic fluttering of the mitral valve is specific but not sensitive for detection of AR.

■ Left ventricular diameters and fractional shortening are less reproducible by 2D echo than by M-mode.

■ Left ventricular and left atrial dimensions and volumes frequently do not separate mild from moderate AR.

■ Other valvular or myocardial diseases can affect left ventricular and left atrial dimensions.

Doppler Echocardiography for Assessment of the Severity of Aortic Regurgitation

Pulsed Wave Doppler

Best Imaging Planes

■ TTE three-chamber and five-chamber views and suprasternal notch for assessment of flow.

■ TTE parasternal long-axis or TEE basal long-axis views for left ventricular outflow tract (LVOT) diameter.

Diagnostic Methods and Formulas

■ *Total stroke volume* = $(D^2/4$ *or* $\pi \times r^2)_{LVOT} \times VTI_{LVOT}$, where D = LVOT diameter, r = LVOT radius, and VTI = velocity time integral.

■ *Forward stroke volume* = $(D^2/4$ *or* $\pi \times r^2)_{RVOT} \times VTI_{RVOT}$, where D = right ventricular outflow tract diameter, and VTI is obtained from the

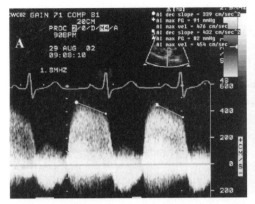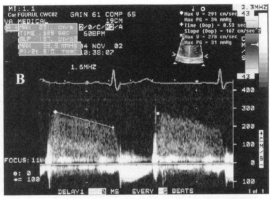

FIG. 8-2. A: Continuous wave Doppler in a patient with severe aortic regurgitation (AR) demonstrates a deceleration slope >3 m/sec^2 and similar diastolic and systolic spectral signal intensities. The AR end-diastolic velocity of 3.9 m/sec corresponds to an end-diastolic pressure of 61 mm Hg. The patient's diastolic blood pressure was 80 to 85 mm Hg. Therefore, the estimated left ventricular end-diastolic pressure was 20 to 25 mm Hg. **B:** Continuous wave Doppler of a patient with moderate AR by color Doppler demonstrates a pressure half-time of >500 msec and a deceleration slope <2 m/sec^2 consistent with mild AR. Note the AR jet peak velocity of only 2.7 to 2.9 m/sec is equivalent to a peak diastolic pressure of 31 to 34 mm Hg. The patient's diastolic blood pressure was 70 mm Hg. Therefore, this is a misalignment of the ultrasound beam with the AR jet, leading to underestimation of AR severity.

parasternal short-axis view at the pulmonic valve level. Mitral annulus diameter and mitral VTI can be used if less than moderate MR present.

- *Regurgitant volume* = total stroke volume – forward stroke volume.
- *Regurgitant fraction* = regurgitant volume ÷ total stroke volume.
- *Regurgitant orifice area* = regurgitant volume ÷ AR continuous wave Doppler *VTI*.
- *Flow velocity reversal in the aortic arch or descending aorta.* Short-lasting diastolic flow reversal is normal in the aorta. Diastolic retrograde flow is proportional to AR severity.
- *High left ventricular end-diastolic pressure* from moderate or worse AR is suggested by a pseudonormalization or restrictive mitral inflow and diastolic predominance on the pulmonary veins' inflow.

Continuous Wave Doppler

Best Imaging Planes

- TTE apical three-chamber and five-chamber views and right parasternal view.
- TEE transgastric three-chamber or five-chamber views.

Diagnostic Methods

- *Pressure half-time ($P_{1/2}$ time) in msec* = time it takes the initial pressure gradient between aorta and left ventricle (LV) (transvalvular pressure gradient) to decrease by 50%. The faster the decline in aortic pressure or decline of AR jet velocity (the shorter the $P_{1/2}$ time), the faster the rise in left ventricular end-diastolic pressure and the worse the AR (Fig. 8-2).
- *Deceleration slope (m/sec^2)* = the rate of decline of aortic diastolic pressure or AR jet velocity is also related to the severity of AR (Fig. 8-2).
- *Signal intensity of the AR* spectral display is also related to the severity of AR (Fig. 8-2).
- *Left ventricular end-diastolic pressure* = patients' diastolic blood pressure – 4 × (end-diastolic AR velocity)^2. The higher the pressure, the worse the AR (Fig. 8-2).

Color Doppler

Best Imaging Planes

- TTE parasternal long-axis and short-axis views and apical three-chamber and five-chamber views.

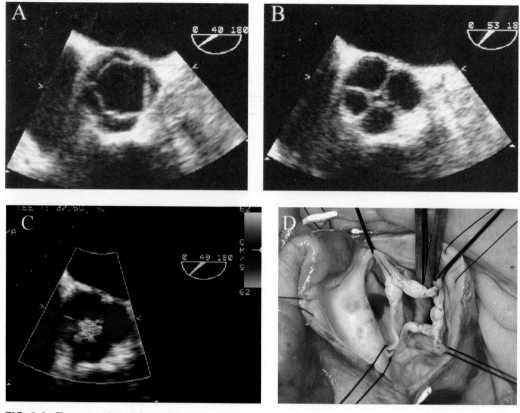

FIG. 8-3. Transesophageal echocardiographic basal short-axis view of a quadricuspid aortic valve during systole **(A)** and diastole **(B)**. The planimetered end-diastolic anatomic regurgitant orifice was >0.4 cm². **C:** Color Doppler demonstrated an aortic regurgitation jet vena contracta width and area of >6 mm and 7.5 mm², respectively. **D:** Surgical confirmation of the quadricuspid aortic valve.

■ TEE basal short-axis and long-axis views.

Diagnostic Methods and Formulas

■ *Ratio of jet height* (at the junction of LVOT and aortic annulus) to LVOT height from TTE parasternal or TEE basal long-axis views (Figs. 8-3 and 8-4).

■ *Ratio of jet area to LVOT area* from TTE parasternal or TEE short-axis views.

■ *Vena contracta* (narrowest portion of AR jet measured at or just distal to its orifice) *width and area* correlate well with the effective regurgitant orifice area and separate severe from nonsevere AR (Figs. 8-3, 8-4, and 8-5) (7,8).

■ *Proximal isovelocity surface area (PISA)* or acceleration zone proximal to the regurgitant orifice is used to calculate the regurgitant flow rate and effective regurgitant orifice area (9).

◆ *Regurgitant flow rate* (cm³/sec) = $2 \times \pi \times r^2 \times Vr$ (Figs. 8-4 and 8-5)
  • Where *r* is the radius of the PISA measured in early diastole and
  • *Vr* is the color Doppler aliasing velocity or Nyquist limit (cm/sec).

◆ *Regurgitant orifice area (cm²) = regurgitant flow rate ÷ maximal AR velocity by continuous wave*

■ *Color M-mode flow propagation velocity* is obtained from apical five-chamber or long-axis view with M-mode cursor placed parallel to AR flow and with the narrowest sector angle. A flow propagation velocity cut point of 80 cm/sec separates severe from mild or moderate AR. A cut point of 40 cm/sec separates mild from moderate or severe AR (10).

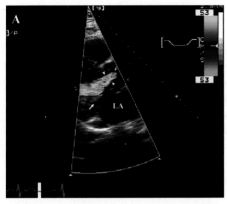
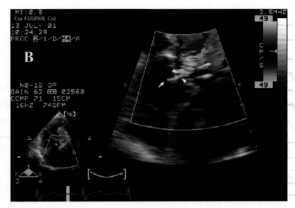

FIG. 8-4. A: Transthoracic echocardiographic (TTE) parasternal long-axis view in a patient with severe aortic regurgitation (AR) demonstrates a ratio of the jet height to left ventricular outflow tract height of >65%, a vena contracta width of >6 mm (*arrowheads*), and a large (1 cm) flow convergence zone or proximal isovelocity surface area (PISA) (*small arrow*). By PISA method with a measured peak AR velocity by continuous wave of 5 m/sec, the effective regurgitant orifice was 0.66 cm². Note the premature closure of the mitral valve (*large arrow*). **B:** Apical TTE close-up view and color Doppler in a patient with mild AR demonstrates a small vena contracta width of 3 mm (*arrowheads*) and a small flow convergence zone of 4 mm (*arrow*). LA, left atrium.

■ In summary, an accurate assessment of the severity of AR requires integration of all Doppler echo parameters with those of left ventricular size and function (Table 8-2) (11).

■ Color Doppler is less accurate for defining moderate AR than mild or severe AR.

■ Color Doppler parameters are dependent on the regurgitant orifice size and also on the

Pitfalls

■ Errors in estimating stroke or regurgitant volume and regurgitant fraction are predominantly related to overestimation or underestimation of LVOT or RV outflow tract diameters.

■ Mitral valve stroke volume is less accurate due to the complex morphology of its annulus.

■ Flow velocity reversal in the aortic arch or descending aorta is not easy to obtain and can be mistaken for flow in the takeoff of the arch branches.

■ If AR peak velocity jet is not well-defined or is obtained at a cosine >20 degrees, peak velocity, $P_{1/2}$ time, deceleration slope, and severity of AR are underestimated (Fig. 8-2B).

■ AR jet depth (extension into LV) and area correlate poorly with angiographic AR severity.

■ The ratio of AR jet to LVOT height in eccentric jets more commonly leads to underestimation of AR severity.

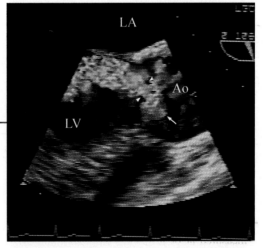

FIG. 8-5. Longitudinal transesophageal echocardiographic view of the aortic valve and root in a patient with severe aortic regurgitation demonstrates a vena contracta width of >6 mm (*arrowheads*) and a large (1.3 cm) flow convergence zone (*arrow*). By proximal isovelocity surface area method, the effective regurgitant orifice area was 1.2 cm². Ao, aorta; LA, left atrium; LV, left ventricle.

TABLE 8-2. *Echocardiography Parameters of the Severity of Aortic Regurgitation*

Method	Mild	Moderate	Moderate to severe	Severe
Left ventricular or left atrial enlargement[a]	None	None or mild	Mild to moderate	Moderate to severe
Planimetered anatomic regurgitant area (cm^2)	≤0.2	>0.2–≤0.4	—	>0.4
Regurgitant fraction (%)	<30	30–39	40–49	>50
Regurgitant volume (mL/beat)	<30	30–44	45–59	≥60
Pressure half-time (msec)	>500	350–500	200–350	<200
Deceleration slope (m/sec^2)	<2	2–3	—	>3
Jet/LVOT width ratio (%)	<25	25–45	46–64	≥65
Jet/LVOT area ratio (%)	<5	5–20	21–59	≥60
Vena contracta width (mm)[b]	3	3–6	—	>6
Vena contracta area (mm^2)[b]	—	<7.5	—	>7.5
Effective regurgitant orifice (cm^2)	<0.10	0.10–0.19	0.2–0.29	≥0.30
Color M-mode flow propagation velocity (cm/sec)	≤40	>40–60	—	≥80

LVOT, left ventricular outflow tract.
[a]Applies to chronic aortic regurgitation.
[b]By transesophageal echocardiography, a vena contracta width of >6 mm^2 or area of >7.5 mm^2 predicts a regurgitant fraction of >50% or a regurgitant volume of >40 mL.

transvalvular pressure gradient. A high or low aortic diastolic pressure or systemic vascular resistance can result in overestimation or underestimation of the severity of AR. Thus, patients' blood pressure must be recorded and taken into account when assessing the severity of AR.

■ Similarly, a high left ventricular end-diastolic pressure due to hypertension or coronary or myocardial disease leads to shortening of $P_{1/2}$ time and overestimation of AR severity (Fig 8-6).

■ Color Doppler is dependent on gain, pulsed repetition frequency, and differences in displays. If no attention is given to these settings, AR severity can be overestimated or underestimated (12).

Diagnostic Accuracy for Assessing the Severity of Aortic Regurgitation

■ A planimetered anatomic regurgitant orifice area by 2D TEE of <0.2 cm^2, >0.2 and ≤0.4 cm^2, and >0.4 cm^2, predict angiographic mild, moderate, and severe AR, respectively, with sensitivity, specificity, and predictive values of 81% to 97% (4).

■ Regurgitant fraction by pulsed Doppler correlates highly (0.91) with that obtained by left ventricular angiography and thermodilution.

■ A $P_{1/2}$ time <400 msec by continuous wave Doppler separates moderately severe or severe AR from mild or moderate AR, with a specificity of 92% and a predictive value of 90%.

■ AR jet deceleration slope correlates highly (0.93) with angiographic AR severity and accurately separates mild, moderate, and severe AR.

■ The ratios of AR jet height to LVOT height and jet area to LVOT area correctly predict angiographic severity of AR in 79% and 96% of cases, respectively.

■ By TTE, a vena contracta width ≥6 mm predicts a regurgitant orifice area of ≥30 mm^2 by quantitative Doppler and 2D echo, with a 95% sensitivity and 90% specificity (7).

■ By TEE, a vena contracta width of >6 mm or area of >7.5 mm^2 predicts a regurgitant volume of >40 mL assessed intraoperatively with a 67% and 94% accuracy, respectively (8).

■ The PISA method predicts a regurgitant orifice area with a high (0.90) correlation coefficient when tested against quantitative Doppler or 2D echo.

■ Color M-mode flow propagation velocity correlates highly (0.93) with angiographic AR severity. A cut point of 80 cm/sec separates severe from mild or moderate AR, with sensitivity, specificity, and predictive values of 85% to 100%. A cut point of 40 cm/sec separates

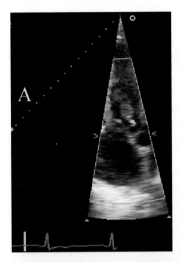

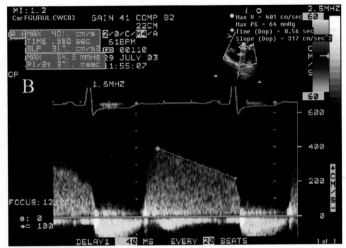

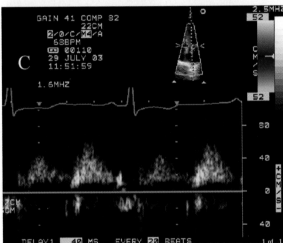

FIG. 8-6. A: This apical transthoracic echocardiographic five-chamber view demonstrates unequivocally mild aortic regurgitation (AR) by color Doppler. B: By continuous wave Doppler, a pressure half-time of 340 msec and a deceleration slope of >3 m/sec^2 suggest moderate to severe AR; however, the severity of AR is overestimated by continuous wave Doppler due to high left ventricular end-diastolic pressure, as suggested by blunted systolic and predominant diastolic flow velocities of the pulmonary vein inflow (C).

mild AR from moderate or severe AR, with sensitivity, specificity, and predictive values of 100% (10).

Use in the Pregnant Patient with Aortic Regurgitation

■ In normal pregnancy, the prevalence of physiologic AR is that of healthy nonpregnant women (<2%), and its prevalence or severity does not increase throughout pregnancy.

■ During pregnancy, a low systemic vascular resistance and diastolic blood pressure balance the physiologic volume overload and aortic dilatation. Therefore, the physiologic increase in left ventricular size and widening of pulsed pressure should not be mistaken as worsening AR.

■ Mild or moderate AR due to primary valve disease poses low risk to mother and fetus. Thus, there is no need for echo monitoring during pregnancy or the postpartum period.

■ Patients with asymptomatic severe AR due to primary valve disease generally tolerate well an uncomplicated pregnancy, labor, and delivery. In symptomatic patients, the need for medical or surgical interventions is determined by clinical rather than echo data.

■ In patients with Marfan syndrome, the prevalence of aortic root dilatation and AR are approximately 75% and 25%, respectively (13). Pregnant patients with Marfan syndrome

TABLE 8-3. *Echocardiography Follow-Up in Patients with Aortic Regurgitation (AR)*

Clinical scenario	Echocardiography
Asymptomatic patients with moderate or worse AR of unknown duration	Within 3 mo
Asymptomatic patients with severe AR, LVEDD >70 mm or ESD >50 mm but normal LVEF	Every 4–6 mo
Patients with known mild or worse AR with progressive left ventricular dilatation or declining LVEF	Every 6 mo
Asymptomatic patients with severe AR, normal LVEF, and LVEDD >60 mm	Every 6–12 mo
Asymptomatic patients with mild AR, normal or mildly dilated LV, and normal LVEF	Every 2–3 yr; every yr if worsens

ESD, left ventricular end-systolic diameter; LV, left ventricle; LVEDD, left ventricular end-diastolic diameter; LVEF, left ventricular ejection fraction.

are at increased risk of aortic dissection (10–60%) and mortality (up to 50%) (14). Their risk is proportional to the degree of root dilatation and AR.

■ Therefore, patients with Marfan syndrome without or with root dilatation or AR of any degree may need echo during each trimester of pregnancy and the peripartum period. No specific guidelines are currently available, however.

Follow-Up in Patients with Aortic Regurgitation

■ Serial echo is aimed at detection of asymptomatic left ventricular dilatation or dysfunction.
■ The frequency of echo is determined by the patient's symptoms, initial severity of AR, and degree of left ventricular dilatation or systolic dysfunction, or both (Table 8-3) (1,2,14).
■ Repeat echo is indicated in a patient with new-onset symptoms, equivocal change in symptoms or exercise tolerance, or clinically suspected worsening AR or left ventricular dilatation.
■ In patients with aortic root dilatation and any degree of AR, serial echo is indicated to eval-

uate root size and left ventricular size and function; however, the degree of root dilatation that warrants serial and interval frequency of echo has not been defined.

Indicators of Poor Prognosis in Aortic Regurgitation

Asymptomatic Patients

■ Asymptomatic patients with chronic severe AR develop symptoms or asymptomatic left ventricular systolic dysfunction and require valve replacement at a yearly rate of 1.3% to 3.5%.
■ Patients with a left ventricular end-systolic diameter >50 or >55 mm have a 65% or 80% rate of valve replacement at 3 or 4 years, as compared to 0% or 20% of those with a left ventricular end-systolic diameter <50 or <55 mm, respectively (Table 8-4).

Symptomatic Patients

■ Patients with an EF <50% have a 3- to 5-year survival of 54% to 64% after valve replace-

TABLE 8-4. *Echocardiographic Predictors of Death, Persistent Left Ventricular Dilatation and Dysfunction, and Decreased Exercise Tolerance after Aortic Valve Replacement in Patients with Aortic Regurgitation*

Left ventricular ejection fraction	<50%
Left ventricular end-diastolic diameter	>72 mm
Left ventricular end-diastolic diameter index	>38 mm/m^2
Left ventricular end-systolic diameter	>50 mm
Left ventricular end-systolic diameter index	>26 mm/m^2
Left ventricular shortening fraction	<28%
Left ventricular end-systolic volume	>200 mL
Left ventricular end-systolic volume index	>90 mL/m^2
Left ventricular radius to wall thickness ratio	>3.2
End-systolic wall stress	>235 mm Hg
Left ventricular end-diastolic pressure	>20 mm Hg

ment, as compared to 87% to 91% survival in those with an EF ≥50% (Table 8-4).

■ Patients with left ventricular systolic dysfunction for ≥18 months have a 4-year to 5-year postoperative survival of 45%, as compared to 100% survival of those with left ventricular dysfunction for <14 months.

■ The 5-year postoperative survival rates in patients with left ventricular shortening fraction of >35%, 31% to 35%, and <30% are 100%, 91%, and 78%, respectively.

■ Patients with a left ventricular end-systolic dimension of <55 mm or a shortening fraction >26% have a 2.5-year to 3.5-year postoperative survival of 83% to 90%, as compared to 42% to 70% in those with a left ventricular end-systolic dimension of >55 mm or fractional shortening <25%.

■ Those with a left ventricular end-diastolic dimension ≥70 mm or end-systolic volume index >90 mL/m² have a high risk for postoperative death, persistent left ventricular systolic dysfunction, or heart failure.

■ Finally, patients with an end-diastolic radius to wall thickness ratio of >3.2 or >4 have persistent postoperative left ventricular dilatation.

TABLE 8-5. *Indications for Aortic Valve Replacement in Symptomatic Patients with Chronic Severe Aortic Regurgitation*

Patients with normal resting EF (≥50%) and NYHA functional class III or IV symptoms.

New onset of mild dyspnea in patients with increasing left ventricular chamber size or declining LVEF into the low normal range.

Patients with NYHA functional class II–IV symptoms and LVEF of 25–49%.

In patients with NYHA functional class II–III symptoms if (a) symptoms and left ventricular dysfunction are of recent onset and (b) short-term vasodilator, diuretic, and/or IV positive inotropic therapy result in substantial improvement in hemodynamics or systolic function.

Patients with NYHA functional class II symptoms and EF ≥50% at rest but with progressive left ventricular dilatation or declining EF at rest on serial studies or declining exercise tolerance.

Patients with greater than class II Canadian Heart Association angina with or without coronary artery disease.

Patients undergoing coronary artery bypass surgery or surgery of the aorta or other heart valve.

LVEF, left ventricular ejection fraction; NYHA, New York Heart Association.

Parameters That Indicate Need for Aortic Valve Replacement or Repair in Aortic Regurgitation

■ Symptoms are the most important indication, but asymptomatic patients with left ventricular dilatation or dysfunction, or both, also need valve replacement (Tables 8-5 and 8-6).

■ Asymptomatic patients with preserved left ventricular function but severely dilated LV should be considered for surgery. They are at increased risk of sudden cardiac death, and their surgical results are excellent. Operative mortality is higher once symptoms develop or EF decreases.

■ Elderly patients with associated aortic stenosis or coronary artery disease develop symptoms of left ventricular dysfunction at earlier stages or left ventricular dilatation and have more persistent left ventricular dysfunction,

heart failure, and worse postoperative survival rates than younger patients or those with isolated AR.

Intraoperative Use during Aortic Valve Replacement or Repair

■ The cost-effectiveness of routine intraoperative TEE is debatable. Data suggest that TEE changes the operation or immediate postoperative treatment in only 1.6% of patients (15). TEE detects 15% to 50% of trivial to mild degrees of valvular bioprosthetic and 5% to 15% of paravalvular prosthetic or bioprosthetic regurgitation. More than 95% of these regurgitant lesions resolve or persist unchanged, and <5% progress (16,17).

■ TEE is indicated in patients with AR associated with proximal aortic dissection, aneurysmal root disease, annular or root aortic abscesses, and aortic trauma. In these patients, TEE can detect pseudoaneurysms of the composite aortic graft, aortic annulus or coronary artery dehiscence, and compression of the aortic graft by a hematoma.

TABLE 8-6. *Indications for Aortic Valve Replacement in Asymptomatic Patients*

Patients with an LVEF below 50% at rest or 50% on two consecutive measurements.

Patients with LVEDD >75 mm or ESD >55 mm, even if LVEF is normal.

Patients with an LVEDD of 70–75 mm or ESD of 50–55 mm with evidence of declining exercise tolerance or abnormal hemodynamic responses to exercise.

In patients with disease of the proximal aorta and AR of any degree if root dilatation ≥50 mm (valve replacement and aortic root reconstruction), independent of left ventricular size or function.

Asymptomatic patient with a resting LVEF of 25–49%.

ESD, end-systolic diameter; LVEF, left ventricular ejection fraction; LVEDD, left ventricular end-diastolic diameter.

■ In patients with proximal aortic dissection, TEE defines the success of replacement of the ascending aorta with resuspension of the aortic valve; composite graft replacement; separate aortic valve and ascending aorta replacement; or aortic root or valve repair, or both.

■ TEE can define the success of valve repair, such as free-edge aortic cusp extension using pericardium in rheumatic, infective or postvalvuloplasty AR; aortic annuloplasty in aortic root dilatation; and direct suture or patch repair of ruptured sinus of Valsalva aneurysm (18–20).

Use after
Aortic Valve Replacement

■ A baseline echo should be performed at the first outpatient evaluation to assess valve function and left ventricular size and function. Eighty percent reduction in left ventricular end-diastolic dimension occurs within 10 to 14 days after valve replacement.

■ Patients with normally functioning mechanical valves should have follow-up echo at 5, 10, 12, and 15 years. After 15 years, patients should have yearly studies.

■ Patients with normally functioning bioprosthetic valves should undergo echo at 2 to 3 and 5 years after replacement, every 2 years after 5 years since replacement, and every year after 10 years since replacement.

■ Patients with persistent left ventricular dilatation on initial study should have echo to assess left ventricular size and function at 6 and 12 months. If left ventricular dysfunction persists beyond this time, echo is repeated as clinically indicated.

■ If patient is asymptomatic and postoperative echo demonstrates significant reduction in left ventricular end-diastolic diameter and left ventricular function is normal, serial studies are not indicated.

■ Repeat echo is warranted in patients with a new murmur or question of prosthetic or left ventricular dysfunction.

REFERENCES

1. Cheitlin MD, Armstrong WF, Aurigemma GP, et al. ACC/AHA/ASE guideline update for the clinical application of echocardiography: summary article. *J Am Coll Cardiol* 2003;42:954–970.

2. Bonow RO, Carabello B, De Leon AC, et al. ACC/AHA guidelines for the management of patients with valvular heart disease. *J Am Coll Cardiol* 1998;32: 1486–1588.

3. Crawford MH, Roldan CA. Quantitative assessment of valve thickness in normal subjects by transesophageal echocardiography. *Am J Cardiol* 2001;87:1419–1423.

4. Ozkan M, Ozdemir N, Kaymaz C, et al. Measurement of aortic valve anatomic regurgitant area using transesophageal echocardiography: implications for the quantitation of aortic regurgitation. *J Am Soc Echocardiogr* 2002;15:1170–1174.

5. Tolstrup K, Crawford MH, Roldan CA. Morphologic classification of aortic valve sclerosis: its importance for the prediction of coronary artery disease. *Cardiology* 2002;98:154–158.

6. Roldan CA, Chavez J, Weist P, et al. Aortic root disease and valve disease associated with ankylosing spondylitis. *J Am Coll Cardiol* 1998;32:1397–1404.

7. Tribouilloy CM, Enriquez-Sarano M, Bailey KR, et al. Assessment of severity of aortic regurgitation using the width of the vena contracta: a clinical color Doppler imaging study. *Circulation* 2000;102:558–564.

8. Willet DL, Hall SA, Jessen ME, et al. Assessment of aortic regurgitation by transesophageal color Doppler imaging of the vena contracta: validation against an intraoperative aortic flow probe. *J Am Coll Cardiol* 2001;37:1450–1455.

9. Tribouilloy CM, Enriquez-Sarano M, Fett SL, et al. Application of the proximal flow convergence method to calculate the effective regurgitant orifice area in aortic regurgitation. *J Am Coll Cardiol* 1998;32:1032–1039.

10. Onsbasili OA, Tekten T, Ceyhan C, et al. A new echocardiographic method for the assessment of the severity of aortic regurgitation: color M-mode flow propagation velocity. *J Am Soc Echocardiogr* 2002;15:1453–1460.

11. Zoghbi WA, Enriquez-Sarano M, Foster E, et al. Recommendations for evaluation of the severity of native valvular regurgitation with two-dimensional and Doppler echocardiography. *J Am Soc Echocardiogr* 2003;16: 777–802.

12. Sahn DJ. Instrumentation and physical factors related to visualization of stenotic and regurgitant jets by color Doppler flow mapping. *J Am Coll Cardiol* 1998;12:1354–1365.

13. Mayet J, Steer P, Somerville J. Marfan's syndrome, aortic dilatation, and pregnancy. *Obstet Gynecol* 1998; 92:713.

14. Gopal K, Hudson IM, Ludmir J, et al. Homograft aortic root replacement during pregnancy. *Ann Thorac Surg* 2002;74:243–245.

15. Borer JS, Hochreiter C, Herrold EM, et al. Prediction of indications for valve replacement among asymptomatic or minimally symptomatic patients with chronic aortic regurgitation and normal left ventricular performance. *Circulation* 1998;97:525–534.

16. Ionescu AA, Proudman C, Butchart G, et al. Prospective study of routine perioperative transesophageal echocardiography for elective valve replacement: clinical impact and cost-saving implications. *J Am Soc Echocardiogr* 2001;14:659–667.

17. Morehead AJ, Firstenberg MS, Shiota T, et al. Intraoperative echocardiographic detection of regurgitant jets after valve replacement. *Ann Thorac Surg* 2000;69:135–139.

18. Grinda JM, Latremouille C, Berrebi AJ, et al. Aortic cusp extension valvuloplasty for rheumatic aortic valve disease: midterm results. *Ann Thorac Surg* 2002;74:438–443.

19. Murashita T, Rubota T, Kamikubo Y, et al. Long-term results of aortic valve regurgitation after repair of rupture sinus of Valsalva aneurysm. *Ann Thorac Surg* 2002;73:1466–1471.

20. O'Rourke DJ, Palac RT, Malenka DJ, et al. Outcome of mild periprosthetic regurgitation detected by intraoperative transesophageal echocardiography. *J Am Coll Cardiol* 2001;38:163–166.

9

Aortic Valve Sclerosis and Aortic Valve Stenosis

Kirsten Tolstrup and Carlos A. Roldan

The physical examination cannot accurately differentiate between aortic valve sclerosis and stenosis, commonly underestimates or overestimates the severity of aortic stenosis, and cannot accurately assess the impact of aortic stenosis on the left ventricle.

DEFINITION

- *Aortic valve sclerosis:* Thickened and hyper-reflectant cusps without causing obstruction to left ventricular outflow.
- *Aortic stenosis:* Obstruction to left ventricular outflow at the valvular (most common), sub-

valvular, or supravalvular levels. This chapter focuses on valvular aortic stenosis.

COMMON ETIOLOGIES AND PREVALENCE

Aortic Valve Sclerosis

- Aortic valve sclerosis is an atherosclerotic process that occurs mainly in the elderly.
- Affects 21% to 29% of the general population >65 years of age, 40% of a veteran population >50 years old, and up to 55% of those in the ninth to tenth decade (1–3).

Aortic Valve Stenosis

Valvular Aortic Stenosis

- The most common forms of aortic valve stenosis are degenerative, congenital, and rheumatic.
- In subjects >65 years old, degeneration associated with atherosclerosis of an inherently normal trileaflet valve is the most common etiology, with a prevalence of 2% to 4% (1,4).
- In patients >50 years old, isolated aortic stenosis due to a congenital bicuspid valve is the most common etiology, with a prevalence of 1% to 2% of the general population (5). In a familial form, the prevalence among first-degree relatives has been reported to be 9% to 21% (6).
- Rheumatic heart disease is more likely to be the cause if rheumatic mitral valve disease coexists. Rheumatic heart disease is an uncommon cause in the United States.

Supravalvular Aortic Stenosis

Supravalvular aortic stenosis occurs as an isolated lesion or as part of the Williams syndrome (caused by mutation in the gene encoding elastin) (7). It accounts for <5% of left ventricular outflow obstructions in children.

Subvalvular Aortic Stenosis

Subvalvular aortic stenosis often is associated with other congenital heart disease (25–60%), most commonly ventricular septal defects. Accounts for 10% to 20% of left ventricular outflow obstructions in pediatric patients.

TABLE 9-1. *Class I Indications for Echocardiography in Patients with Aortic Stenosis*

Diagnosis and assessment of the severity of aortic stenosis

Assessment of left ventricular function, size, and/or hemodynamics

Reevaluation of patients with known aortic stenosis with changing symptoms or signs

Assessment of changes in hemodynamic severity and ventricular function in those with known aortic stenosis in pregnancy

Reevaluation of asymptomatic patients with severe aortic stenosis

ECHOCARDIOGRAPHY

Class I Indications for Echocardiography

- There are no guidelines for echocardiography (echo) in subjects with aortic valve sclerosis. We suggest transthoracic echo (TTE) in asymptomatic middle-aged or older subjects with risk factors for atherosclerosis and a II to III/VI systolic ejection murmur at the aortic area. The presence of aortic valve sclerosis suggests underlying atherosclerosis.
- Table 9-1 depicts the class I indications for echo in patients with aortic valve stenosis (8,9).
- Transesophageal echo (TEE) for planimetry of the valve to assess the severity of aortic stenosis is uncommonly indicated when TTE is inconclusive or equivocal.
- TEE is the test of choice for the diagnosis of supravalvular aortic stenosis.

M-Mode and Two-Dimensional Echocardiography: Morphology of the Sclerotic and Stenotic Aortic Valve

Best Imaging Planes

- TTE parasternal long-axis and short-axis and apical three-chamber and five-chamber views.
- TEE basal short-axis (usually 35–55 degrees) and long-axis (usually 120–140 degrees) views.

Key Diagnostic Features

Degenerative Aortic Valve Disease

Aortic Valve Sclerosis

- In aortic valve sclerosis, one or more cusps are hyperreflectant and thickened (>2 mm). Mobil-

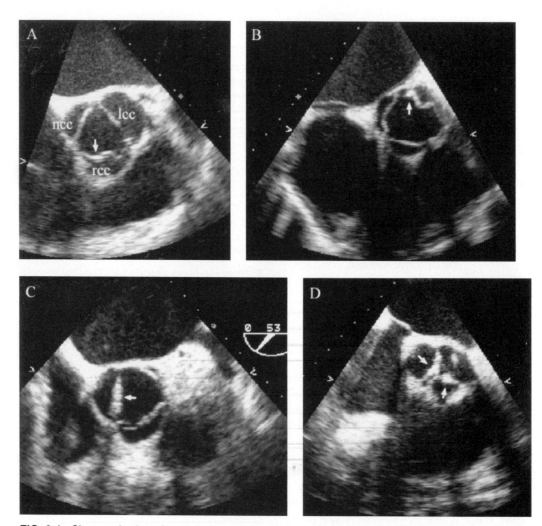

FIG. 9-1. Characterization of aortic valve sclerosis by transesophageal echocardiography. **A:** Localized nonnodular sclerosis (*arrow*) of the right coronary cusp (rcc). **B:** Localized nodular sclerosis (*arrow*) of the left coronary cusp (lcc). **C:** Diffuse sclerosis (*arrow*) of the noncoronary cusp (ncc). **D:** Mixed, diffuse sclerosis of the noncoronary cusp (*long arrow*) and nodular sclerosis (*short arrow*) of the right coronary cusp.

ity is usually normal, but it can be mild or moderately decreased. Valve sclerosis can be diffuse, localized, nodular, or mixed; it can affect all areas of the cusps, but it most frequently affects the margins and basal portions (Fig. 9-1).

■ Cusp separation ≥1 cm by M-mode indicates valve sclerosis or noncritical stenosis.

Aortic Valve Stenosis

■ In aortic valve stenosis, the cusps are hyperreflectant, thickened, calcified, and nonmobile with a decrease in orifice area. The fibrosis, nodular deposits, and calcification are more severe at the base of the cusps, extend to the cusps' margins and commissural regions, and then progress to the free edge (Fig. 9-2A). The base of the leaflets may become fixed and immobile. Commissural fusion rarely occurs.

■ Aortic annulus and root sclerosis and calcification are common.

Congenital Bicuspid Aortic Valve Disease

■ A bicuspid valve demonstrates two cusps of unequal size and a single linear commissure

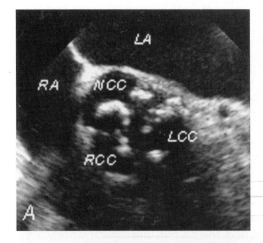

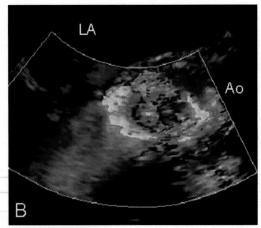

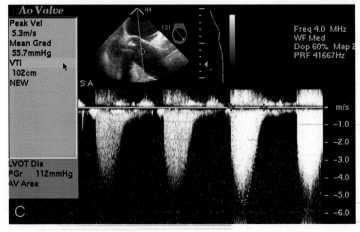

FIG. 9-2. A: Degenerative aortic valve stenosis by two-dimensional transesophageal echocardiography. **B:** Color Doppler flow across the stenotic valve. **C:** Continuous wave Doppler tracings of severe aortic stenosis. Ao, aorta; LA, left atrium; LCC, left coronary cusp; NCC, noncoronary cusp; RA, right atrium; RCC, right coronary cusp.

with increased echogenicity due to calcific deposits (Fig. 9-3A). A raphe makes the bicuspid valve appear tricuspid-like, but two cusps become apparent in systole.

■ The long-axis views show the eccentric closure of the bicuspid valve (Fig. 9-3B).

■ An early sign of bicuspid valve stenosis is systolic doming of the cusps, which means that the edges of the leaflets are curved toward the center of the aorta (Fig. 9-3B). This finding suggests pliable cusps with restricted mobility of the tips relative to the body of the cusps. Domed but thickened and sclerotic cusps suggest aortic stenosis.

■ In late stages, it is difficult to separate a bicuspid from a trileaflet degenerative valve.

■ Aortic root dilatation out of proportion to the degree of stenosis is common due to associated cystic medial necrosis.

Rheumatic Aortic Valve Disease

■ The hallmark of rheumatic aortic valve disease is commissural fusion, thickening of the tip portions, and retraction of the cusps with focal thickening of the edges. Often, all commissures are affected. Retraction of leaflets with associated aortic regurgitation is common.

■ Secondary calcification is common, and, at the extreme, it is difficult to discern between chronic, healed rheumatic stenosis and the degenerative form. Associated mitral stenosis helps in diagnosing rheumatic disease.

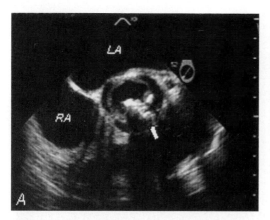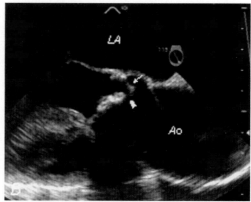

FIG. 9-3. Bicuspid aortic valve stenosis. Two-dimensional echocardiographic images **(A)** demonstrate two cusps and a raphe (*arrow*). **B:** Eccentric closure (*thick arrow*) and doming mobility of the cusps (*thin arrow*). Ao, aorta; LA, left atrium; RA, right atrium.

Supravalvular Aortic Stenosis

- Three types of supravalvular aortic stenosis exist. The most common is a discrete fibrous membrane near the sinotubular junction in a normal-sized aorta (Fig. 9-4A); other types include fibromuscular thickening above the coronary sinuses causing an hourglass-shaped narrowing, and diffuse hypoplasia of the ascending aorta.
- Supravalvular diffuse or discrete narrowing is associated with dilated coronary ostia and aortic valve cusps' thickening and sclerosis.

Subvalvular Aortic Stenosis

- The most common type of subvalvular aortic stenosis is a fibrous membrane located just below the aortic valve extending from the anterior septum to the anterior mitral leaflet; it appears on echo as a discrete linear structure in the left ventricular outflow tract (LVOT) from the TTE apical long-axis view (ultrasound beam is perpendicular to the membrane).
- The second, less common type is a fibromuscular ridge or tunnel causing diffuse

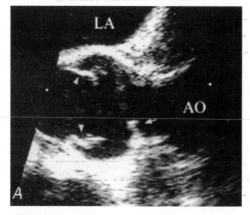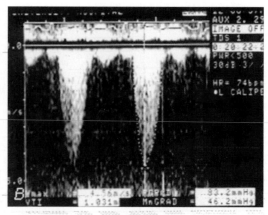

FIG. 9-4. Supravalvular aortic stenosis. **A:** Transesophageal echocardiographic long-axis view demonstrates a membrane at the sinotubular junction (*arrow*). The valve is shown by the arrowheads. **B:** Continuous wave Doppler velocity profile of severe supravalvular aortic stenosis. AO, aorta; LA, left atrium.

thickening and narrowing of the LVOT; it appears on echo as a thick, ill-defined membrane.

- In both forms, a characteristic, coarse systolic flutter of the aortic cusps and a mid-systolic partial closure of the valve can be seen.
- Associated aortic regurgitation is common.

Pitfalls

- Underestimation of the LVOT diameter is the most common error leading to underestimation of the aortic valve area (AVA).
- Aortic valve cusps' separation is decreased and mimics aortic stenosis in low stroke volume states, such as left ventricular dysfunction or severe mitral regurgitation.
- Planimetry of the aortic valve can overestimate or underestimate the valve area.
- Cusp separation of >1 cm by M-mode lacks specificity for assessment of the severity of bicuspid and rheumatic aortic stenosis.
- The coarse systolic fluttering and mid-systolic closure of the aortic valve seen in subvalvular aortic stenosis is also seen in hypertrophic obstructive cardiomyopathy.

Doppler Echocardiography for the Assessment of the Severity of Aortic Stenosis

Pulsed and Continuous Wave Doppler

Best Imaging Planes

- TTE left parasternal, right parasternal, apical, suprasternal notch, and, in children, the subcostal approach are necessary to find the highest peak velocity.
- In >90% of cases, the highest velocity is obtained from the apical views.

Diagnostic Methods and Formulas

Peak and Mean Gradients

- Peak velocities across the aortic valve reflect the systolic pressure difference between the left ventricle and aorta, and are directly related to the severity of aortic stenosis.
  - The simplified Bernoulli equation $\Delta P = 4v^2$ using V_{max} and $V_{integral}$ to calculate peak and

mean gradients, respectively (Figs. 9-2C and 9-4B).
  - If LVOT gradient (V_1) becomes significant, use $\Delta P = 4(v_2^2 - v_1^2)$.

Aortic Valve Area

- The continuity equation is based on the fact that flow before the valve equals flow after the valve ("what goes in must come out"). The continuity equation is as follows:

$$\text{Valve area} = \text{Area}_{LVOT} \ (cm^2) \times \text{velocity time integral (VTI)}_{LVOT} \ (cm) = \text{Area}_{AV} \ (cm^2) \times VTI_{AV} \ (cm)$$

$$\text{Area}_{LVOT} = \pi r^2 = 3.14 \ (\text{LVOT diameter}/2)^2 \ (cm^2)$$

- LVOT diameter is measured from TTE parasternal or TEE long-axis views at the onset of T wave on the electrocardiogram.

Ratio of Outflow Tract to Aortic Valve Peak Velocities

- A ratio <0.25 is consistent with severe stenosis and AVA <1 cm^2.

Key Diagnostic Features

Aortic Valve Sclerosis

- Peak velocity and gradient across the valve are >1.2 to ≤2.0 m/sec and >6 to <16 mm Hg, respectively.

Aortic Valve Stenosis

- Peak velocity and gradient across the valve are >2 m/sec and >16 mm Hg, respectively. Valve area is <2.0 cm^2.
- Integration of peak and mean gradients and valve area and index are necessary to define the severity of aortic stenosis (Table 9-2).

Color Doppler

Best Imaging Planes

- TTE parasternal long-axis, apical three-chamber and five-chamber views.
- TEE transgastric and basal long-axis views.

Key Diagnostic Features

- Turbulent color flow aliasing suggests obstruction (Fig. 9-2B).

TABLE 9-2. *Severity of Aortic Sclerosis and Stenosis by Echocardiography*

Severity	Valve morphology	Peak gradient (mean gradient)	Valve area (valve area index)
Sclerosis	Thickened and hyperreflectant cusps	<16 mm Hg (<10 mm Hg)	>2.0 cm² (>1.1 cm²/m²)
Mild stenosis	Thickened/Ca^{2+} cusps with 1+ decreased mobility	16–<25 mm Hg (<20 mm Hg)	1.5–2.0 cm² (0.9–1.1 cm²/m²)
Moderate stenosis	Thickened/Ca^{2+} cusps with 2–3+ decreased mobility	25–64 mm Hg (20–45 mm Hg)	1.0–1.5 cm² (0.6–0.9 cm²/m²)
Severe stenosis	Heavily thickened/Ca^{2+} and fixed cusps	>64 mm Hg (>45 mm Hg)	< 1.0 cm² (<0.6 cm²/m²)

- Identify the direction and location of the systolic jet to direct the continuous wave Doppler beam as parallel as possible to the vena contracta.
- Can detect concomitant subaortic valve obstruction.
- Useful for evaluation of coexisting aortic and mitral regurgitation.

Pitfalls

Underestimation or overestimation of the severity of aortic stenosis can occur (Table 9-3).

Diagnostic Accuracy for Detection of Aortic Sclerosis and Stenosis

General

- Two-dimensional TTE or TEE provides an accurate morphologic characterization of the sclerotic and stenotic aortic valve and, in their earlier stages, can accurately define their etiology.

TABLE 9-3. *Pitfalls of Doppler Echocardiography in the Assessment of Aortic Valve Stenosis*

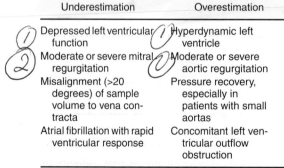

Underestimation	Overestimation
Depressed left ventricular function	Hyperdynamic left ventricle
Moderate or severe mitral regurgitation	Moderate or severe aortic regurgitation
Misalignment (>20 degrees) of sample volume to vena contracta	Pressure recovery, especially in patients with small aortas
Atrial fibrillation with rapid ventricular response	Concomitant left ventricular outflow obstruction

- Doppler echo accurately separates aortic valve sclerosis from stenosis.
- Doppler echo is highly accurate and currently the method of choice to define the presence and severity of aortic valve stenosis. The correlation coefficients for the measurement of peak and mean gradients and valve area as compared with cardiac catheterization are 0.91 to 0.97. The highest correlation is seen in severe lesions.
- Peak to peak gradients in the catheterization laboratory measure the difference between peak left ventricular pressure and aortic pressure. Echo Doppler measures the maximum instantaneous pressure gradient across the valve, which occurs before the peak aortic pressure (Fig. 9-5). Therefore, Doppler overestimates peak gradient and severity of aortic stenosis (10).
- The mean pressure gradients (average pressure difference during the systolic ejection period) from both Doppler and cardiac catheterization are true gradients and are better for comparison purposes (Figs. 9-2C and 9-4B).

Pressure Recovery

- As the aortic jet decelerates and expands beyond the vena contracta, the associated turbulence results in an increase in aortic pressure (*pressure recovery*). Thus, by cardiac catheterization, the left ventricular pressure to aortic pressure difference is less than if aortic pressure would be measured in the vena contracta.
- Therefore, Doppler gradients and valve area severity are overestimated by Doppler as compared to catheterization (11). The magni-

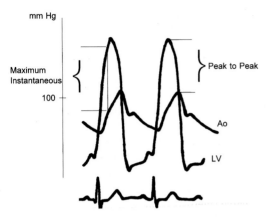

mm Hg

Maximum
Instantaneous

Peak to Peak

100

Ao

LV

FIG. 9-5. Echocardiographic Doppler maximum instantaneous gradient and catheter-based peak to peak gradient of aortic stenosis. Ao, aortic pressure curve; LV, left ventricular pressure curve.

tude of pressure recovery is greater in those patients with small aortic roots and moderate stenosis (12).

Low-Gradient Aortic Stenosis

■ Low-gradient aortic stenosis applies to patients with sclerotic and frequently calcified aortic cusps with decreased mobility, a low transvalvular mean gradient (≤30 mm Hg), and a calculated AVA ≤1 cm² in the presence of a decreased left ventricular systolic function (ejection fraction <35%). True AVAs tend to be underestimated in these patients.

■ Resting Doppler echo cannot separate patients with left ventricular dysfunction due to severe aortic valve stenosis (low-gradient aortic stenosis) from those with mild or moderate aortic stenosis and an unrelated cardiomyopathy (pseudostenosis). Dobutamine echo has proven to be of important diagnostic and prognostic value in these patients (13,14).

■ Patients with contractile reserve show an improvement in wall motion score or index of ≥20% and ejection fraction of ≥10%, or an increase in stroke volume of >50%. An increase in peak velocity of >0.6 m/sec, or an increase in peak gradient of ≥20 mm Hg or >25% from baseline, but no change or <20% change in valve area indicates severe aortic stenosis.

■ Patients with contractile reserve but with an increase in peak gradient <20 mm Hg and a >25% increase in valve area have mild or moderate stenosis or pseudostenosis. In a small proportion of patients with no contractile reserve, a separation will not be possible.

Stratification of the Severity of Aortic Valve Sclerosis and Stenosis

■ Sclerosis is *mild* when cusp mobility is normal or minimally reduced, and the cusp thickening is <4 mm; *moderate* when cusp sclerosis is 4 to 6 mm and is associated with decreased mobility; and *severe* when in addition to sclerosis and decreased mobility, there is an increase in velocity across the valve but <2 m/sec (2).

■ Stratification of aortic valve stenosis severity requires the integration and, generally, concordance of peak and mean gradients and valve area and valve area index (Table 9-2).

■ In a patient with a normal stroke volume, an aortic valve peak velocity of ≥4 m/sec or <2.5 m/sec (but ≥2 m/sec) determines the presence of severe or mild aortic stenosis, respectively (10).

■ Finally, a V_1/V_2 ratio <0.25 is consistent with severe aortic stenosis and AVA ≤1 cm².

Prognostic Value in Aortic Valve Sclerosis and Stenosis

■ Aortic valve sclerosis is associated with atherogenic risk factors and an increased risk of myocardial infarction, stroke, heart failure, and cardiovascular death (1,15–17).

■ Aortic valve sclerosis progresses to aortic valve stenosis.

■ A mixed, nodular, and diffuse aortic valve sclerosis is associated with coronary artery disease (Fig. 9-1D) (16).

■ Aortic valve sclerosis is highly associated with aortic atheromatous disease (2).

■ The extent of aortic valve calcification in combination with a rapid increase in aortic jet velocity of ≥0.3 m/sec per year identifies asymptomatic patients with aortic stenosis at high risk for adverse outcomes (18).

■ A ratio of AVA at mid-acceleration and mid-deceleration to valve area at peak velocity of

TABLE 9-4. *Recommendations for Valve Replacement*

Clinical scenario	Class
Symptomatic patients with severe aortic stenosis	I
Patients with severe stenosis undergoing CABG	I
Patients with severe stenosis undergoing surgery on the aorta or other heart valves	I
Patients with moderate stenosis undergoing CABG or surgery on the aorta or other heart valves	IIa
Asymptomatic patients with severe stenosis and left ventricular systolic dysfunction or abnormal response to exercise (e.g., hypotension)	IIa

CABG, coronary artery bypass grafting.

≥1.25 has 80% positive predictive value for rapid progression of stenosis (19).

■ Patients with low-gradient aortic stenosis and negative contractile reserve during dobutamine infusion have high operative and overall mortality.

Indicators for Valve Replacement or Valvuloplasty

■ Indeterminate AVA or gradients by echo in symptomatic patients indicates the need for cardiac catheterization if the patient is a candidate for valve surgery.

■ Class I indications for aortic valve replacement in aortic stenosis, according to the American College of Cardiology/American Heart Association guidelines, include symptomatic severe stenosis and patients with moderate to severe asymptomatic stenosis undergoing coronary artery bypass grafting or surgery of the aorta or other valve (Table 9-4).

■ Balloon valvuloplasty in severe aortic stenosis is indicated in a high surgical risk symptomatic patient without significant concomitant aortic regurgitation.

■ Indications for percutaneous aortic valve replacement are still undefined.

Use in the Pregnant Patient with Aortic Stenosis

■ Aortic stenosis in a pregnant patient is usually due to a congenitally abnormal valve. As stroke volume increases during pregnancy, an increase in valve gradient is seen (20).

■ Asymptomatic patients with severe stenosis before pregnancy may decompensate due to an increase in metabolic demand and heart rate, reduced left ventricular compliance due to left ventricular hypertrophy, and limited ability to increase stroke volume.

■ Thus, echo is indicated during the first and third trimester in a pregnant patient with known aortic stenosis for assessment of changes in hemodynamic severity and ventricular function.

Role of Stress Echocardiography in Aortic Stenosis

■ Regular exercise testing should not be performed in *symptomatic* patients with moderate or severe aortic stenosis.

■ In asymptomatic patients, exercise testing is probably safe and may add information to the initial evaluation by quantifying patients' functional capacity and symptoms, and providing information regarding hemodynamic severity of aortic stenosis.

■ Dobutamine echo is indicated for the diagnosis and assessment of prognosis in patients with low-gradient aortic stenosis.

Intraoperative Use in Aortic Stenosis

■ Although TEE may be of diagnostic value to surgeons at the time of or immediately after valve replacement, it is not recommended to be routinely performed.

■ When TEE is performed, the following parameters are of greatest interest to surgeons:
  ◆ Aortic annulus diameter for sizing the valve.
  ◆ Aortic root and ascending aorta diameter to evaluate if root repair or replacement is indicated. This is of particular interest in cases of bicuspid aortic valve stenosis in which the aortic root may be dilated out of proportion to the degree of stenosis.
  ◆ Proximal aorta calcification and degree of atheromatous disease can guide the cross-clamping technique and site.

TABLE 9-5. *Echocardiography Follow-Up in Patients with Asymptomatic Aortic Stenosis*

Stenosis severity	Echo follow-up
Mild	Every 5 yr
Moderate	Every 2 yr
Moderate-severe	Every 1–2 yr
Severe	Yearly

◆ Concomitant lesions of other valves and evaluation of the presence of systolic anterior motion of the mitral valve apparatus.
◆ Degree of left ventricular hypertrophy and left ventricular systolic function.
■ For balloon valvuloplasty, echo is used to evaluate preprocedure and postprocedure AVA and gradients as well as aortic regurgitation.

Follow-Up in Patients with Aortic Stenosis

■ The average rate of decrease in AVA in aortic stenosis is 0.12 cm²/year.
■ More than one-half of patients show little or no progression over a 3-year to 9-year period, but others may have rapid progression, with increases in pressure gradients of 15 to 19 mm Hg/year and a decrease of AVA of 0.1 to 0.3 cm²/year.
■ Therefore, echo follow-up is advised in asymptomatic patients with aortic stenosis (Table 9-5) (8,16), with increasing frequency in those with moderate or worse disease and especially if development of symptoms is suspected.
■ Patients with a newly diagnosed severe aortic stenosis by echo should have a follow-up study 6 months after diagnosis. If no changes in left ventricular systolic function and size are noted, then yearly studies are recommended.
■ Follow-up echo of asymptomatic patients with mild to moderate aortic stenosis, stable physical signs, and normal left ventricular size and function lack supportive data.

REFERENCES

1. Otto CM, Lind BK, Kitzman DW, et al. Association of aortic valve sclerosis with cardiovascular mortality and morbidity in the elderly. *N Engl J Med* 1999;341: 142–147.
2. Tolstrup K, Roldan CA, Qualls CR, et al. Aortic valve sclerosis, mitral annular calcification, and aortic root sclerosis are markers of atherosclerotic disease. *J Am Coll Cardiol* 2000;35:282A.
3. Agmon Y, Khanderia BK, Tajik AJ, et al. Aortic valve sclerosis and aortic atherosclerosis: different manifestations of the same disease? Insights from a population based study. *J Am Coll Cardiol* 2001;38:827–834.
4. Wierzbicki A, Shetty C. Aortic stenosis: an atherosclerotic disease? *J Heart Valve Dis* 1999;8:416–423.
5. Ward C. Clinical significance of the bicuspid aortic valve. *Heart* 2000;83:81–85.
6. Fedak PW, Verma S, David TE, et al. Clinical and pathophysiological implications of a bicuspid aortic valve. *Circulation* 2002;106:900–904.
7. Metcalfe K, Rucka AK, Tassabehji M, et al. Elastin: mutational spectrum in supravalvular aortic stenosis. *Eur J Hum Genet* 2000;8:955–963.
8. Brown RO, Carabello B, Leon AC, et al. ACC/AHA guidelines for the management of patients with valvular heart disease. *J Am Coll Cardiol* 1998;32:1486–1588.
9. Cheitlin MD, Armstrong WF, Aurigemma GP, et al. ACC/AHA/ASE guideline update for the clinical application of echocardiography: summary article. *J Am Coll Cardiol* 2003;42:954–970.
10. Otto CM. Valvular aortic stenosis: Which measure of severity is best? *Am Heart J* 1998;136:940–942.
11. Garcia D, Dumesnil JG, Pibarot P, et al. Discrepancies between catheter and Doppler estimates of valve effective orifice area can be predicted from the pressure recovery phenomenon. *J Am Coll Cardiol* 2003;41:435–442.
12. Crawford MH, Roldan CA. Prevalence of aortic root dilatation and small aortic roots in valvular aortic stenosis. *Am J Cardiol* 2001;87:1311–1313.
13. Lin SS, Roger VL, Pascoe R, et al. Dobutamine stress Doppler hemodynamics in patients with aortic stenosis: feasibility, safety, and surgical considerations. *Am Heart J* 1998;136:1010–1016.
14. Monin JL, Quere JP, Gueret P, et al. Low-gradient aortic stenosis: operative risk stratification and predictors for long-term outcome: a multicenter study using dobutamine stress hemodynamics. *Circulation* 2003; 108:319–324.
15. Aronow WS, Ahn C, Shirani J, Kronzon I. Comparison of frequency of new coronary events in older subjects with and without valvular aortic sclerosis. *Am J Cardiol* 1999;83:599–600.
16. Tolstrup K, Crawford MH, Roldan CA. Morphologic characteristics of aortic valve sclerosis by transesophageal echocardiography: importance for the prediction of coronary artery disease. *Cardiology* 2002;98:154–158.
17. Jeong D, Atar S, Siegel RJ. Association of mitral annulus calcification, aortic valve sclerosis and aortic root calcification with abnormal myocardial perfusion single photon emission tomography in subjects age ≤65 years old. *J Am Coll Cardiol* 2001;38:1988–1993.

18. Rosenhek R, Binder T, Porenta G, et al. Predictors of outcome in severe, asymptomatic aortic stenosis. *N Engl J Med* 2000;343:611–617.

19. Lester SJ, McElhinney DB, Miller JP, et al. Rate of change in aortic valve area during a cardiac cycle can predict the rate of hemodynamic progression of aortic stenosis. *Circulation* 2000;101:1947–1952.

20. Reimold SC, Rutherford JD. Clinical practice. Valvular heart disease in pregnancy. *N Engl J Med* 2003; 349:52–59.

10

Tricuspid and Pulmonic Valve Disease

Dara K. Lee and Carlos A. Roldan

- The physical examination remains the primary screening method for detection of tricuspid or pulmonic valve disease.
- However, the sensitivity of the physical examination for detection and determining the etiology, severity, and prognosis of right-sided valve disease is low.
- The limitations of the physical examination in the assessment of right-sided valve disease stem largely from the fact that the right-sided (venous) heart is a low-pressure system, the transvalvular gradients are low, and, therefore, the audibility of tricuspid and pulmonic murmurs is low.
- Tricuspid regurgitation (TR) can be mistaken for eccentric mitral regurgitation, and pulmonic regurgitation (PR) or pulmonic stenosis (PS) can be mistaken for aortic regurgitation or aortic stenosis, respectively.
- As with left-sided lesions, acute right-sided regurgitant lesions may be clinically silent.
- Finally, the physical examination cannot distinguish if valve regurgitation is due to a structurally abnormal valve (primary valve disease) or secondary to pulmonary hypertension or right ventricular or annular dilatation (secondary or functional valve disease).

COMMON ETIOLOGIES

Primary Right-Sided Valve Disease

Acquired Lesions

- Rheumatic heart disease affects the right-sided valves in 30% to 50% of cases.
- TR and/or tricuspid stenosis (TS) are predominantly caused by rheumatic heart disease (>90% of all cases).
- Only 3% to 5% of cases of rheumatic heart disease have significant TR or TS, however.
- Carcinoid or anorectic drugs rarely cause TS.
- Infective endocarditis occurs in intravenous drug abusers.
- Carcinoid tumors with metastasis to the liver resulting in elevated serotonin levels can cause thickening and retraction of the valve leaflets.
- Ergotamine alkaloids and diet pills containing fenfluramine-phentermine mimic the effects of carcinoid on the heart valves (1,2).

- Severe PR is rare and is generally due to primary valve disease.
- Rarely, blunt chest trauma is associated with primary right-sided valve disease.
- The pulmonic valve is the least affected by rheumatic disease, carcinoid disease, or endocarditis.

Congenital Lesions

- Congenital lesions include myxomatous valve degeneration or floppy valve syndrome.
- Ebstein's anomaly is characterized by apical displacement and dysplasia of the septal and posterior tricuspid leaflets.
- Congenital pulmonic valve stenosis may be due to a unicuspid, bicuspid, or, rarely, a quadricuspid valve.
- Most cases of congenital PS are valvular (approximately 90%) and rarely are subvalvular or supravalvular.
- Congenital PS is usually an isolated anomaly, but it may be associated with a ventricular septal defect or secondary hypertrophic subpulmonic stenosis.

Functional Right-Sided Valve Disease

- Mild TR and PR is seen in up to 75% of healthy individuals.
- It is most commonly caused by pulmonary hypertension due to pulmonary vascular or parenchymal disease, or transmission of elevated left-heart pressures.
- Pulmonary hypertension leads to high right ventricular systolic pressure; right ventricular hypertrophy; right ventricular and tricuspid annular dilatation; right ventricular outflow tract, pulmonic valve annular, and main pulmonary artery (PA) dilatation; and, consequently, to TR or PR, or both.
- Right ventricular volume overload (due to left to right intracardiac shunt or primary TR) may result in right ventricular dilatation and functional TR or PR.
- Right ventricular ischemia or infarction and right ventricular arrhythmogenic cardiomyopathy can cause TR or PR.

ECHOCARDIOGRAPHY

Class I Indications for Echocardiography

■ The American College of Cardiology/American Heart Association (ACC/AHA) guidelines recommend echocardiography (echo) in patients with signs or symptoms of possible right-sided valve disease, such as dyspnea of unclear etiology, elevated central venous pressures, acute or chronic pulmonary hypertension and its response to therapy, unexplained hypotension, and suspected pulmonary embolism (Table 10-1) (3,4).

■ Echo determines the presence and severity of right ventricular enlargement, hypertrophy, or dysfunction, which may be the result of, or a cause of, tricuspid or pulmonic valve disease.

■ Transesophageal echo (TEE) is of important diagnostic value in patients with suspected right-sided endocarditis or chest trauma.

Tricuspid Valve Regurgitation

Two-Dimensional Echocardiography: Valve Morphology

Best Imaging Planes

■ Transthoracic echo (TTE) parasternal long-axis view of the right ventricle (RV), parasternal basal short-axis view, and apical and subcostal four-chamber views.

■ TEE transgastric short-axis and long-axis views of the RV, mid-esophageal four-chamber view, and basal short-axis view longitudinal to right ventricular outflow tract.

Key Diagnostic Features

■ Mild or worse TR in a valve with thin leaflets, normal coaptation, and normal-appearing supporting structures, suggests regurgitation is physiologic or functional (5).

■ In rheumatic disease, leaflets' tip thickening, leaflet retraction, leaflet tethering from chordal or papillary muscle thickening, fusion and retraction, and commissural fusion cause both stenosis and regurgitation.

■ With endocarditis, valvular vegetations or perforations, or both, are often seen.

TABLE 10-1. *Class I Indications for Echocardiography in Tricuspid or Pulmonic Valve Disease*

For distinguishing cardiac vs. noncardiac etiology of dyspnea in patients in whom clinical and laboratory clues are ambiguous.

Edema with clinical signs of elevated central venous pressure when a potential cardiac etiology is suspected or when central venous pressure cannot be estimated with confidence and clinical suspicion of heart disease is high.

Dyspnea with clinical signs of heart disease.

Patient with unexplained hypotension, especially in the intensive care unit.

Diagnosis and assessment of hemodynamic severity of valvular stenosis or regurgitation.

Assessment of left and right ventricular size, function, and/or hemodynamics in a patient with valvular stenosis or regurgitation.

Assessment of changes in hemodynamic severity and ventricular compensation in patients with known valvular stenosis or regurgitation during pregnancy.

Assessment of the effects of medical therapy on the severity of regurgitation and ventricular compensation and function when it might change medical management.

Assessment of valvular morphology and regurgitation in patients with a history of anorectic drug use or the use of any drug known to be associated with valvular heart disease who are symptomatic, have cardiac murmurs, or have a technically inadequate auscultation.

Reevaluation of asymptomatic patients with severe stenosis or severe regurgitation.

Reevaluation of patients with mild to moderate valvular regurgitation with changing symptoms.

Reevaluation of patients with mild to moderate valvular regurgitation with ventricular dilatation without clinical symptoms.

Assessment of the effects of medical therapy on the severity of regurgitation and ventricular compensation and function.

Adapted from Cheitlin MD, Armstrong WF, Aurigemma GP, et al. ACC/AHA/ASE 2003 guideline update for the clinical application of echocardiography: summary article. *J Am Coll Cardiol* 2003;42:954–970; and Bonow RO, Carabello AC, De Leon AC, et al. ACC/AHA guidelines for the management of patients with valvular heart disease. *J Am Coll Cardiol* 1998;32:1486–1588.

■ Imaging of the tricuspid valve by TEE is especially useful in infective endocarditis when small vegetations or valve perforations are suspected.

■ In carcinoid disease, the leaflets are thickened and retracted with a fixed orifice usually leading to predominant regurgitation and less severe stenosis (Fig. 10-1) (6).

■ Approximately 30% of patients with mitral valve prolapse have redundancy and prolapse of the tricuspid valve, leading to TR.

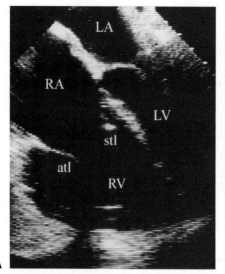
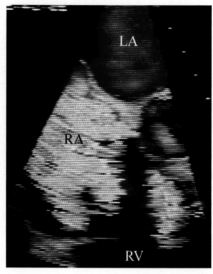

A   **B**

FIG. 10-1. Tricuspid regurgitation due to carcinoid syndrome. **A:** Transesophageal echocardiographic four-chamber view during systole (note the closed mitral valve) demonstrates severe dilatation of the right heart chambers and thickened and fixed open anterior (atl) and septal (stl) tricuspid leaflets. **B:** Color Doppler demonstrates a large regurgitant jet occupying the entire atria consistent with severe tricuspid regurgitation. LA, left atrium; LV, left ventricle; RA, right atrium; RV, right ventricle.

- More than 1 cm apical displacement and dysplasia of the septal tricuspid leaflet is consistent with Ebstein's anomaly.
- Significant thickening or calcification of the annulus or leaflets may be seen in patients with tricuspid valve dysplasia.

Doppler Echocardiography for the Assessment of the Severity of Tricuspid Regurgitation

Pulsed and Continuous Wave Doppler: Key Diagnostic Features

- Pulsed Doppler is highly sensitive for the detection of TR but not for defining its severity.
- Pulsed wave Doppler of the hepatic veins can be used for assessment of the severity of TR. In moderate TR, there is reduction in the normal systolic flow; in severe TR, absent or reversed systolic flow is seen (Table 10-2).
- In severe TR, the continuous wave Doppler envelope is as dense as the tricuspid inflow signal. Also, a V wave (reduction in velocity or concave configuration during the latter half of systole of the Doppler envelope) is seen as

right ventricular and right atrial pressures equalize (7).
- A tricuspid inflow velocity ≥1.0 m/sec also suggests severe TR.

Color Doppler: Diagnostic Methods and Key Diagnostic Features

- The indices of severity used for assessment of mitral regurgitation cannot be applied to TR because of the lower pressures in the right heart.
- The size and length of a regurgitant jet are related to momentum, which is the product of mass and velocity. Velocity increases relative to the pressure gradient across a valve. Because the RV is a low-pressure chamber, regurgitation of a similar volume of blood appears smaller in the right atrium (RA) than in the left atrium.
- In severe pulmonary hypertension, a regurgitant jet may appear larger and longer in relation to the RA, despite a smaller regurgitant volume (8).
- The TR jet area and proximal flow convergence zone on echo, as compared to right

TABLE 10-2. *Stratification of Tricuspid and Pulmonic Valve Diseases*

	Mild	Moderate	Severe
Parameter	Tricuspid valve regurgitation		
Valve morphology	Normal	Normal/abnormal	Abnormal
RV, RA, IVC size	Normal	Normal or dilated	Dilated unless acute TR; TV annulus ≥4 cm
CW jet	Less intense than inflow	Almost as dense as inflow	As dense as inflow with late delay
Jet area	<5 cm^{2a}	5–10 cm^2	>10 cm^2
Jet/RA area	<20%	20–40%	>40%
Vena contracta width	Small^a	Probably <7 mm	≥7 mm
Proximal isovelocity surface area radius	≤5 mm	0.6–0.9 mm	>10 mm for a Nyquist limit of 30 cm/sec; ≥7 mm for a Nyquist limit of 40 cm/sec Other feature: jet length >5.3 cm^a
Hepatic vein flow	Systolic dominance	Systolic blunting	Systolic reversal
	Tricuspid valve stenosis		
Mean gradient	<2 mm Hg	2–5 mm Hg	>5–7 mm Hg
	Pulmonic valve regurgitation		
Valve morphology	Normal	Normal or abnormal	Abnormal
RV size	Normal	Normal or mildly dilated	Moderately dilated
Pulsed Doppler	Slightly increased pulmonic flow compared to systemic flow	Intermediate	Greatly increased
CW Doppler density	Less dense than systolic flow	Almost as dense as systolic flow	As dense as systolic flow; dense
CW pressure half-time	>100 msec	Variable but most commonly <100 msec	<100 msec
Jet length	<10 mm with narrow origin	10–20 mm	>20 mm
	Pulmonic valve stenosis		
Peak gradient	<50 mm Hg	50–80 mm Hg	>80 mm Hg
Valve area	1–2 cm^2/m^2	0.5–1.0 cm^2	RV pressure >100 mm Hg

CW, continuous wave; IVC, inferior vena cava; RA, right atrium; RV, right ventricle; TR, tricuspid regurgitation; TV, tricuspid valve.
^{a}Jet area and length and vena contracta width are assessed with a Nyquist limit at 50–60 cm/sec.
Adapted from references 3, 4, and 7–14.

ventricular angiography, differentiates mild to moderate (grade 1–2) TR from severe (grade 3 or 4) TR.

■ The proximal isovelocity surface area (PISA) radius at an aliasing velocity of 28 or 41 m/sec is comparable to jet area or jet length, but all are better than the ratio of jet area to right atrial area.

■ The following parameters are consistent with severe TR (8–11):

1. A jet length of 5.3 cm.
2. A jet area of 10.6 cm^2.
3. A jet area to right atrial area ratio of >40% (Fig. 10-1B).
4. A PISA radius of >10 mm for a Nyquist limit of 30 cm/sec.
5. A PISA radius of ≥7 mm for a Nyquist limit of 40 cm/sec.
6. A vena contracta width of ≥7 mm.

Pitfalls

■ The color Doppler area of a TR jet is related to the jet momentum. Thus, a similar volume

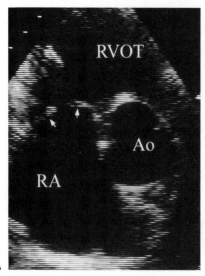
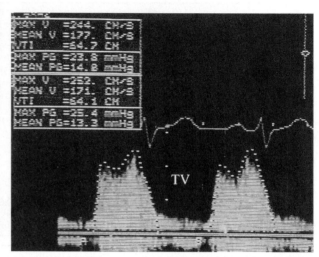

A   B

FIG. 10-2. Tricuspid stenosis due to carcinoid syndrome. **A:** Transthoracic echocardiographic short-axis view demonstrates diffusely thickened, retracted leaflets with doming (*arrows*) of the anterior and septal tricuspid leaflets. **B:** Continuous wave Doppler tracing confirmed the presence of severe tricuspid stenosis with peak and mean gradients of 25 mm Hg and 13 mm Hg, respectively. Ao, aorta; RA, right atrium; RVOT, right ventricular outflow tract; TV, tricuspid valve.

of regurgitation appears as a larger jet if the right ventricular pressure is elevated.

- Because of the potential pitfalls in assessing the severity of TR by Doppler imaging alone, it is important to complement it with morphologic characteristics of the RV and RA (Table 10-2).

Tricuspid Valve Stenosis

Two-Dimensional Echocardiography: Valve Morphology

Best Imaging Planes

- TTE parasternal long-axis view of the RV, parasternal basal short-axis views, and apical and subcostal four-chamber views.
- TEE transgastric short-axis and long-axis views of the RV, mid-esophageal four-chamber view, and basal short-axis view longitudinal to the right ventricular outflow tract.

Key Diagnostic Features

- In rheumatic TS, leaflets' tip thickening, retraction, and tethering are seen (12).

- An uncommon cause of TS is carcinoid syndrome, which may cause mixed stenosis and predominant regurgitation. The leaflets appear diffusely thickened, retracted, and fixed (Fig. 10-2A).
- Loeffler's disease also causes diffuse thickening of the tricuspid leaflets, resulting in stenosis and regurgitation.
- TEE can be used to assess a patient's eligibility for percutaneous valvuloplasty using similar criteria to those described earlier for mitral valvuloplasty (see Table 7-2).
- Indirect indicators of TS include right atrial enlargement and inferior vena cava (IVC) plethora in cases of moderate or severe TS. With significant coexisting TR, right ventricular dilatation can be seen.

Pitfalls

- TS can be missed on routine TTE because the degree of leaflet thickening may appear subtle, even with significant TS.
- Planimetry of the tricuspid valve orifice by two-dimensional (2D) images is difficult and unreliable.

Doppler Echocardiography for the Assessment of the Severity of Tricuspid Stenosis

Pulsed and Continuous Wave Doppler: Diagnostic Methods and Key Diagnostic Features

- Assessment of the mean transvalvular gradient, pressure half-time, and valve area are essential for defining the severity of TS because valves that appear severely stenotic by 2D images may have low gradients and vice versa.
- TS is significant if the mean transvalvular gradient is ≥ 4 mm Hg (in the absence of significant TR). A mean gradient of ≥ 5 to 7 mm Hg suggests severe TS (Table 10-2) (Fig. 10-2B).
- A pressure half-time ≥ 190 msec suggests severe TS (6,12).
- Valve area is less often used for determining TS severity, but an area <1.3 to 1.5 cm^2 is generally considered significant enough to cause symptoms.

Color Doppler: Key Diagnostic Features

Color Doppler echo is of limited use for the assessment of TS; however, the presence of an acceleration zone is suggestive of underlying valve stenosis and helps to direct the sample volume for assessment of valve gradients and pressure half-time.

Pulmonic Valve Regurgitation

Two-Dimensional Echocardiography: Valve Morphology

Best Imaging Planes

- TTE parasternal and subcostal short-axis views.
- TEE deep transgastric view and mid-esophageal short-axis view with the imaging plane longitudinal to the right ventricular outflow tract.

Key Diagnostic Features

- In primary PR, the valve leaflets are structurally abnormal.
- In rheumatic disease, the leaflets are thickened, retracted, and tethered.
- In carcinoid syndrome, the valve leaflets appear thickened and fixed with incomplete closure.

- With endocarditis, a mass or vegetation is seen on one or more leaflets.
- In PR secondary to pulmonary hypertension with PA and annulus dilatation, the valve leaflets are normal.
- With mild or moderate PR, right ventricular size and function are normal.
- With moderate to severe PR, right ventricular dilatation and systolic dysfunction and TR may occur.

Pitfalls

- The pulmonic valve is often difficult to visualize by TTE because of its anterosuperior location and interference by the lungs.
- By TEE, interference from the bronchus may limit the visualization of the pulmonic valve.

Doppler Echocardiography for the Assessment of the Severity of Pulmonic Valve Regurgitation

Pulsed and Continuous Wave Doppler: Diagnostic Methods and Key Diagnostic Features

- *Regurgitant volume:* In the absence of significant left-sided valve disease, forward left ventricular outflow tract stroke volume subtracted from total right ventricular outflow tract stroke volume is equal to right ventricular regurgitant volume.
- *Pressure half-time:* In the presence of PR, the pressure half-time (time it takes for the pressure gradient between PA and right ventricular to decrease by 50%) is a useful indicator of the severity of PR (12,13).
  - A pressure half-time >100 msec indicates mild PR.
  - In moderate or severe PR, pressure half-time is variable but most commonly <100 msec.
  - A pressure half-time <100 msec is consistent with severe PR (13,14).

Color Doppler: Diagnostic Methods and Key Diagnostic Features

- An indicator of the severity of PR is the width of the regurgitant jet relative to the width of the right ventricular outflow tract, but specific cutoff values have not been defined (Fig. 10-3C).

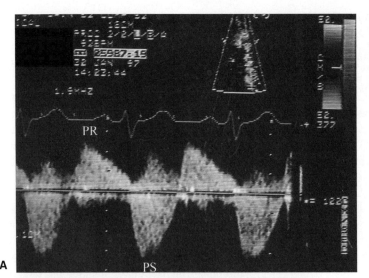

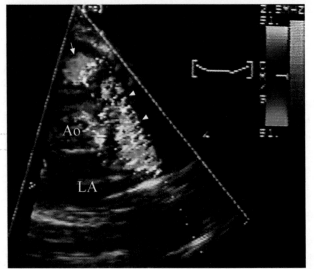

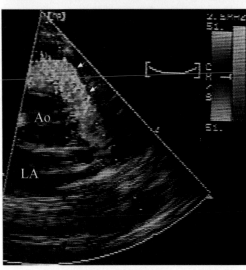

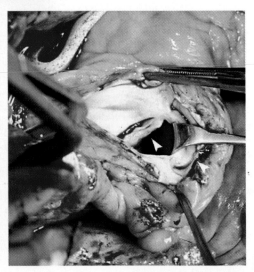

FIG. 10-3. Pulmonic valve stenosis and regurgitation due to carcinoid syndrome. **A:** At the pulmonic valve level, continuous wave Doppler demonstrates significant pulmonic valve stenosis (PS) (peak velocity, 3.5 m/sec and gradient of 49 mm Hg) and regurgitation (short pressure half-time). **B:** Color Doppler above the pulmonic valve level demonstrates an acceleration zone (*arrow*) and, at the valve level, a high turbulence or mosaic pattern (*arrowheads*). These features suggest pulmonic valve stenosis. **C:** At the pulmonic valve level, color Doppler demonstrates a regurgitant jet width that occupies the entire right ventricular outflow tract. This feature is consistent with severe pulmonic regurgitation (PR). **D:** Pulmonic valve demonstrates a shaggy appearance, severe thickening, and marked stiffness (*arrowhead*). Ao, aorta; LA, left atrium.

- The length of the PR jet is also a rough indicator of severity. A jet length of <10 mm is consistent with insignificant PR; a jet of >20 mm suggests significant PR (Table 10-2).
- Significant PR may also be suggested by a jet area >1.5 cm².
- The regurgitant jet area indexed to body surface area correlates well with pulmonic regurgitant fraction.
- Mild PR is predicted by an index of <0.64 ± 0.60 cm/m², and severe PR is predicted by an index of 2.2 ± 1.67 cm/m².

Pitfalls

- Because of limitations in measuring the diameter of the right ventricular outflow tract, the right ventricular regurgitant volume is not routinely performed, and specific cut-off values have not been determined.
- The color Doppler jet length of PR is also dependent on the pressure gradient between the PA and RV, and therefore is not a reliable indicator of the severity of PR.
- Significant variability and overlap of PR jet area to body surface area ratio limit this method's accuracy for assessing the severity of PR.

Pulmonic Valve Stenosis

M-Mode and Two-Dimensional Echocardiography: Valve Morphology

Best Imaging Planes

- TTE parasternal and subcostal short-axis views.
- TEE transgastric and mid-esophageal short-axis view longitudinal to the right ventricular outflow tract.

Key Diagnostic Features

- On M-mode, PS is associated with an exaggerated A wave, but there is no mid-systolic closure. Associated signs of right ventricular pressure overload can be seen.
- On 2D images, congenital PS appears as thin and pliable leaflets with commissural fusion and characteristic systolic doming appearance with a central orifice.

- Left PA dilatation may occur because the post-stenotic jet is directed toward the left. Dilatation is usually mild and rarely requires surgical repair.
- Acquired PS is generally not associated with poststenotic dilatation.
- Dysplastic pulmonic valve, which accounts for 10% to 15% of congenital PS, is sometimes associated with Noonan's syndrome.
  - ◆ A dysplastic stenotic pulmonic valve is characterized by thickened, fixed, and deformed leaflets; small annulus; and a concentric orifice. Systolic doming of the leaflets is generally absent. The proximal PA may be dysplastic as well.
  - ◆ A dysplastic stenotic valve is less amenable to valvuloplasty than a congenitally stenosed valve.
- In carcinoid disease, the valve cusps are thickened, retracted, and nonmobile or fixed.

Pitfalls

- Visualization of the pulmonic valve cusps can be technically difficult, and PS can be missed on a routine study.
- Because of the limitations of M-mode and 2D echo in visualizing the pulmonic valve, assessment of the presence and severity of PS is mainly based on Doppler parameters.

Doppler Echocardiography for the Assessment of the Severity of Pulmonic Valve Stenosis

Continuous and Pulsed Wave Doppler: Diagnostic Methods and Key Diagnostic Features

- Using the simplified Bernoulli equation ($\Delta P = 4V^2$, where P = pressure and V = peak TR velocity), the gradient between the RV and RA is determined. An estimate of right atrial pressure is added to this gradient to obtain the right ventricular systolic pressure, which is equal to the peak gradient of PS.
- In mild PS, the peak gradient is <50 mm Hg.
- PS is considered severe when the gradient is >80 mm Hg (Table 10-2) (Fig. 10-3A).
- Pulmonic valve area can also be assessed using the continuity equation (see Chapter 9 for further discussion).

Color Doppler: Key Diagnostic Features

■ Color Doppler is useful for identifying an acceleration zone, the vena contracta (the narrowest jet height or width), and a poststenotic jet (Fig. 10-3B).
■ Color Doppler can also be helpful for localizing prevalvular and postvalvular stenosis secondary to bands that are difficult to visualize with 2D echo.

Pitfalls

■ The largest source of error in calculating the pulmonic valve area using the continuity equation is the measurement of the diameter of the right ventricular outflow tract because of dropout in its distal anterior portion.
■ Another potential source of error is that patients with PS can have a dynamic right ventricular outflow tract gradient as a result of right ventricular hypertrophy. This gradient decreases the accuracy of the continuity equation for assessment of the pulmonic valve area.

Hemodynamic Impact of Tricuspid or Pulmonic Valve Disease on the Right Heart

■ *Right ventricular volume overload* leads to an increased right ventricular diastolic pressure, flattening or inversion of the septum during mid-diastole, and a diastolic D shape of the left ventricle (LV). During systole, the pressure difference reverses, and the septum shows a rapid anterior movement.
■ *Right ventricular pressure overload* due to PS leads to a prolonged right ventricular upstroke. As a result, the pressure in the RV exceeds the pressure in the LV during late systole and early diastole. This leads to flattening of the septum toward the LV (D-shaped LV). The septum resumes its usual shape during mid-diastole and late diastole.
■ Chronic right ventricular pressure overload also leads to right ventricular dilatation and, consequently, to functional TR. Therefore, a mixed pattern of pressure and volume overload is often present.
■ *Right atrial hypertension* and enlargement result from right ventricular pressure or vol-

ume overload. Right atrial pressure is estimated as follows:
◆ Low (<5 mm Hg) if the IVC is small (<1.5 cm) and collapses with inspiration.
◆ Normal (5–10 mm Hg) if IVC is normal in size (1.5–2.5 cm) and collapses >50% with inspiration.
◆ Mildly elevated (10–15 mm Hg) if IVC is normal and collapses <50% with inspiration.
◆ Moderately elevated (15–20 mm Hg) if IVC is >2.5 cm and collapses <50%.
◆ Right atrial pressure is markedly elevated (>20 mm Hg) if the hepatic veins are dilated and IVC does not collapse with a sniff.
■ In patients with right atrial hypertension, systolic, diastolic, and atrial reversal of hepatic vein inflow show similar changes to those seen in the pulmonary vein inflow of left atrial hypertension.
■ Right ventricular diastolic dysfunction may develop as a result of chronic pressure or volume overload.
◆ Abnormal right ventricular relaxation is suggested by a decrease in E wave and an increase in A wave of the tricuspid valve inflow.
◆ With worsening right ventricular diastolic function, E wave velocity increases, and a restrictive pattern with an elevated E wave and a decreased A wave may occur (15).
■ Right ventricular systolic function is normal if systolic annular excursion toward right ventricular apex is >2 cm. A right ventricular annular systolic excursion ≤1 cm indicates right ventricular dysfunction.

Diagnostic Accuracy in Tricuspid and Pulmonic Valve Disease

■ In TR, PISA radius at an aliasing velocity of 28 or 41 m/sec is comparable to either jet area or jet length, but both are better than the ratio of jet area to right atrial area (87% accuracy vs. 79% accuracy).
■ A vena contracta width of >7 mm predicts severe TR with 88% sensitivity and 93% specificity.
■ In PR, a pressure half-time <100 msec has a sensitivity of 76% and a specificity of 94%

for predicting a significant regurgitant fraction of $\geq$20% (13).

Use in the Pregnant Patient with Tricuspid or Pulmonic Valve Disease

- Beginning in the middle to late second trimester and continuing until shortly after delivery, the circulating blood volume of the pregnant woman increases by approximately 50%.
- Echo findings in the normal pregnancy include mild dilation of heart chambers and annular dilatation with resultant mild to mild/moderate TR and PR.
- Pregnant patients generally tolerate well even severe TR or PR.
- Women with baseline moderate to severe TS or PS before pregnancy may decompensate with the rise in circulating volume during pregnancy and delivery. In these patients, balloon valvuloplasty should be considered.
- The ACC/AHA guidelines recommend against pregnancy in patients with severe TS or PS (4).

Follow-Up of Patients with Tricuspid or Pulmonic Valve Disease

- Patients found to have significant right-sided valve lesions on routine echo should have serial studies, even in the absence of symptoms (Table 10-1).
- Untreated severe PR and TR can lead to progressive right ventricular dilatation over time, with resulting annular dilatation in increased regurgitation.
- Although specific guidelines do not exist, annual echo for the asymptomatic patient with significant right-sided valve regurgitation is appropriate.
- The development of symptoms should prompt earlier imaging and intervention.

Indicators of Poor Prognosis in Tricuspid or Pulmonic Valve Disease

- Patients with long-standing untreated lesions of the tricuspid or pulmonic valves are subject to chronic pressure or volume overload, or both, of the RV.
- Development of right ventricular dilatation and systolic dysfunction generally predict a poor prognosis.
- Once right ventricular failure develops, it is often irreversible, even with medical and mechanical or surgical correction of the underlying valve lesion.

Indicators for Tricuspid or Pulmonic Valve Replacement, Valvuloplasty, or Valve Repair

- The ACC/AHA guidelines recommend annuloplasty for severe TR in patients with pulmonary hypertension (PA pressure $\geq$60 mm Hg) and mitral valve disease undergoing mitral valve surgery (class I) (4,16–18).
- Severe and symptomatic TR with PA pressure <60 mm Hg is considered a relative indication for tricuspid valve surgery (class IIa).
- When annuloplasty or repair is not technically feasible, valve replacement for severe TR may be warranted to prevent the development of right ventricular dysfunction (class IIa).
- Biologic prostheses are preferred to mechanical valves because of the high rate of thromboembolic complications seen in valves in the low-pressure tricuspid valve position (16–18).
- Pulmonic valve balloon valvotomy or replacement is recommended in patients with symptoms and mild or worse stenosis and for asymptomatic patients with gradients >50 mm Hg.
- There is disagreement about the treatment of asymptomatic patients with pulmonic valve gradients between 30 to 50 mm Hg.

Intraoperative Use in Patients Undergoing Tricuspid or Pulmonic Valve Replacement or Repair

The value of intraoperative echo in patients undergoing right-sided valve replacement, valvuloplasty, or repair is similar to that described for those undergoing mitral or aortic valve replacement or repair not really needed.

Use after Tricuspid or Pulmonic Valve Surgery

- ACC/AHA guidelines recommend a baseline echocardiogram, usually at the first postoperative visit 3 to 4 weeks after discharge.
- This study is performed to assess for prosthetic stenosis, valvular or paravalvular regurgitation, and pericardial effusion, and to determine PA pressures and chamber dimensions.
- The ACC/AHA does not offer specific guidelines for the ongoing evaluation of the asymptomatic patient with a mechanical valve, as subclinical valve dysfunction in these prostheses is unusual.
- Biologic valves, however, may begin to show evidence of deterioration after 5 to 8 years, and therefore, close clinical follow-up is important.
- For all patients with prosthetic valves, annual clinic visits are recommended; any decrease in functional capacity or new murmur should prompt echo.
- If mild regurgitation is detected, follow-up echo every 3 to 6 months may be warranted.

REFERENCES

1. Connolly HM, Crary JL, McGoon MD, et al. Valvular heart disease associated with fenfluramine-phentermine. *N Engl J Med* 1997;337:581–588.
2. Roldan CA, Shively BK, Gelgand E, et al. Morphology of anorexigen-associated valve disease by transthoracic and transesophageal echocardiography. *Am J Cardiol* 2002;90:1269–1273.
3. Cheitlin MD, Armstrong WF, Aurigemma GP, et al. ACC/AHA/ASE 2003 guideline update for the clinical application of echocardiography: summary article. *J Am Coll Cardiol* 2003;42:954–970.
4. Bonow RO, Carabello AC, De Leon AC, et al. ACC/AHA guidelines for the management of patients with valvular heart disease. *J Am Coll Cardiol* 1998;32:1486–1588.
5. Singh JP, Evans JC, Levy D. Prevalence and clinical determinants of mitral, tricuspid, and aortic regurgitation (the Framingham Heart Study). *Am J Cardiol* 1999;83:892–902.
6. Blaustein AS, Ramanathan A. Tricuspid valve disease. *Cardiol Clin* 1998;16:551–672.
7. Schiller NB. Echocardiographic evaluation of the severity of tricuspid valve regurgitation: 29 considerations useful in recognizing hemodynamically important lesions. *Isr J Med Sci* 1996;32:853–867.
8. Zoghbi WA, Enriquez-Sarano M, Foster E, et al. Recommendations for evaluation of the severity of native valvular regurgitation with two-dimensional and Doppler echocardiography. *J Am Soc Echocardiogr* 2003; 16:777–802.
9. Nagueh SF. Assessment of valvular regurgitation with Doppler echocardiography. *Cardiol Clin* 1998;16:405–419.
10. Grossman G, Stein M, Kochs M, et al. Comparison of the proximal flow convergence method for the assessment of the severity of tricuspid regurgitation. *Eur Heart J* 1998;19:652–659.
11. Tribouiloy CM, Enriquez-Sarano M, Bailey KR, et al. Quantification of tricuspid regurgitation by measuring the width of the vena contracta with Doppler color flow imaging: a clinical study. *J Am Coll Cardiol* 2000;36:472–478.
12. Pearlman AS. Role of echocardiography in the diagnosis and evaluation of severity of mitral and tricuspid stenosis. *Circulation* 1991;84[Suppl 10:I-193–I-197.
13. Silversides CK, Veldtman GR, Crossin J, et al. Pressure half-time predicts hemodynamically significant pulmonary regurgitation in adult patients with repaired tetralogy of Fallot. *J Am Soc Echocardiogr* 2003;16:1057–1062.
14. Lei MH, Chen JJ, Ko YL, et al. Reappraisal of quantitative evaluation of pulmonary regurgitation and estimation of pulmonary artery pressure by continuous wave Doppler echocardiography. *Cardiology* 1995;86:249–256.
15. Ozer N, Tokgozoglu L, Coplu L, et al. Echocardiographic evaluation of left and right ventricular diastolic function in patients with chronic obstructive pulmonary disease. *J Am Soc Echocardiogr* 2001;14:557–561.
16. Scully HE, Armstrong CS. Tricuspid valve replacement: fifteen years of experience with mechanical prostheses and bioprostheses. *J Thorac Cardiovasc Surg* 1995;109:1035–1041.
17. Mcgrath LB, Chen C, Bailey BM, et al. Early and late events following tricuspid valve replacement. *J Card Surg* 1992;7:245–253.
18. Arbulu A, Asfaw I. Tricuspid valvulectomy without prosthetic replacement: ten years of clinical experience. *J Thorac Cardiovasc Surg* 1981;82:684–691.

11

Prosthetic Valve Dysfunction

Michael H. Crawford

- There are two basic types of prosthetic valves: bioprosthetic and mechanical (1).
- Bioprosthetic valves rarely alter the normal cardiovascular physical examination, and disease of bioprosthetic valves presents with the same physical examination findings as are seen with native valves. Thus, significant regurgitation and stenosis can be detected, but the severity of these lesions can be difficult to assess by physical examination alone.
- Mechanical prosthetic valves alter the normal cardiac physical examination. Mechanical prosthetic valve closure sounds are accentu-

ated, and certain types of mechanical prosthetic valves may produce opening sounds, which are not normally heard with native valves.
- Because mechanical valves often have smaller orifices than native valves, flow murmurs are frequent and do not necessarily indicate stenosis. Regurgitant murmurs are almost always pathologic, but valvular leaks cannot be differentiated from perivalvular leaks by physical examination.
- The baseline physical examination can be confusing in patients with prosthetic valves.

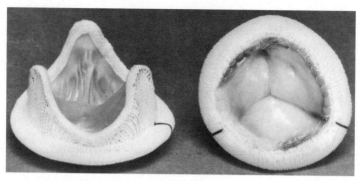

FIG. 11-1. Stented porcine bioprosthetic valve showing the cloth-covered stents and sewing ring surrounding the porcine leaflets. (From Crawford MH. The patient with prosthetic heart valves. In: Roldan CA, Abrams J, eds. *Evaluation of the patient with heart disease: integrating the physical examination and echocardiography*. Philadelphia: Lippincott Williams & Wilkins, 2002:252, with permission.)

The physical examination is most valuable when changes in auscultation of the valve are detected during follow-up. Such changes would suggest valve dysfunction and indicate an echocardiogram (echo) is needed.

■ By the time significant alterations in the cardiac physical examination are detected, often valve dysfunction is marked and the patient is not doing well.

■ The physical examination is therefore of limited value for early detection of prosthetic valve dysfunction. This makes routine echo an attractive option.

CLASSIFICATION OF PROSTHETIC VALVES

Bioprosthetic Valves

■ Stented valves are fashioned from animal valves or pericardial tissue and supported by a synthetic framework (Fig. 11-1).
■ Stentless valves are created from unsupported animal tissue (2,3).
■ Homographs are human valves and are autografts (from the same patient) or allografts (from another human).

Mechanical Valves

■ Bileaflet valves have two semicircular leaflets attached by hinges to the supporting apparatus and sewing ring (Fig. 11-2) (4,5).

■ Single-tilting disk valves are constrained by a series of struts.
■ Ball valves are contained by a cage.

NORMAL HEMODYNAMICS OF PROSTHETIC VALVES

The peak and mean velocity and valve area of normally functioning prosthetic valves vary according to their position, type, and size (Table 11-1).

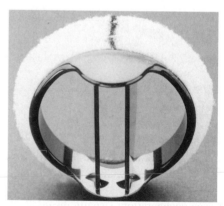

FIG. 11-2. St. Jude bileaflet mechanical prosthetic valve showing the two semicircular leaflets in the open position. Note the three flow channels and the leaflet hinges at the bottom. (From Crawford MH. The patient with prosthetic heart valves. In: Roldan CA, Abrams J, eds. *Evaluation of the patient with heart disease: integrating the physical examination and echocardiography*. Philadelphia: Lippincott Williams & Wilkins, 2002:252, with permission.)

TABLE 11-1. *Normal Hemodynamics of Prosthetic Valves*

Prosthesis/size	Peak velocity (m/sec)	Mean gradient (mm Hg)	Valve area (cm²)
Aortic valve			
Mechanical bileaflet			
21–23 mm	2.6 ± 0.4	10–30	1.3
25 mm	2.5 ± 0.4	5–30	1.8
27 mm	2.4 ± 0.4	5–20	2.4
29 mm	2.4 ± 0.4	5–15	2.7
Stented porcine			
21–23 mm	2.6 ± 0.4	13 ± 6	1.8–2.1 ± 0.2
25 mm	2.5 ± 0.4	11 ± 2	—
27 mm	2.4 ± 0.4	10 ± 1	—
29 mm	2.4 ± 0.4	—	—
Stentless porcine	2.2 ± 0.4	3 (2–20)	1.8–2.3
Homograft	1.8 ± 0.4	7 ± 3	1.7–3.1
Mitral valve[a]			
Mechanical bileaflet	1.6 ± 0.3	5 ± 2	2.9 ± 0.6 (1.8–4.4)
Stented porcine			
Hancock	1.5 ± 0.3	4.3 ± 2.1	1.3–2.7
Carpentier Edwards	1.8 ± 0.2	6.5 ± 2.1	1.6–3.5
Homograft	1.8 ± 0.4	6.4 ± 3	1.9–2.9

[a]Pressure half-time for mechanical and bioprosthetic mitral valves is generally <100 msec and <130 msec, respectively.

PROSTHETIC VALVE DYSFUNCTION

Definition

Prosthetic valve dysfunction is performance less than expected due to surgical complications, valve component failure, valve tissue degeneration, thrombus formation, or pannus ingrowth.

Mechanisms of Prosthetic Valve Dysfunction

- Surgical complications: Partial or complete valve dehiscence resulting in paravalvular leak or valve escape.
- Mechanical failures: Stent fracture, disk or poppet escape, stuck disk (usually in an open position).
- Tissue degeneration: Usually results in regurgitation, but stenosis can occur due to an accelerated immune reaction.
- Valve regurgitation: Usually results from tissue degeneration, endocarditis, thrombus, or pannus ingrowth.
- Valvular stenosis: A less common complication due to tissue degeneration or pannus ingrowth (Fig. 11-3).

- Valve thrombosis: Occurs with mechanical prosthesis, usually with subtherapeutic anticoagulation, and may result in regurgitation or obstruction.
- Pannus ingrowth: Occurs with mechanical and bioprosthetic valves and may result in regurgitation or obstruction.
- Infective endocarditis: Usually results in regurgitation, but large vegetation can obstruct the valve.
- Patient prosthesis mismatch: Prosthetic valve area is too small for the patient's size, which results in relative stenosis.

ECHOCARDIOGRAPHY

Indications for Use in Patients with Prosthetic Heart Valves

Transthoracic echo (TTE) or transesophageal echo (TEE) is performed in patients after valve replacement, according to different clinical scenarios and American College of Cardiology/American Heart Association/American Society of Echocardiography guidelines (Table 11-2).

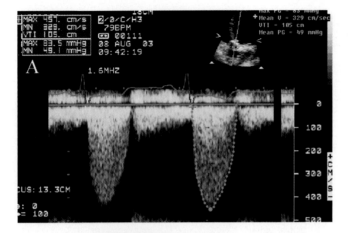

A

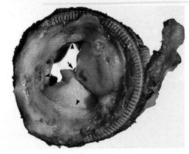

B

FIG. 11-3. Bioprosthetic valve stenosis due to pannus ingrowth. **A:** Continuous wave Doppler demonstrating a peak and mean gradients of 84 mm Hg and 49 mm Hg, respectively. **B:** Note the pannus ingrowth on the ventricular side of the valve (*arrowheads*) and the normal-appearing leaflets (*arrow*). (Courtesy of Carlos A. Roldan, M.D.)

Characterization of Mechanisms of Prosthetic Valve Dysfunction

M-Mode Transthoracic or Transesophageal Echocardiography

Best Imaging Planes

- TTE: Parasternal long-axis for aortic, mitral, and pulmonic valves; parasternal right ventricular inflow view for tricuspid valve.
- TEE: Basal four-chamber view for mitral valve and tricuspid valve, and basal long-axis view for aortic and pulmonic valves.

Key Diagnostic Features

- Abnormal leaflet disk or poppet motion with regard to cardiac cycle; for example, late opening or closing or failure to close or open.
- Thickened prosthetic valve or periprosthetic valve tissue.
- Flail bioprosthetic valve leaflet.

Pitfall

The poor lateral resolution of M-mode echo may superimpose adjacent structures in the image and give the appearance of abnormalities.

Two-Dimensional Transthoracic or Transesophageal Echocardiography

Best Imaging Planes

- TTE: Parasternal long-axis and short-axis, and right ventricular inflow and apical views.
- TEE: Basal four-chamber, long-axis, and short-axis views.

Key Diagnostic Features

- Valve dehiscence: Rocking motion of entire prosthetic valve.
- Bioprosthetic valve: Thickened or flail leaflets (see Fig. 11-6).
- Abnormal tissue masses, thrombi, or vegetations. Pannus is more dense than thrombus or

TABLE 11-2. *Indications for Echocardiography in Patients with Prosthetic Valves and Prosthetic Valve Dysfunction*

Baseline TTE 1–3 mo after valve replacement
New regurgitant murmur (TTE)
Development of new or changing cardiovascular symptoms (TTE)
Lack of improvement or deterioration of functional capacity or cardiovascular symptoms after valve replacement (TTE)
Every 6 mo in asymptomatic patients with bioprosthetic valve degeneration and ± mild regurgitation (TTE)
Patients with suspected valve obstruction caused by thrombus or pannus ingrowth (TEE)
Patients with suspected prosthetic valve endocarditis (TEE)

TEE, transesophageal echocardiography; TTE, transthoracic echocardiography.
Adapted from Cheitlin MD, Armstrong WF, Aurigemma GP, et al. ACC/AHA/ASE 2003 guidelines update for the clinical application of echocardiography: summary article. *J Am Coll Cardiol* 2003;42:954–970, and Bonow RO, Carabello B, De Leon AC, et al. ACC/AHA guidelines for the management of patients with valvular heart disease. *J Am Coll Cardiol* 1998;32:1486–1588.

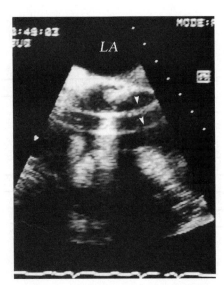

FIG. 11-4. Transesophageal echocardiographic basal short-axis view of a bileaflet mechanical aortic prosthetic valve. Note the side lobes (*arrowheads*) from the leaflets in the open position. LA, left atrium. (From Crawford MH. The patient with prosthetic heart valves. In: Roldan CA, Abrams J, eds. *Evaluation of the patient with heart disease: integrating the physical examination and echocardiography.* Philadelphia: Lippincott Williams & Wilkins, 2002:256, with permission.)

vegetation, which can be detected as hard versus soft echoes (Fig. 11-3) (6,7).

■ Abnormal leaflet, poppet, or disk motion.
■ Analysis of chamber sizes and function.

Pitfalls

■ Poor lateral resolution may exaggerate the thickness of valve-related structures in apical views and create side lobes emanating from the valve (Fig. 11-4).
■ Cannot reliably differentiate histology of masses (i.e., pannus, thrombus, or vegetation).
■ Intense echo reflections from prosthetic valve structures result in reverberations, which obscure details of other valve-adjacent structures. In stented bioprosthetic valves reverberations from the struts obscure the valve leaflets (Fig. 11-5).
■ The material in ball valves is denser than tissue or blood, so ultrasound waves travel through it slowly, resulting in a magnification of the apparent size of the ball, which overwhelms other valve details and adjacent structures.
■ Small filamentous echoes can be observed attached to prosthetic valves (8). Whether these represent the ends of sutures or other structures

is controversial, but they must be distinguished from vegetations, which are usually larger in width. Also, they are not to be confused with the bright, fleeting echoes that sometimes occur with mechanical valve closure. Some believe these are traumatic microcavitations (9,10).

Assessment of Prosthetic Valve Regurgitation and Stenosis

Pulsed and Continuous Wave Doppler

Best Imaging Planes

■ Aortic valve: TTE apical views, suprasternal notch views, and right parasternal views; TEE transgastric apical view.
■ Mitral valve: TTE apical views; TEE basal four-chamber and two-chamber views or transgastric apical view.
■ Tricuspid valve: TTE parasternal right ventricular inflow and short-axis basal views; TEE basal and transgastric apical views.

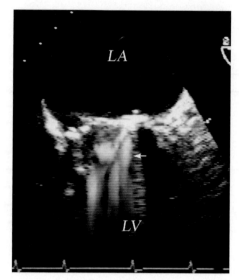

FIG. 11-5. Transesophageal echocardiographic basal four-chamber view of a mitral bileaflet mechanical valve in the closed position. Note the strong reverberations (*arrow*) on the left ventricular side of the valve. LA, left atrium; LV, left ventricle. (From Crawford MH. The patient with prosthetic heart valves. In: Roldan CA, Abrams J, eds. *Evaluation of the patient with heart disease: integrating the physical examination and echocardiography.* Philadelphia: Lippincott Williams & Wilkins, 2002:255, with permission.)

- Pulmonic valve: TTE parasternal right ventricular outflow tract view and subcostal left ventricular short-axis view; TEE basal long-axis view.

Key Diagnostic Features

- Measurement of valve peak flow velocity and estimation of valve gradient and area.
- Aortic stenosis: Increased aortic valve velocity and reduced expected valve area for the size of the prosthesis.
- Aortic regurgitation: Reduced or shorter pressure half-time of regurgitant jet or faster deceleration slope.
- Mitral stenosis: Increased mitral early diastolic flow velocity (E wave), prolonged pressure half-time, and reduced expected valve area for prosthetic size (11).
- Mitral regurgitation detected.
- Tricuspid stenosis: Increased flow velocities across the tricuspid valve.

- Tricuspid regurgitation detected.
- Pulmonic stenosis: Increased velocity and pressure gradient across the pulmonic valve.
- Pulmonic regurgitation detected.

Pitfalls

- Errors in estimating stroke or regurgitant volume and regurgitant fraction are predominantly related to overestimation or underestimation of left or right ventricular outflow tract diameters.
- Bileaflet valves have three flow orifices (Fig. 11-2). The middle channel is the smallest and has the highest flow velocity. If one mainly samples from this channel, the valve gradient may be overestimated. Continuous wave Doppler favors the highest velocity.
- Ball valves result in circumferential flow around the valve, which is difficult to sample accurately by Doppler. Thus, flow velocity may be underestimated, resulting in overestimation of valve area.

Color Doppler

Best Imaging Planes

- Aortic valve: TTE parasternal long-axis and short axis and apical five-chamber views; TEE basal five-chamber, long-axis and short-axis, and transgastric five-chamber and three-chamber views.
- Mitral valve: TTE parasternal long-axis and short-axis and apical views; TEE basal four-chamber and long-axis views and transgastric long-axis views.
- Tricuspid valve: TTE parasternal right ventricular inflow and short-axis views and apical four-chamber view; TEE basal four-chamber view, transgastric short-axis and long-axis views of the right ventricle.
- Pulmonic valve: TTE basal short-axis and subcostal short-axis views; TEE basal long-axis view.

Key Diagnostic Features

Color Doppler allows detection of valvular or perivalvular regurgitation and estimation of severity of valvular regurgitation applying parameters used for native valves (Figs. 11-6 and 11-7).

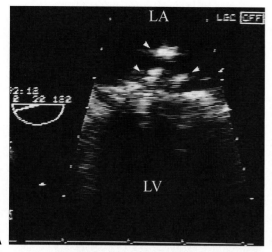 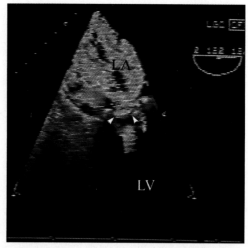

FIG. 11-6. A: Transesophageal echocardiographic basal four-chamber view of a stented mitral bioprosthesis. The lower two arrowheads indicate torn leaflets, and the upper arrowhead points to a vegetation. **B:** Same view with color jet exhibiting severe central mitral regurgitation. Arrowheads show large acceleration zone. LA, left atrium; LV, left ventricle. (From Crawford MH. The patient with prosthetic heart valves. In: Roldan CA, Abrams J, eds. *Evaluation of the patient with heart disease: integrating the physical examination and echocardiography.* Philadelphia: Lippincott Williams & Wilkins, 2002:259, with permission.)

Pitfalls

- Regurgitant jets that hit the cardiac walls may result in underestimation of regurgitation severity. When such jets swirl in a chamber, severity is usually at least moderate.
- Shadowing of regurgitation jets by dense prosthetic material—for example, mitral regurgitation in the apical four-chamber view on TTE—may be obliterated by shadowing from the mitral prosthesis. A proximal flow acceleration zone may provide a clue to the presence of significant regurgitation, however.
- Bileaflet valves normally exhibit trivial regurgitation at the two hinge points. This is normal and may help reduce thrombus formation at the hinges. This normal regurgitation must be distinguished from paravalvular leaks and mirror-image artifacts from the left ventricular outflow tract exhibited behind a mitral prosthesis (12).
- Periprosthetic leaks must be distinguished from fistulous tracts. This is relatively easy when they end in adjacent rather than contiguous chambers (i.e., mitral annulus to right heart).

Diagnostic Accuracy for Detection of Prosthetic Valve Dysfunction

- Prosthetic valve dehiscence is usually readily detectable by TTE.
- Mechanical prosthesis valve structural failure is almost always detectable by TTE because such abnormalities are dramatic.
- Bioprosthetic valve tissue degeneration may be difficult to diagnose on TTE, but it should be readily detected by TEE.
- Prosthetic valve regurgitation is usually detected by TTE, except in cases of multiple valve replacement in which one valve shadows the other (e.g., prosthetic mitral regurgitation in patients with an aortic valve prosthesis as well).
- Distinguishing valvular from perivalvular regurgitation by TTE can be difficult, but it is easily distinguished by TEE.
- Prosthetic valve stenosis is almost always detected by TTE, but TEE may help better define the mechanism of stenosis (e.g., bioprosthetic valve degeneration vs. pannus formation).
- Prosthetic valve thrombosis, pannus, vegetations, and abscesses are better defined by TEE.

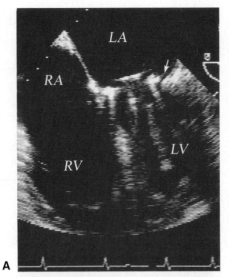

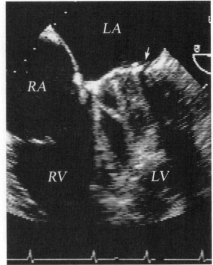

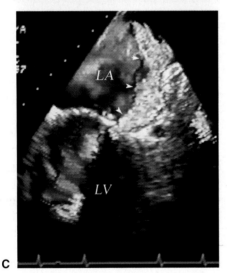

FIG. 11-7. Transesophageal echocardiographic basal four-chamber view of a mitral bileaflet mechanical valve. **A:** Open position. **B:** Closed position. Note reverberations (*white lines*) and shadowing (*dark spaces*) on the left ventricular side and the perivalvular defect or dehiscence (*arrow*). **C:** Color flow jet (*arrowheads*) of the eccentric regurgitation through the dehiscence effect. LA, left atrium; RA, right atrium; RV, right ventricle. (From Crawford MH. The patient with prosthetic heart valves. In: Roldan CA, Abrams J, eds. *Evaluation of the patient with heart disease: integrating the physical examination and echocardiography.* Philadelphia: Lippincott Williams & Wilkins, 2002:257, with permission.)

- Interrogating the motion of both leaflets in a bileaflet aortic mechanical valve is best accomplished by TEE (13).

Severity of Prosthetic Valve Dysfunction

- The criteria for regurgitation severity in native valves apply to prosthetic valves.
- Because normally functioning prosthetic valves are mildly stenotic, the criteria for moderate and severe stenosis in native valves apply to prosthetic valves.

Prognostic Value in Prosthetic Valve Dysfunction

- Valve dehiscence, mechanical failure, severe bioprosthetic valve tissue degeneration, thrombosis, or suspected infectious endocarditis augur for a poor prognosis, and surgery should be considered.
- In selected patients, thrombolytic therapy may dissolve a valve thrombus.
- Some patients with prosthetic valve infectious endocarditis can be cured by antibiotics,

especially if the infection occurs late after surgery (>60 days).

■ Prosthetic valvular stenosis or regurgitation follows the same prognostic factors as native valve disease, except that repeat surgery carries a higher risk than initial surgery.

Indicators for Therapeutic Interventions

■ Valve thrombosis: Thrombolytic therapy in selected cases and surgery in others.
■ Mechanical prosthetic valve failure indicates need for surgery.
■ Severe bioprosthetic valve degeneration indicates need for surgery.
■ Severe regurgitation: Surgery if symptomatic or if left ventricular function deteriorates.
■ Severe stenosis: Surgery if symptomatic or if left ventricular function deteriorates.
■ Perivalvular leak: Surgery if symptomatic or if left ventricular function deteriorates.
■ Valve dehiscence: Surgery usually is indicated.
■ Prosthetic valve infectious endocarditis: surgery usually indicated. Some patients with late infections (>60 days postoperative) and nonvirulent microbes may respond to aggressive antibiotic therapy.

Use in the Pregnant Patient with Normal and Dysfunctional Prosthetic Valves

■ The rate of bioprosthetic valve degeneration in young patients (16–40 years old) is high (approximately 50% at 10 years and 90% at 15 years) and can be manifested as early as 2 to 3 years after implantation.
■ In patients who have been pregnant, the rate of bioprosthetic valve degeneration at 10 years is even higher (55–75%), and the incidence of reoperation is 60% to 80% (14).
■ During pregnancy, the incidence of bioprosthetic valve degeneration is as high as 24%.
■ Thus, in patients with bioprosthetic valves who are or have been pregnant, echo should be performed during the second to third trimester and every 2 to 3 years.
■ Another major issue in pregnant patients with prosthetic valves is anticoagulation management.

TABLE 11-3. *Echocardiography (Echo) Follow-Up in Patients with Prosthetic Valves*

Clinically normally functioning bioprosthetic valves: Transthoracic echo 1–3 mo after surgery. At this point, the heart is healed, anemia is corrected, and serum catecholamine levels are reduced.

For bioprosthetic valves and unless symptoms occur, follow-up echo every 2–3 yr and then at 5 yr. After 5 yr, every 2 yr, and after 10 yr, annual echo should be done.

Clinically normal mechanical prosthetic valves: baseline echo at 1–3 mo. Follow-up echo at 5 yr and 10 yr and then every 2 yr until 15 yr, then yearly. If there are suspected abnormalities, the frequency of follow-up echo should be increased.

If abnormalities of bioprosthetic or mechanical valves are suspected or detected, the frequency of follow-up echo should be increased, depending on the type and severity of the lesion and the expected course.

In patients with bioprosthetic valves who are or have been pregnant, echo should be performed during the second to third trimester of pregnancy and every 2–3 yr thereafter.

ment. Valve thrombosis would be a serious complication in a pregnant patient because thrombolysis is precluded, and surgery would likely result in fetal loss.

◆ Careful management of the patient therefore is indicated, with a baseline echo and follow-up echoes for any lapse in anticoagulant coverage or suspected problems.

■ A new murmur during pregnancy may occur due to increased flow, but if valve dysfunction is suspected, an echo is indicated.
■ During the high-flow state of pregnancy, prosthetic valve/patient mismatch may occur with a relatively small prosthetic valve. Although usually not an indication for surgery, it complicates management of the patient. Echo is useful in this diagnosis during the second and third trimesters when cardiac output is maximal.

Stress Echocardiography in Patients with Suspected or Known Prosthetic Valve Dysfunction

■ There is little experience with stress echo in patients with prosthetic valves.
■ If prosthetic valve/patient mismatch is suspected, stress echo may identify problems by

increasing the cardiac output and detecting increased filling pressures or prosthetic valve pressure gradients.

- In patients with symptoms but no signs of prosthetic valve dysfunction, stress echo may help clarify the problem.

Intraoperative Use in Patients with Prosthetic Valve Dysfunction

- TEE is very useful for defining the precise anatomy of prosthetic valve dysfunction before surgery.
- Whether TEE is useful during surgery depends on the situation. Most dysfunctioning prosthetic valves are replaced, and TEE would be of little use in such cases.
- If valve repair is attempted, TEE may be useful to assure normal valve function immediately after repair before the chest is closed.

Follow-Up in Patients with Normal and Dysfunctional Prosthetic Valves

Echo has important diagnostic value in the follow-up of normal functioning or dysfunctional mechanical and bioprosthetic valves (Table 11-3).

REFERENCES

1. Wernly JA, Crawford MH. Choosing a prosthetic heart valve. *Cardiol Clin* 1998;16:491–504.
2. Williams RJ, McLean AD, Pathi J, et al. Six-year follow-up of the Toronto stentless porcine valve. *Semin Thorac Cardiovasc Surg* 2001;13:168–172.
3. Morocutti G, Gelsomino S, Spedicato L, et al. Intraoperative transesophageal echo-Doppler evaluation of stentless aortic xenografts. Incidence and significance of moderate gradients. *Cardiovasc Surg* 2002;10: 328–332.
4. Moidl R, Simon P, Wolner E, et al. The On-X prosthetic heart valve at five years. *Ann Thorac Surg* 2002;74:S1312–1317.
5. Niinami H, Aomi S, Tomioka H, et al. A comparison of the in vivo performance of the 19-mm St. Jude medical hemodynamic plus and 21-mm standard valve. *Ann Thorac Surg* 2002;74:1120–1124.
6. Barbetseas J, Nagueh SF, Pitsavos C, et al. Differentiating thrombus from pannus formation in obstructed mechanical prosthetic valves: an evaluation of clinical, transthoracic and transesophageal echocardiographic parameters. *J Am Coll Cardiol* 1998;32:1410–1417.
7. Aoyagi S, Nishimi M, Tayama E, et al. Obstruction of St. Jude medical valves in the aortic position: a consideration for pathogenic mechanism of prosthetic valve obstruction. *Cardiovasc Surg* 2002;10: 339–344.
8. Ionescu AA, Moreno de la Santa P, Dunstan FD, et al. Mobile echoes on prosthetic valves are not reproducible. Results and clinical implications of a multicentre study. *Eur Heart J* 1999;20:140–147.
9. Girod G, Jaussi A, Rosset C, et al. Cavitation versus degassing: *in vitro* study of the microbubble phenomenon observed during echocardiography in patients with mechanical prosthetic cardiac valves. *Echocardiography* 2002;19:531–536.
10. Kaymaz C, Ozkan M, Ozdemir N, et al. Spontaneous echocardiographic microbubbles associated with prosthetic mitral valves: mechanistic insights from thrombolytic treatment results. *J Am Soc Echocardiogr* 2002;15:323–327.
11. Fernandes V, Olmos L, Nagueh SF, et al. Peak early diastolic velocity rather than pressure half time is the best index of mechanical prosthetic mitral valve function. *Am J Cardiol* 2002;89:704–710.
12. Linka AZ, Barton M, Jost CA, et al. Doppler mirror image artifacts mimicking mitral regurgitation in patients with mechanical bileaflet mitral valve prostheses. *Eur J Echocardiogr* 2000;1:138–143.
13. Shapira Y, Vaturi M, Perlmuter M, et al. Feasibility of two-dimensional bileaflet valve imaging: a prospective transthoracic echocardiographic study. *J Heart Valve Dis* 2002;11:576–582.
14. Hung L, Rahimtoola S. Prosthetic heart valves and pregnancy. *Circulation* 2003;107:1240–1246.

12

Common Adult Congenital Heart Diseases

Carlos A. Roldan

- Common adult congenital heart diseases (CHDs) include atrial septal defect (ASD), ventricular septal defect (VSD), patent ductus arteriosus (PDA), and coarctation of the aorta (1).
- The history and physical examination are valuable in the detection of CHD but are limited in defining the type, location, severity, and therapy of a defect.

INDICATIONS FOR ECHOCARDIOGRAPHY

- Transthoracic echocardiography (TTE), transesophageal echocardiography (TEE), and intracardiac echocardiography (ICE) are essential in the diagnosis, characterization, severity assessment, and management of CHD (Table 12-1) (2,3).
- The diagnostic accuracy of echocardiography (echo) has decreased the need for cardiac catheterization procedures, and in some centers, patients with ASD, VSD, PDA, or coarctation of the aorta undergo surgical or transcatheter closure of defects with the diagnosis and guidance of echo (4,5).

ATRIAL SEPTAL DEFECT

Definition and Classification

- An ASD is a >5 mm discontinuity of the interatrial septum and is classified into secundum ASD, primum ASD, sinoseptal ASD, and patent foramen ovale (PFO). A PFO is usually <5 mm in diameter.
- Secundum ASD, the most common defect (70% of all defects), is caused by a deficient septum primum that fails to cover the ostium secundum; is located centrally in the fossa ovalis area; and is usually single.
- Primum ASD, which accounts for approximately 20% of defects, is caused by failure of the endocardial cushions to meet the atrial septum; is always associated with a cleft anterior mitral leaflet; and is located posteroinferior to the aortic root (1).
- Sinoseptal defects include the sinus venosus defect and the unroofed coronary sinus.
  - ◆ The superior vena cava (SVC) sinus venosus ASD, the most common (5–10% of all defects) sinoseptal defect, occurs at the most

TABLE 12-1. *Class I Indications for Echocardiography in the Adult with Suspected Congenital Heart Disease (CHD)*

Atypical or pathologic murmur or other abnormal cardiac finding

Cardiomegaly on chest radiography

Patients with a known CHD to assess timing of medical or surgical therapy or to monitor pulmonary artery pressure

Selection, placement, patency, and monitoring of endovascular devices, as well as identification of intracardiac or intravascular shunting before, during, and after interventional cardiac catheterization

Immediate assessment after percutaneous interventional cardiac catheterization procedure

Immediate preoperative evaluation for cardiac surgery of a patient with known CHD to guide surgical management and to inform the patient and family of the risks of surgery

Patient with known CHD and change in physical findings

Postoperative CHD with suspected residual or recurrent abnormality, poor ventricular function, pulmonary artery hypertension, thrombus, sepsis, or pericardial effusion, or obstruction of conduits and baffles

Presence of a syndrome associated with CHD and dominant inheritance or multiple affected family members (e.g., Marfan or Ehlers–Danlos syndrome)

Exercise-induced precordial chest pain or syncope

Identification of site of origin and initial course of coronary arteries (TEE may be needed)

Follow-up echocardiography after surgical treatment of CHD if there is a change in clinical status or reassessment of ventricular function and pulmonary artery pressure

TEE, transesophageal echocardiography.
Modified from Cheitlin MD, Armstrong WF, Aurigemma GP, et al. ACC/AHA/ASE 2003 guideline update for the clinical application of echocardiography: summary article. *J Am Coll Cardiol* 2003;42:954–970.

superior portion of the atrial septum at the junction of the SVC with the right atrium (RA), and it is almost always associated with anomalous drainage of the right upper and, commonly, the lower pulmonary veins into the SVC or RA.
  - ◆ Inferior vena cava (IVC) sinus venosus defects are rare, are associated with anomalous drainage of the right lower pulmonary vein, and are found inferior to the fossa ovalis at the IVC/RA junction.
    - ◆ An unroofed coronary sinus is a rare defect of the coronary sinus in the left atrium (LA), allowing flow from the LA to the RA and often associated with a persistent left SVC (Raghib anomaly).

■ A PFO is present in up to 20% of the general population, is generally small (<5 mm), and of no hemodynamic significance.

Prevalence

ASD accounts for approximately 10% of children's CHD and approximately 40% of adults CHD, with a female to male ratio of 2:1 (1,2).

Echocardiography

Morphology of Atrial Septal Defects on M-Mode and Two-Dimensional Transthoracic, Transesophageal, or Intracardiac Echocardiography

Best Imaging Planes

■ TTE parasternal short-axis view at the aortic level and apical and subcostal four-chamber views to identify secundum and primum ASD (from the apical view, the atrioventricular valves are at the same level and perpendicular to the imaging plane).

■ TTE right parasternal long-axis and short-axis and subcostal views to identify sinus venosus ASD. From the right parasternal long-axis view, the SVC and IVC are aligned, and then a rightward sweep may identify a defect at the entry of the SVC or IVC.

■ TEE mid-esophageal four-chamber view allows optimal visualization of the entire interatrial septum, the atrioventricular valves, and the subvalvular apparatus. From this view, a careful multiplane interrogation of the entire septum allows for identification of all types of ASD.

■ TEE four-chamber view with clockwise rotation to focus on the RA and with the multiplane sector scan at 30 to 60 degrees to assess the atrial septum, IVC (on the left), and SVC (on the right) to identify sinus venosus defects.

■ ICE longitudinal view to assess atrial septum from cranial to distal margins, and the perpendicular short-axis view to assess the anterior septum and its transition to the ascending aorta. ICE is best suited for detection of secundum ASD and PFO (6).

Key Diagnostic Features

■ TTE or TEE M-mode is limited in the diagnosis of ASD but provides information on right ventricular volume or pressure overload, or both; hypertrophy; and dilatation.

◆ In volume overload, the septum is displaced posteriorly or toward the left ventricle (LV) during diastole. In pressure overload, the septum is displaced posteriorly during late systole and early diastole.

■ By TTE, TEE, or ICE two-dimensional (2D) echo, an ASD appears as an area of focal dropout or discontinuity in the interatrial septum with some broadening of the edges of the defect (Figs. 12-1, 12-2, 12-3, and 12-4) (2–6).

■ Atrial septal tissue above the base of the atrioventricular valves suggests a secundum ASD (Fig. 12-1).

■ Absence of septal tissue in the most anterior portion of the interatrial septum (at the level of the atrioventricular valves) is diagnostic of an ostium primum defect (Fig. 12-3).

■ In ostium primum, ASD is always associated with a cleft anterior mitral leaflet, which should be identified and assessed for severity. Also in these patients, chordal attachments of the anterior leaflet to the interventricular septum can be seen, causing left ventricular outflow obstruction.

■ TEE or ICE 2D determines location and diameter of an ASD and the relation of the ASD to adjacent heart valves and veins, and defines tissue availability for appropriate transcatheter closure device position and deployment (3,4,6).

■ TEE 2D and ICE are more accurate than TTE in the detection of sinus venosus ASD and associated anomalous pulmonary venous return (100% with sinus venosus ASD and 9% with secundum ASD) (Fig. 12-4). In these patients, right ventricular dilatation out of proportion to the size of the ASD suggests the presence of anomalous pulmonary venous return.

■ TEE and ICE are more accurate than TTE in defining the size of an ASD as PFO (<5 mm), small defect (5–10 mm in diameter), or large ASD (2–3 cm) (Figs. 12-1 through 12-4 and Fig. 14-6).

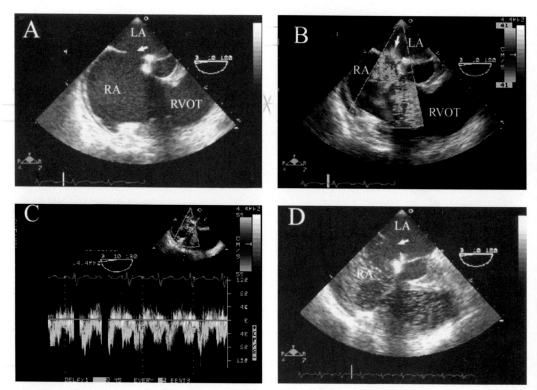

FIG. 12-1. Secundum atrial septal defect in a 31-year-old woman. **A:** Two-dimensional mid-esophageal transesophageal echocardiographic view longitudinal to the right ventricular outflow tract (RVOT) demonstrates a large (1.5 cm in diameter) secundum atrial septal defect (*arrow*). **B:** Color Doppler at the atrial septal defect demonstrates significant left to right atrial shunting (*arrow*). **C:** Pulse wave Doppler at the atrial septal defect demonstrates left to right atrial flow predominantly during late diastole and early systole. **D:** Saline contrast study demonstrates a marked negative contrast effect in the right atrium (RA) due to left to right shunting blood jet (*arrow*). LA, left atrium.

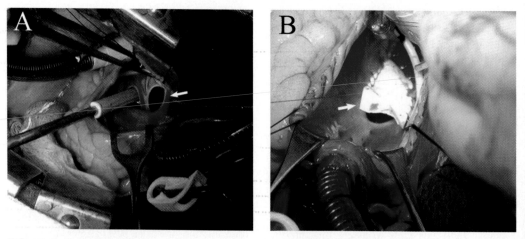

FIG. 12-2. Surgical confirmation and correction of a secundum atrial septal defect. These surgical views from a right atriotomy in the patient described in Figure 12-1 demonstrate **(A)** a large atrial septal defect (*arrow*) and **(B)** a partially patched atrial septal defect (*arrow*).

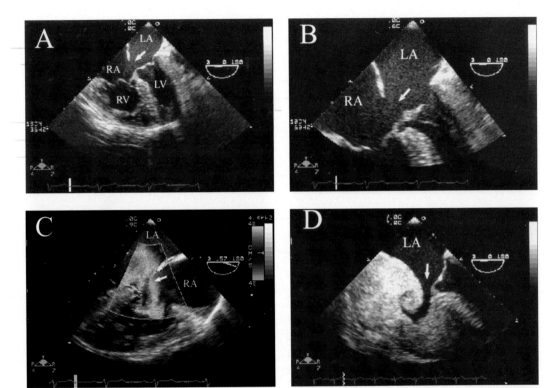

FIG. 12-3. Ostium primum atrial septal defect in a 35-year-old man. **A,B:** Two-dimensional midesophageal transesophageal echocardiographic views demonstrate a large ostium primum atrial septal defect (*arrows*). Note the absence of ostium primum above the atrioventricular valves. **C:** Color Doppler at the atrial septal defect demonstrates significant left to right shunting (*arrow*). Mild to moderate mitral regurgitation and cleft anterior mitral leaflet also were demonstrated. **D:** Saline contrast study demonstrates a marked swirling negative contrast effect in the distal right atrium (RA) (*arrow*). LA, left atrium; LV, left ventricle; RV, right ventricle.

■ TEE or ICE 2D images guide transcatheter closure device positioning and deployment. After closure of the ASD, the presence and degree of residual defect and the need for device reposition or redeployment can be detected (3,4,6–8).

■ TEE and ICE are highly accurate in the detection of atrial thrombi (incidence of 1.2% in ASD and 2.5% in PFO; 70% detected within 4 weeks of device deployment) after transcatheter closure of ASD or PFO (8).

■ ICE is the technique of choice for guidance of transcatheter closure of secundum ASD and PFO. The technique is safe (<1% complication rate) and has contributed to a 98% success rate of transcatheter closures. The technique prevents or minimizes patients' exposure to radiation and precludes them from the discomfort and need for sedation, as with TEE (6,7).

■ Periprocedural TEE or ICE can detect complications of surgical closure of an ASD (i.e., closure of the os of the coronary sinus or part of the IVC instead of the septal defect).

■ Finally, TTE three-dimensional echo measurement of secundum ASD diameter and rims has demonstrated good correlation with measurements obtained using a balloon (r = 0.78) (9).

Saline Contrast Echocardiography: Key Diagnostic Features

■ Shunting in ASD is predominantly left to right, but most defects have right to left or bidirectional shunting. Thus, saline contrast echo is sensitive in detecting ASD or PFO.

■ Bubbles enter the LA during early systole, inspiration, Valsalva maneuver, or coughing (right atrial pressure is transiently higher than left atrial

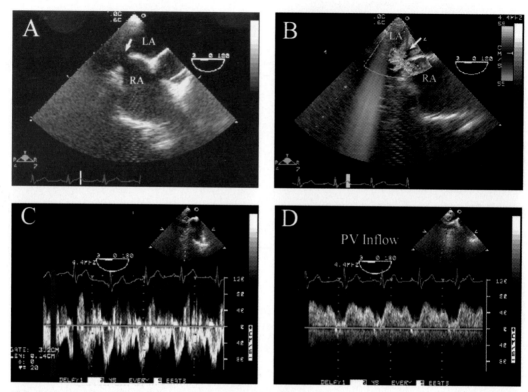

FIG. 12-4. Sinus venosus atrial septal defect in a 29-year-old man. **A:** Two-dimensional transesophageal echocardiographic mid-esophageal view demonstrates a large proximal atrial septal defect (*arrow*) near the junction with the superior vena cava. **B:** Color Doppler demonstrates significant left to right atrial shunting (*arrow*). **C:** Pulsed wave Doppler with the sample volume in the right atrium (RA) demonstrates continuous flow predominantly after atrial contraction. **D:** Pulsed wave Doppler demonstrates anomalous connection of the right upper pulmonary vein (PV) and RA. LA, left atrium.

pressure), and within three cardiac cycles of their appearance in the RA (≥four cardiac cycles suggests a pulmonary arteriovenous fistula).

- The predominant left to right shunting is seen as a negative contrast effect or washout of bubbles in the right atrial side of the septum by the shunting blood jet (Figs. 12-1D and 12-3D).

Assessment of the Severity of Atrial Septal Defects with Doppler Echocardiography

Pulsed Wave Doppler: Diagnostic Methods and Key Diagnostic Features

- Pulsed wave Doppler and 2D echo are used to estimate the ratio of right heart or pulmonary (Qp) to left heart or systemic (Qs) stroke volume as follows:

$$Qp = CSA_{PA} \times VTI_{PA}$$

$$Qs = CSA_{LVOT} \times VTI_{LVOT}$$

$$Qp/Qs = CSA_{PA} \times VTI_{PA}/CSA_{LVOT} \times VTI_{LVOT}$$

where CSA_{PA} and CSA_{LVOT} = cross-sectional area of pulmonary artery (PA) and left ventricular outflow tract (LVOT) as = $\pi(d/2)^2$ and VTI = velocity time integral at the PA and LVOT.

- Pulsed wave Doppler interrogation of the interatrial septum from TTE subcostal four-chamber or TEE mid-esophageal longitudinal view to the right ventricular outflow tract (RVOT) helps to identify an ASD and differentiate it from an artifactual echo dropout.

- Continuous but phasic flow predominantly after atrial and ventricular systole and during expiration or apnea (when right atrial pressure is lowest) is demonstrated (Figs. 12-1C and 12-3C).

■ Sinus venosus ASDs are associated with anomalous pulmonary venous return, especially of the right lower pulmonary vein. Therefore, pulsed wave Doppler can detect the flow of a pulmonary vein entering the RA (Fig. 12-3D).

Color Doppler:
Key Diagnostic Features

■ Bidirectional with predominant left atrial to right atrial shunt is demonstrated (Figs. 12-1B, 12-3C, and 12-4B).
■ With a Nyquist limit at 30 to 40 cm/sec, connection of the pulmonary veins into the LA, SVC, or IVC can be defined from the suprasternal notch view (the "crab view").
■ The width of the color Doppler jet through the ASD correlates well with the anatomic or surgical defect. Color Doppler helps exclude other associated lesions.
■ Color Doppler also increases the detection of small ASD and helps to separate ASD from PFO. From the mid-esophageal four-chamber view and with a low Nyquist limit (30 cm/ sec), minimal flow from RA to LA is consistent with a PFO.

Pitfalls

■ TTE 2D images from the apical four-chamber view are parallel to the septum and may lead to a false dropout in the area of the thin fossa ovalis, suggestive of an ostium secundum ASD.
■ With TTE, visualization of the pulmonary veins can be very difficult due to the distance of the veins from the transthoracic window.
■ Visualization of the more anterior cardiac structures is limited with TEE. Multiplane TEE allows optimization of the image plane between the horizontal and vertical planes.
■ During a saline contrast study, inadequate opacification of the RA may miss small ASDs. Also, a negative contrast effect has low specificity.
■ Doppler Qp/Qs estimate assumes laminar flow through a rigid tube, similar PA and aor-

tic compliance, and adequate measurement of the outflow tract.

VENTRICULAR SEPTAL DEFECT

Definition

■ VSD is a communication between the ventricles of variable size located at the inlet or atrioventricular septum, the muscular or sinus septum, or conoventricular septum (Fig. 12-5).
■ The inlet defects, located beneath the septal tricuspid leaflet, are associated with atrioventricular valve abnormalities, ranging from a cleft anterior mitral leaflet to a common annulus for both atrioventricular valves. These defects account for 8% to 10% of VSDs.
■ Muscular defects are located in the mid- or apical portions of the septum, are often multiple, are most likely to close spontaneously early in life, and account for 5% to 20% of cases.
■ Conoventricular defects account for 75% of VSDs and are divided into paramembranous, subpulmonic, and misaligned (Fig. 12-5).
  ◆ Defects adjacent to the tricuspid valve are termed *paramembranous* and those adjacent to the pulmonary valve are termed *subpulmonic*.
  ◆ Anterior misalignment of the conal septum narrows the right ventricular outflow, resulting in tetralogy of Fallot. Posterior misalignment narrows the LVOT, causing subaortic stenosis or coarctation or interruption of the aortic arch.
■ In subpulmonic and, less commonly, in paramembranous defects, the muscular support below the aortic valve may be deficient, allowing the right coronary cusp to prolapse and occasionally herniate and obliterate the VSD. The associated aortic regurgitation (AR) may be severe or progressive and outweigh the consequences of the VSD itself.

Prevalence

VSD is the most common congenital anomaly in children (30% of all isolated defects), but it is the anomaly most often recognized early and treated. Also, VSDs frequently close spontaneously [overall closure rate of 30–55%, 5–30%

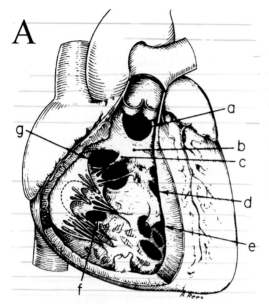

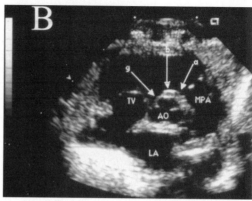

FIG. 12-5. Anatomic and echocardiographic location of ventricular septal defects. **A:** Location of ventricular septal defects viewed from the right ventricle: (*a*) subpulmonic, (*b*) crista supraventricularis, (*c*) papillary muscle of the conus, (*d*) anterior muscular defect, (*e*) apical muscular defect, (*f*) inlet defect, and (*g*) paramembranous defect. **B:** Transthoracic parasternal short-axis view at the aortic valve level and corresponding anatomic areas of septal defects: (*a*) subpulmonic area, (*b*) crista supraventricularis, and (*g*) paramembranous defect. AO, aorta; LA, left atrium; MPA, main pulmonary artery; TV, tricuspid valve.

for paramembranous defects, and 55–65% for muscular defects (10)]. Thus, isolated VSDs account for up to 10% of adult CHD.

Echocardiography

Morphology of Ventricular Septal Defects on M-Mode and Two-Dimensional Transthoracic or Transesophageal Echocardiography

Best Imaging Planes

■ TTE parasternal long-axis view of the septum to assess the infundibular and muscular portions. By sweeping this plane anteriorly and to the left, the conal septum and RVOT can be seen. By sweeping the plane posteriorly and to the right, the paramembranous and inlet septum are imaged.

■ TTE parasternal short-axis view images portions of the conoventricular, muscular, and atrioventricular septum. By directing the ultra-

sound beam toward the base of the heart, the membranous septum defect is seen beneath the tricuspid septal leaflet and to the right of the aortic right coronary cusp (10 o'clock position). The conal septum is seen left of the aortic left coronary cusp and adjacent to the pulmonic valve (2 o'clock position) (Figs. 12-5, 12-6, 12-7, and 12-8).

■ TTE parasternal short-axis view through the two atrioventricular valves allows visualization of the inlet defects (located posteriorly between the atrioventricular valves), as well as mid-muscular and anterior muscular defects (located leftward).

■ TTE parasternal short-axis view at the level of the papillary muscles detects posterior, mid-muscular, and anterior muscular defects. Inferior to this view, apical muscular defects may be identified.

■ TTE apical four-chamber view provides a posterior projection through the atrioventricular valves and muscular septum. Inlet defects are seen in the superior one-third, mid-muscular

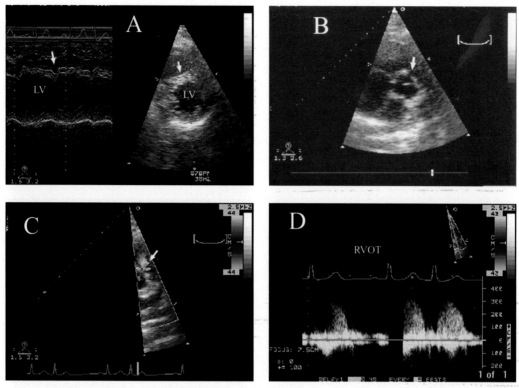

FIG. 12-6. Subpulmonic ventricular septal defect in a 42-year-old man by transthoracic echocardiography (TTE). **A:** TTE parasternal short-axis view of the left ventricle (LV) demonstrates on M-mode a posterior septal displacement during late systole and early diastole (*arrow*) and corresponding diastolic septal flattening on two-dimensional images consistent with right ventricular volume and pressure overload. **B:** Two-dimensional basal short-axis view demonstrates a septal discontinuity left of the left aortic coronary cusp and just above the pulmonic valve suggestive of a subpulmonic ventricular septal defect (*arrow*). **C:** Color Doppler demonstrates high systolic flow from the left ventricular outflow to the right ventricular outflow tract (RVOT) (*arrow*). Note the acceleration zone in the lateral left ventricular outflow tract. **D:** Continuous wave high systolic flow velocity at the subpulmonic ventricular septal defect.

defects are seen in the middle one-half, and apical defects are distal to the moderator band.

■ TTE subcostal four-chamber view allows evaluation of the entire ventricular septum as the ultrasound plane is swept from a posterior to anterior position. The short-axis view can identify anterior muscular VSD and misalignment of the conal septum.

■ In a TEE mid-esophageal four-chamber view with a gradual sweep of the septum, neutral or slight transducer retroflexion allows assessment of the posterior septum. With anteflexion, the anterior septum is visualized.

Slow withdrawing of the transducer with anteflexion provides an *en face* view of the aortic valve and the conoventricular septum (Figs. 12-6 and 12-7).

■ TEE longitudinal view of the RVOT is helpful in identifying misalignment of the conal septum, residual VSD, or postoperative RVOT obstruction.

Key Diagnostic Features

■ M-mode echo is useful for assessment of ventricular dilatation and volume or pressure overload, as well as atrial dilatation (Fig. 12-6A).

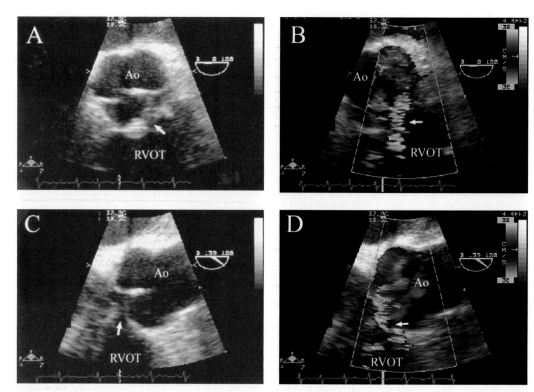

FIG. 12-7. Subpulmonic ventricular septal defect by transesophageal echocardiography (TEE). **A,C:** TEE basal short-axis and long-axis close views at the aortic valve level in the patient in Figure 12-6 demonstrate a subpulmonic ventricular septal defect (*arrows*). **B,D:** Corresponding color Doppler confirmed the subpulmonic communication between the left ventricular and right ventricular outflow tracts (RVOT) (*arrows*). Because of the patient's dyspnea on exertion, moderate pulmonary hypertension, and right heart enlargement, he underwent surgical closure of the defect. Ao, aorta.

- From multiple 2D planes, a VSD is characterized by an area of tissue discontinuity of variable size (Figs. 12-6B, 12-7A, and 12-7C). Muscular defects can have a serpiginous course.
- A VSD is small if it measures <1 cm, moderate if it measures 1 to 2 cm or is less than one-half of the aortic valve area, and large if it is >2 cm or greater than or equal to the aortic valve area.
- In adults, detection of isolated VSD by 2D images ranges from 74% to 88% in prospective studies and 88% to 100% in patients known to have a VSD.
- Aortic valve prolapse is seen in 12% of cases and, more commonly, in patients with subpulmonic and paramembranous VSD (21% and 17%, respectively) (10).

- Features of underlying AR include aortic cusp override of the septum from the apical five-chamber and subcostal coronal views (highly sensitive but low specificity) and aortic cusp prolapse (present in >70% of patients with AR) (11).
- Detect aneurysmal transformation of VSD (55–60% of cases) and subaortic ridge (6%).
- TTE or TEE 2D images can assist in the surgical or transcatheter closure of VSD (12,13).

Saline Contrast Echocardiography: Key Diagnostic Features

- In VSD, the high pressure gradient between ventricles and unidirectional flow from the LV to the right ventricle does not allow saline contrast into the LV. A less specific negative-

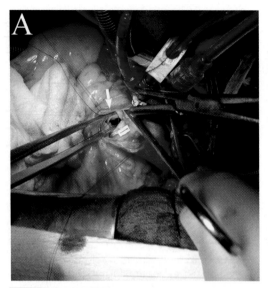 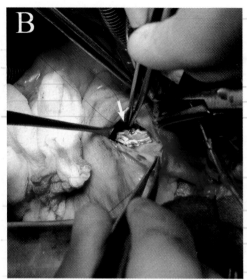

FIG. 12-8. Surgical confirmation **(A)** and closure **(B)** of the subpulmonic ventricular septal defect of the patient described in Figures 12-6 and 12-7.

contrast effect in the right ventricle is usually seen. Thus, saline contrast echo is of limited value in the detection of VSD.

■ Cavity-enhancing contrast agents may help to define endocardial borders of a VSD, orient to the site of Doppler sampling, and improve signal intensities (14).

Doppler Echocardiography for the Assessment of the Location and Severity of Ventricular Septal Defects

Pulsed and Continuous Wave Doppler: Key Diagnostic Features

■ Documentation of highly turbulent and wraparound systolic pulsed wave Doppler velocities through or at the right ventricular side of a suspected VSD by 2D images is highly diagnostic of a VSD, with a sensitivity of 90% and specificity of 98% (Fig. 12-6B,D).

■ Pulsed Doppler is used to estimate the Qp/Qs ratio; however, right ventricular or LVOT turbulent velocities caused by the VSD may not be suitable for analysis (Figs. 12-6C,D and 12-7B,D). Mitral and tricuspid inflows are alternative sites, but the atrioventricular annulus is elliptical in shape, and the simplified

Bernoulli equation (πr^2) may not reflect true valve areas.

■ Patients with VSD may have impaired left ventricular relaxation manifested in the mitral inflow as a decreased early diastolic transmitral velocity (E wave)/atrial filling transmitral velocity (A wave) ratio, increased deceleration time, and increased isovolumic relaxation time.

■ Guided by 2D or pulsed wave Doppler, or both, continuous wave Doppler velocities at the site of a VSD reflect the left ventricular to right ventricular pressure difference, and the spectral signal mimics MR.

■ Because an LV greater than right ventricular diastolic gradient is present, a low-velocity spectral Doppler mimicking that of mitral stenosis can be obtained. This flow ceases if right ventricular diastolic pressure is elevated.

■ In a large VSD with systemic right ventricular pressure, systolic velocities may be <2.5 m/ sec. Also, right ventricular systolic pressure can be estimated as equal to systolic blood pressure minus $4(V$ of VSD jet$)^2$.

Color Doppler: Key Diagnostic Features

■ Color Doppler detects small VSDs frequently missed by other imaging modalities, defines the location and size of a VSD, and can detect additional shunts (Figs. 12-6C and 12-7B,D).

■ Detects and stratifies AR associated with sub-pulmonic and paramembranous VSD. Color flow across the ventricular septum in the parasternal long-axis view is predictive of AR (11).

■ Moderate to severe tricuspid regurgitation associated with a paramembranous VSD is due to dysplasia of the leaflets, clefts of the tricuspid leaflets, or forward displacement of the anterior leaflet by a moderate-sized, restrictive VSD with low right ventricular pressure (15).

■ Identifies residual defects in patients postsurgical or percutaneous closure of a VSD.

Pitfalls

■ False dropout of the septum may lead to mis-diagnosis of a VSD.

■ As with ASD, many assumptions are made when using the Qp/Qs shunt ratio.

■ A VSD turbulent flow may preclude accurate assessment of right ventricular or LVOT velocities.

■ The size of a VSD can be underestimated when the aortic valve prolapses into the VSD.

PATENT DUCTUS ARTERIOSUS

Definition and Classification

PDA, a vascular structure connecting the aorta and PA, is necessary in the fetal circulation to allow right ventricular output to be diverted away from the unexpanded lungs into the descending aorta. The PDA constricts physiologically in response to oxygen and withdrawal of placental prostaglandins in the first hours and days of life.

Prevalence

PDA constitutes 5% to 10% of CHD at birth and is more common in premature infants, children born at high altitude, and females, with a 2:1

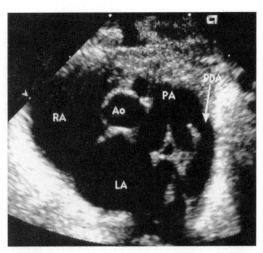

FIG. 12-9. Patent ductus arteriosus (PDA). Transthoracic high parasternal short-axis view of the right pulmonary artery, left pulmonary artery, and a PDA ("three-legged pant" view). The aortic arch is out of the plane, and the left atrium (LA) is dilated. Ao, aorta; PA, pulmonary artery; RA, right atrium. (Courtesy of M. Beth Goens, M.D.)

female to male ratio. Most PDA that escape detection in childhood are small, but its true prevalence in adults is uncertain.

Echocardiography

Morphology of Patent Ductus Arteriosus on M-Mode and Two-Dimensional Transthoracic or Transesophageal Echocardiography

Best Imaging Planes

■ TTE high left parasternal view with the sector scan rotated clockwise or superior and left-ward angulation (to avoid the lungs) to obtain the "three-legged pant" view of the right and left PA and PDA inserting into the proximal left PA (Fig. 12-9).

■ TTE suprasternal notch long-axis view with angulation toward the left PA to define the ductal insertion into the descending aorta and aortic isthmus and to define the aortic arch arterial branches. A short-axis sweep from this position shows the innominate artery branching into the subclavian and right carotid arteries.

- TEE imaging is limited by the left bronchus lying between the esophagus and the PDA.

Key Diagnostic Features

- In most cases, M-mode is normal. With a large PDA, nonspecific findings of chamber enlargement and hypertrophy and patterns of volume or pressure overload can be detected.
- By 2D imaging, the length, width, and constriction of the ductus at the PA (most common) or aortic end should be noted when planning for percutaneous coil closure of the PDA.
- Assessment of the aortic arch anatomy and branching is important. The innominate artery should direct to the right and divide into the subclavian and right carotid arteries. If directed to the left, a right or double aortic arch may be present, with a right PDA entering the right PA. Bilateral ductus are rare.
- TTE 2D echo measurements of PDA minimal diameter, diameter at the aortic ostium, and classification of PDA correlate highly with angiography (r = 0.88, r = 0.72, and r = 0.86, respectively) (16).
- 2D echo can be used to monitor PDA patency with prostaglandin therapy.
- In adults, a PDA may show atheromatous disease, sclerosis, and calcification. Also, 2D echo can detect an aneurysmal PDA or a rarely associated dissection or rupture.
- Finally, 2D echo can detect infective endocarditis (incidence of 0.45%/year), aneurysm of the ductus, and thrombus or dissection of a large ductal aneurysm. A small ductal diverticulum at the aortic end is not abnormal after spontaneous constriction of the ductus.
- TTE has been used to guide the transcatheter closure of a PDA. Complete closure is demonstrated in 65%, minimal residual shunt with a PDA diameter <1 mm, and no flow is detected in 19%, and a residual PDA >1 mm with continuous flow is detected in 15%. At 12 months, no shunt is demonstrated in 90% and in 88% of those with initial residual shunts (17).
- Periprocedural TTE echo during transcatheter closure with coils of PDA <3 mm versus >3

mm have demonstrated closure rates of 72% to 100% versus 35% to 96%, respectively (*p* = 0.01). Therefore, PDA >3 mm in size may require surgical closure (17,18).

- Periprocedural echo has also been used to assess the initial or immediate results of video-assisted thoracoscopic surgical closure of PDA.

Assessment of the Severity of Patent Ductus Arteriosus with Doppler Echocardiography

Pulsed and Continuous Wave Doppler: Key Diagnostic Features

- Diastolic flow along the anterior and lateral wall of the PA has a sensitivity of 96% and a specificity of 100% for the diagnosis of PDA.
- From the suprasternal notch view, holodiastolic flow reversal (as in AR) can be seen.
- Multiplane TEE has high diagnostic accuracy in the assessment of the Qp/Qs ratio, as compared with cardiac catheterization (r = 0.87) (18).

Color Doppler: Key Diagnostic Features

- From the suprasternal notch or right parasternal views, retrograde diastolic flow hugging the anterior and lateral wall of the main PA (red color or toward the transducer) contrast with the normal antegrade PA systolic PA flow (blue color or away from the transducer).
- The proximal isovelocity surface area is of complementary diagnostic value in the calculation of the effective shunt orifice area and volume of a PDA (19).
- Right to left flow in a PDA is unusual and is seen when the pulmonary vascular resistance exceeds the systemic vascular resistance or when there is critical coarctation of the aorta.

Pitfalls

- Estimation of Qp/Qs from the mitral and tricuspid annuli is probably imprecise because these annuli are not circular and may lead to errors in area calculations.
- On TTE images, the lung obscures visualization of a PDA. Also, the left bronchus lies

between the ductus and the esophagus and produces an air artifact.

- Pulsed and continuous wave Doppler are limited in the diagnosis and assessment of the severity of a PDA because difficulties in 2D imaging and frequently long, tortuous, or small defects preclude assessment of flow characteristics.
- Normal color Doppler flow of the PA and descending aorta can give the false impression of right to left flow in the ductus.
- The size of the color Doppler is more dependent on the relative resistance in the systemic and pulmonary vascular beds than the size of the PDA.

COARCTATION OF THE AORTA

Definition

- Coarctation of the aorta is characterized by narrowing in the descending thoracic aorta by a shelf of media protruding into the lumen of the aorta from the posterior and lateral aortic wall, proximal and opposite to the insertion of the ligamentum arteriosus, and distal to the left subclavian artery. Because thickness of the intima increases with aging, coarctation of the aorta may be progressive.
- There are two types: (a) discrete or focal narrowing of a short segment and (b) long tubular narrowing.
- Associated cardiac defects include bicuspid aortic valve (>10%), discrete subaortic stenosis (>10%), supravalvular aortic stenosis (<2%), mitral stenosis (>10%), and VSD or PDA.
- Patients with unoperated coarctation of the aorta are at increased risk of death due to cerebral hemorrhage from berry aneurysms, aortic dissection or rupture, endarteritis, and heart failure. Women are at risk for dissection during late pregnancy, labor, and early postpartum.

Prevalence

Coarctation of the aorta constitutes approximately 7% of cases of CHD at birth; is more common in males (>2:1 ratio); and in approximately two-thirds of cases, is associated with other left-sided obstructive lesions (Shone syndrome). Its prevalence in adults is uncertain.

Echocardiography

Morphology of Aortic Coarctation on M-Mode and Two-Dimensional Transthoracic or Transesophageal Echocardiography

Best Imaging Planes

- TTE suprasternal notch and high left parasternal views. The transducer can be rotated counterclockwise from the usual long-axis plane of the aortic arch to image a longer segment of the proximal descending aorta.
- A pillow should be placed behind the patient's shoulders to optimize neck extension and to allow the transducer to be positioned nearly parallel to the long axis of the body.
- TEE at 0-, 90-, and 130-degree views at the level of distal aortic arch and proximal descending thoracic aorta.

Key Diagnostic Features

- M-mode provides data on left ventricular wall thickness, size, and fractional shortening. The presence of aortic root dilatation can be determined and a bicuspid aortic valve suspected.
- TTE or TEE 2D images show a focal or tubular narrowing of the distal aortic arch or descending thoracic aorta, or both; in adults, the narrowing is generally focal (ridge-like) and distal to the ligamentum arteriosum, and in infants, it is commonly diffuse and preductal (Fig. 12-10).
- In adults, the area of coarctation is more echoreflectant due to focal thickening and sclerosis.
- Proximal to the coarctation, aortic branches are dilated and pulsatile. The innominate artery, approximately twice the caliber of the left carotid and subclavian arteries, branches into the right subclavian and carotid arteries. In contrast, the descending aorta at the diaphragm level lacks pulsatility. Poststenotic aortic dilatation is common.
- Transverse arch hypoplasia is associated with a high incidence of recurrent coarctation.
- Associated left SVC connection to the coronary sinus, cor triatriatum, supra or valvular

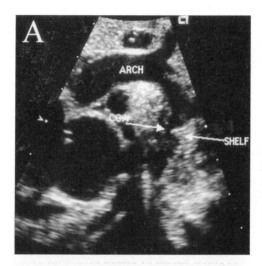
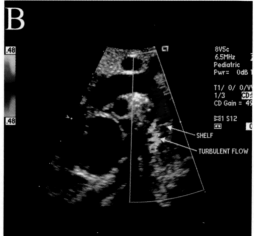
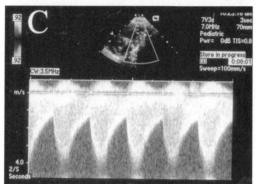
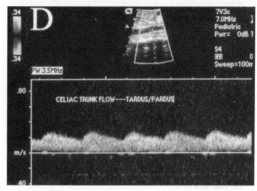

FIG. 12-10. Coarctation of the aorta. **A:** Suprasternal notch view demonstrating a discrete posterior aortic shelf (*arrow*). **B:** Turbulent flow at the shelf. **C:** Classic continuous wave Doppler high-peak velocity, delayed upstroke, and antegrade diastolic flow. **D:** Pulsed wave Doppler of the celiac trunk demonstrates low velocities, slow upstroke, antegrade diastolic flow, and lack of pulsation. COA, coarctation. (Courtesy of M. Beth Goens, M.D.)

mitral stenosis, or subaortic or valvular aortic stenosis can be detected.

■ Post–percutaneous balloon dilatation saccular aneurysm can be detected. Finally, with intravascular ultrasound, precise location and degree of narrowing can be defined for successful endovascular stent placement (20).

Assessment of the Severity of Coarctation of the Aorta on Pulsed, Continuous Wave, and Color Doppler: Key Diagnostic Features

■ Turbulent flow at the coarctation shelf and continuous antegrade flow in diastole distal to the coarctation by pulse wave Doppler.

■ Continuous antegrade systolic and diastolic gradient at the aortic coarctation shelf and a slow, blunted upstroke and decreased peak velocity of the celiac trunk (the latter from the subcostal view) are diagnostic of coarctation of the aorta (Fig. 12-10).

■ Turbulent flow at the coarctation site by color Doppler.

■ Significant transcoarctation gradient (>25 mm Hg), >50% narrowing of the aorta, and hypertension indicate need for intervention in adults.

■ After successful correction of coarctation of the aorta, high Doppler velocities and gradients (2.2 ± 0.4 m/sec and 20 ± 4 mm Hg) are demonstrated at the isthmus in the absence of an arm/leg pressure difference. These persistent gradients are due to mild anatomic aortic narrowing, localized stiffness of the aorta, and pressure/recovery phenomena (21).

- Exercise echo in the postoperative patient with persistent systemic hypertension can demonstrate a pressure gradient not existent at rest. Unless a clear obstruction can be seen on 2D imaging, however, it is unclear that balloon dilatation or surgical augmentation of the aortic arch will abolish this exercise-induced gradient.
- Surgically corrected coarctation in the neonatal period with an end-to-side anastomosis is associated with a 5% to 6% recurrent obstruction (defined as a systolic blood pressure gradient ≥20 mm Hg or a Doppler velocity ≥2.5 m/sec) at 1-year to 2-year follow-up (22).
- Postoperative and probably yearly echo is appropriate in patients post-surgery, after balloon angioplasty, or after stent correction of coarctation to assess absence of complications and residual gradient, and to detect restenosis, aneurysms, dissection, or kinking of the arch (23–25).

Pitfalls

- Precise anatomic and physiologic assessment of coarctation can be difficult by TTE and TEE. Also, on TTE images, the left PA crosses and shadows the aortic coarctation.
- By TEE, the area of a coarctation may be obscured by the left bronchus.
- Precise measurement of the coarctation diameter and length are often difficult.
- Doppler gradients precorrection and postcorrection of coarctation are generally higher than those obtained at cardiac catheterization, probably due to pressure/recovery phenomena.
- With TEE, it is difficult to Doppler at the coarctation site because the interrogation angle is perpendicular to the direction of blood flow.

REFERENCES

1. Hoffman JI, Kaplan S. The incidence of congenital heart disease. *J Am Soc Echocardiogr* 2002;39:1890–1900.
2. Cheitlin MD, Armstrong WF, Aurigemma GP, et al. ACC/AHA/ASE 2003 guideline update for the clinical application of echocardiography. *J Am Coll Cardiol* 2003;42:954–970.
3. Miller-Hance WC, Silverman NH. Transesophageal echocardiography (TEE) in congenital heart disease with focus on the adult. *Cardiol Clin* 2000;18:861–892.
4. Stevenson JG. Utilization of intraoperative transesophageal echocardiography during repair of congenital cardiac defects: a survey of North American centers. *Clin Cardiol* 2003;26:132–134.
5. Sohn S, Kim HS, Han JJ. Pediatric cardiac surgery with echocardiographic diagnosis alone. *J Korean Sci* 2002;17:463–467.
6. Bartel T, Konorza T, Arjumand J, et al. Intracardiac echocardiography is superior to conventional monitoring for guiding device closure of interatrial communications. *Circulation* 2003;107:795–797.
7. Cao QL, Hijazi ZM, Koenig P, et al. Intracardiac echocardiography guidance of transcatheter closure of atrial septal defects and patent foramen ovale: comparison with transesophageal echocardiography and cine fluoroscopy. *J Am Coll Cardiol* 2003;41:437.
8. Krumsdorf U, Ostermayer S, Billinger K, et al. Incidence and clinical course of thrombus formation on atrial septal defect and patent foramen ovale closure devices in 1,000 consecutive patients. *J Am Coll Cardiol* 2004;43:302–309.
9. Acar P, Roux D, Dulac Y, et al. Transthoracic three-dimensional echocardiography prior to closure of atrial septal defects in children. *Cardiol Young* 2003;13:58–63.
10. Eroglu AG, Oztunc F, Saltik L, et al. Evolution of ventricular septal defect with special reference to spontaneous closure rate, subaortic ridge and aortic valve prolapse. *Pediatr Cardiol* 2003;24:31–35.
11. Eapen RS, Lemler MS, Scott WA, et al. Echocardiographic characteristics of perimembranous septal defects associated with aortic regurgitation. *J Am Soc Echocardiogr* 2003;16:209–213.
12. Puchalski MD, Brook MM, Silverman NH. Simplified echocardiographic criteria for decision making in perimembranous ventricular septal defect in childhood. *Am J Cardiol* 2002;90:569–571.
13. Thanopoulos BD, Tsaousis GS, Karanasios E, et al. Transcatheter closure of membranous ventricular septal defects with Amplatzer asymmetric ventricular septal defect occluder: preliminary experience in children. *Heart* 2003;89:918–922.
14. Loyd A, Gordon P, Liu Z, et al. Delineation of intracardiac shunts using contrast echocardiography. *J Am Soc Echocardiogr* 2003;16:770–773.
15. Hagler DJ, Squarcia U, Cabalka AK, et al. Mechanism of tricuspid regurgitation in paramembranous ventricular septal defect. *J Am Soc Echocardiogr* 2002;15:364–368.
16. Ramaciotti C, Lemler MS, Moake L, Zellers TM. Comprehensive assessment of patent ductus arteriosus

by echocardiography before transcatheter closure. *J Am Soc Echocardiogr* 2002;15:1154–1159.

17. Liang CD, Ko SF, Huang SC. Echocardiographic guidance for transcatheter coil occlusion of patent ductus arteriosus in the catheterization laboratory. *J Am Soc Echocardiogr* 2003;16:476–479.

18. Chang ST, Hung KC, Hsieh IC, et al. Evaluation of shunt flow by multiplane transesophageal echocardiography in adult patients with isolated patent ductus arteriosus. *J Am Soc Echocardiogr* 2002;15:1367–1373.

19. Kronzon I, Tunick PA, Rosenzweig BP. Quantification of left-to-right shunt in patent ductus arteriosus with the PISA method. *J Am Soc Echocardiogr* 2002;15:376–378.

20. Hamdan MA, Maheshwari S, Fahey JT, et al. Endovascular stents for coarctation of the aorta: initial results and intermediate-term follow-up. *J Am Coll Cardiol* 2001;38:1518–1523.

21. Verhaaren H, De Mey S, Coomans I, et al. Fixed region of non-distensibility after coarctation repair: in vitro validation of its influence on Doppler peak velocities. *J Am Soc Echocardiogr* 2001;14:580–587.

22. Younoszai AK, Reddy VM, Hanley FL, et al. Intermediate term follow-up of the end-to-side aortic anastomosis for coarctation of the aorta. *Ann Thorac Surg* 2002;74:1631–1634.

23. Roos-Hesselink JW, Scholzel BE, Heijdra RJ, et al. Aortic valve and aortic arch pathology after coarctation repair. *Heart* 2003;89:1074–1077.

24. Lim DS, Ralston MA. Echocardiographic indices of Doppler flow patterns compared with MRI or angiographic measurements to detect significant coarctation of the aorta. *Echocardiography* 2002;19:55–60.

25. Paddon AJ, Nicholson AA, Ettles DF, et al. Long-term follow-up of percutaneous balloon angioplasty in adult aortic coarctation. *Cardiovasc Intervent Radiol* 2000;23:364–367.

13

Infective Endocarditis

Carlos A. Roldan

■ Infective endocarditis (IE) is associated with significant morbidity and mortality if not promptly recognized and treated.
■ General and cardiovascular symptomatology associated with IE is frequently nonspecific.
■ The most common clinical manifestations of IE (fever and heart murmurs) are nonspecific.
■ In patients with acute and severe mitral regurgitation or aortic regurgitation and heart failure, regurgitant murmurs are attenuated or inaudible.

■ Peripheral manifestations of IE, such as Osler nodes and Janeway lesions, are uncommon.
■ Integration of clinical and echocardiography (echo) data, therefore, is critical for the diagnosis, risk stratification, and management of IE.

DEFINITION

■ IE is an infection of the endothelial lining of the heart valves, mitral or tricuspid chorda tendinea, valve annulus, and aortic root.

TABLE 13-1. *Predisposing Heart Diseases in Infective Endocarditis*

Condition	15–60 yr (%)	>60 yr (%)
Rheumatic heart disease	25–30	8
Mitral valve prolapse	10–30	10
Intravenous drug abuse	15–35	10
Congenital heart disease	10–20	2
Degenerative heart disease	Rare	30
Other	10–15	10
None	25–45	25–40

■ It is typically characterized by fever and a heart murmur and confirmed by positive blood cultures or echo or pathologic evidence of valvular or paravalvular infection.

PREEXISTENT HEART DISEASES

■ Preexisting heart disease is found in at least two-thirds of cases of left-sided IE (Table 13-1).

■ Preexisting heart disease is uncommon in right-sided IE.

■ In patients ≤30 years old, rheumatic heart disease (in developing countries) and mitral valve prolapse or intravenous drug abuse (in developed countries) are the most common underlying heart diseases.

■ In patients ≥60 years old, aortic valve sclerosis or stenosis and mitral annular sclerosis with mild or worse regurgitation are common underlying cardiac pathologies.

■ In either age group, at least one-third of patients have normal valves or clinically unrecognized valve disease.

DISTRIBUTION OF TYPES OF INFECTIVE ENDOCARDITIS

■ Subacute and acute IE of native left heart valves constitutes 60% to 75% and 5% to 10% of all cases, respectively.
  ◆ Isolated aortic valve IE is observed in 55% to 60% of cases.
  ◆ Isolated mitral valve IE occurs in 25% to 30% of cases.
  ◆ IE of both valves occurs in 15% of cases.

■ Prosthetic valve IE constitutes 10% to 25% of all cases of IE.
  ◆ Prosthetic valve IE is more common with prosthetic aortic valves, multiple valves, and after replacement of an infected native valve.

■ Right-sided IE, most commonly associated with intravenous drug abuse, constitutes 5% to 10% of all cases.
  ◆ The tricuspid valve is predominantly involved (80% of cases).
  ◆ It also occurs in patients with right heart wires or catheters.

■ Culture-negative IE constitutes 5% to 10% of all cases of IE.

MOST COMMON PATHOGENS

■ Acute native IE: *Staphylococcus aureus*, *Streptococcus pneumoniae* or *pyogenes*, *Haemophilus influenzae*, *Pseudomonas aeruginosa*, and beta-hemolytic streptococci.

■ Subacute native IE: *Streptococcus viridans* and *S. aureus*.

■ Early prosthetic valve IE: *S. aureus* and *Staphylococcus epidermidis*.

■ Late prosthetic valve IE: *S. viridans* and *S. aureus*.

■ Right-sided native IE: *S. aureus*, streptococci, enterococci, gram-negative bacteria, and fungi.

■ Acute right-sided IE related to pacemaker or automatic implantable cardioverter-defibrillator wires: *S. aureus* and *S. epidermidis*.

■ Chronic right-sided IE related to pacemaker or automatic implantable cardioverter-defibrillator wires: *S. epidermidis*, *S. aureus*, and gram-negative bacteria.

■ Culture negative IE: *Candida*; *Aspergillus*; *Coxiella brunetti*; and other fastidious, slow-growing microorganisms.

DIAGNOSIS

Definite Diagnosis

Microorganisms demonstrated by culture or histology in a vegetation or histologic evidence of active vegetation or an intracardiac abscess.

TABLE 13-2. *Duke Diagnostic Criteria for Infective Endocarditis*[a]

Major criteria	Minor criteria
Positive blood cultures for typical microorganisms	Predisposing heart disease
Streptococcus viridans and *bovis*	Mitral valve prolapse
Staphylococcus aureus	Bicuspid aortic valve
Enterococci	Rheumatic heart disease
HACEK group[b]	Congenital heart disease
Persistent bacteremia	Intravenous drug abuse
≥2 positive blood cultures ≥12 h apart or	Fever
≥3 positive cultures ≥1 h apart	Vascular phenomena
70% positive cultures if ≥4 drawn	Major arterial emboli
Evidence of endocardial involvement	Septic pulmonary emboli
Positive echocardiogram	Mycotic aneurysm
Oscillating vegetation	Intracranial hemorrhage
Abscesses	Janeway lesions
New partial dehiscence of prosthetic valve	Immunologic phenomena
New valvular regurgitation	Glomerulonephritis
	Osler nodes
	Roth spots
	Rheumatoid factor
	Other
	Positive blood cultures not meeting major criteria
	Positive echocardiogram not meeting major criteria

[a]Diagnosis: (1) two major criteria, (2) one major and three minor criteria, or (3) five minor criteria.
[b]HACEK group is comprised of *Haemophilus, Actinobacillus, Corynebacterium, Eikenella*, and *Kingella* species. These pathogens uncommonly cause infective endocarditis (<5% of all cases).

Definite Clinical Diagnosis

■ Duke criteria: two major criteria, one major and three minor criteria, or five minor criteria (Table 13-2) (1,2).
  ◆ Other minor criteria [clubbing, splenomegaly, splinter hemorrhages, petechiae, central nonfeeding venous lines, peripheral venous lines, microscopic hematuria, high erythrocyte sedimentation rate (>30 or >50 mm/hour for patients younger than or older than 60 years old, respectively) and C-reactive protein (>100 mg/L)] increase the sensitivity and maintain high specificity of the Duke criteria for diagnosis of native and prosthetic valve IE.

Possible Infective Endocarditis

IE is possible if findings consistent with IE fall short of "definite" but not "rejected."

Rejected Infective Endocarditis

■ IE diagnosis is rejected when an alternate diagnosis explains manifestations suggestive of IE.
■ IE diagnosis also is rejected if clinical manifestations or pathologic evidence of IE were not found after ≤4 days of antibiotics.

ECHOCARDIOGRAPHY

Class I Indications for Use in Infective Endocarditis

■ Transthoracic echo (TTE) and especially transesophageal echo (TEE) are highly accurate and cost-effective for the diagnosis, risk stratification, and therapy of IE (Table 13-3) (1–5).
■ In a patient with a suggestive clinical syndrome, echo confirms the diagnosis of IE by the detection of vegetations (the *sine qua non* of this condition).

TABLE 13-3. *Class I Indications for Echocardiography in Infective Endocarditis of Native and Prosthetic Valves*

Detection and characterization of valvular lesions, their hemodynamic severity, and ventricular compensation[a]

Detection of vegetations and characterization of lesions in patients with congenital heart disease

Detection of abscesses, perforation, or fistulas[a]

Reevaluation studies in patients with complex endocarditis (virulent organism, severe hemodynamic lesion, aortic valve involvement, persistent fever or bacteremia, clinical change or symptomatic deterioration)

In patients with highly suspected culture-negative infective endocarditis[a]

Evaluation of bacteremia without a known source in a patient with a prosthetic valve[a]

---

[a]Transesophageal echocardiography may provide incremental value in addition to information obtained by transthoracic echocardiography.

- In a patient with high pretest likelihood of IE, absence of vegetations on echo does not exclude IE, but it makes the diagnosis unlikely or defines a benign prognosis (6).
- Similarly, in patients with low likelihood of IE, echo has limited additive diagnostic and prognostic value.
- In patients with intermediate likelihood of IE, echo and especially TEE play the most important diagnostic and prognostic role.
- Large (>10 mm) or multiple vegetations or severe valve dysfunction (moderate to severe regurgitation, abscesses, leaflet perforation, fistula, ring dehiscence) predicts high morbidity and mortality and indicates the need for valve surgery (7).
- Echo can also define the mechanism of valve regurgitation and the hemodynamic impact of regurgitant lesions on left ventricular size and function, left atrial size, and left atrial and pulmonary artery pressures.
- Although the diagnosis of IE can be made by clinical and microbiology data alone, the diagnosis of IE frequently relies on the demonstration of endocardial disease by echo.
- Based on the higher diagnostic accuracy of TEE as compared to TTE for the detection of valve vegetations and associated complications, patients with suspected IE should

undergo TEE and, when necessary, a complementary but focused TTE (8,9).

M-Mode and Two-Dimensional Echocardiography: Valve Morphology

Best Imaging Planes

- A systematic approach to the performance and interpretation of TTE and TEE in a patient with suspected IE is essential to the diagnostic accuracy of echo.
- Careful scanning of one heart valve at a time should be performed in multiple planes at short depth settings (12 cm for TTE and 4–8 cm for TEE) and with a narrow sector scan to improve image resolution.
- By TEE, for each valve and especially from the mid-esophageal views, two-dimensional followed by color Doppler imaging should be performed at different valve and subvalvular levels by slowly advancing or withdrawing the probe.
- In the author's laboratory, the following sequence of TEE interrogation of all heart valves are used:
  - Transgastric four-chamber and transgastric short-axis and long-axis views of the mitral and tricuspid valves (allows assessment of the posterior tricuspid leaflet).
  - Transgastric short-axis view of the mitral valve as the TEE probe is withdrawn from the transgastric to the mid-esophageal level.
  - Mid-esophageal four-chamber and two-chamber views, with a sector scan limited to the mitral or tricuspid valve and scanning of the valves at multiple planes and levels.
  - Mid-esophageal short-axis and multiplane interrogation of the aortic and then of the pulmonic valve.
- In addition to characterizing valve vegetations and associated complications, valve and subvalvular apparatus are assessed for thickening, hyperreflectance, retraction, calcification, and mobility. These characteristics categorize a valve morphology as myxomatous, degenerative, rheumatic, or congenital.
- The presence and severity of valve regurgitation is defined according to established color

Doppler echo criteria described in other chapters of this book.

Key Diagnostic Features of Specific Abnormalities

Valve Vegetations

- Vegetations are the *sine qua non* and most common abnormality of IE.
- Vegetations are distinctive masses attached to the leaflets and characterized by their location, size, shape, echoreflectance, mobility, and extent (Fig. 13-1).

Location

- Vegetations are most commonly located at the leaflet coaptation point on the atrial side of atrioventricular valves and ventricular side of semilunar valves.
- Uncommon locations for valve vegetations include mid-portion to distal portion of the anterior mitral leaflet or chordae tendinea as a result of an aortic regurgitant jet lesion or from a contact lesion with the basal septum in patients with obstructive hypertrophic cardiomyopathy (10).
- Also in patients with hypertrophic cardiomyopathy, vegetations can be seen on the basal septum as a result of a contact lesion with the mitral valve.

Size

Vegetations are of variable size, but generally >3 mm. A vegetation is small if it measures <5 mm in diameter, of moderate size if it measures 5 to 10 mm, and large if >10 mm.

Shape

Vegetations are of variable shape; they are most commonly globular but can be polypoid, tubular, frondlike, elongated, pedunculated, and unilobulated or multilobulated.

Echoreflectance

- Echoreflectance of recent vegetations is that of the myocardium (homogeneous soft tissue echoreflectance) and, less frequently, of heterogeneous appearance.
- Infrequently, recent and large vegetations can have discrete areas of echolucency that suggest an *in situ* abscess formation.
- Vegetations denser than the myocardium or partially or completely calcified denote chronicity and are likely healed lesions.

Mobility

- A pedunculated or prolapsing mass has a characteristic independent rotatory mobility.

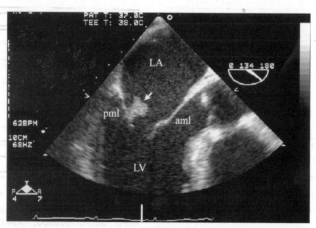

FIG. 13-1. Mitral valve vegetation. This transesophageal echocardiographic long-axis view of the mitral valve demonstrates a large (1.2 cm × 1 cm) vegetation on the distal portion and atrial side of the posterior mitral leaflet (pml) (*arrow*). The soft tissue echoreflectance (similar to that of the myocardium) of the mass suggests a recently formed vegetation. The appearance of the underlying leaflets is unremarkable. aml, anterior mitral leaflet; LA, left atrium; LV, left ventricle.

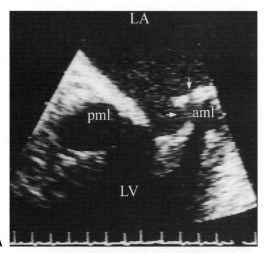
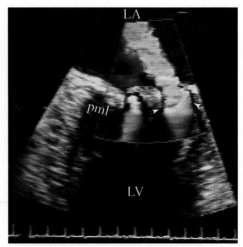

FIG. 13-2. Anterior mitral leaflet perforation. **A:** This transesophageal echocardiographic two-chamber view of the mitral valve demonstrates severe and diffuse thickening of the posterior (pml) and anterior mitral leaflets (aml). Note on the base and mid-portions of the anterior leaflet two discrete areas of tissue discontinuity consistent with leaflet perforations (*arrows*). **B:** Color Doppler confirmed a wide regurgitant jet through the largest perforation (*arrowhead*). LA, left atrium; LV, left ventricle.

- An elongated mass has partial independent mobility.
- A sessile lesion moves with the underlying leaflet.

Detection of Complications

Valve Perforation

- The aortic noncoronary cusp, the aortic-mitral junction or intervalvular fibrosa, and basal to mid-portions of the anterior mitral leaflet are the sites most commonly involved (Figs. 13-2 and 13-3) (11).
- Perforation of the aortic-mitral intervalvular fibrosa or anterior mitral leaflet can also result from ulceration with or without a preceding pseudoaneurysm formation by a metastatic infection from a regurgitant aortic valve (a jet lesion) (Fig. 13-4).
- A perforation can occur on any leaflet portion, but more commonly occurs in the area adjacent to vegetations or leaflet thickening.
- A perforation appears as a leaflet tissue discontinuity of variable size.
- Demonstration by color Doppler of a jet through a leaflet discontinuity highly suggests the diagnosis (Fig. 13-2).

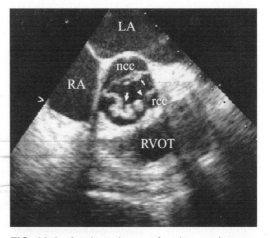

FIG. 13-3. Aortic valve perforation and aneurysm. This transesophageal echocardiographic short-axis view of the aortic valve demonstrates a tissue discontinuity in the lateral portion of the right coronary cusp (rcc) consistent with a perforation (*arrowhead*). Color Doppler confirmed the presence of a perforation. An aneurysmal formation (*large arrow*) in the right coronary cusp was also demonstrated; however, no vegetations were demonstrated in this cusp. A vegetation was noted in the noncoronary cusp (ncc) (*small arrow*). Severe aortic regurgitation was demonstrated. LA, left atrium; RA, right atrium; RVOT, right ventricular outflow tract.

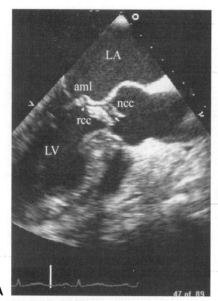 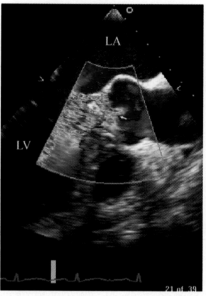

FIG. 13-4. Aortic valve cusp perforation and prolapse. **A:** This transesophageal echocardiographic long-axis view demonstrates lack of coaptation of the aortic valve due to a flail right coronary cusp (rcc) caused by a perforation. The right coronary cusp appears severely and diffusely thickened, but a distinctive vegetation was not demonstrated. On the noncoronary cusp (ncc), a vegetation was demonstrated (*arrow*). Note the thinning and anterior bulging of the mid-anterior to distal anterior mitral leaflet (aml) consistent with a pseudoaneurysm (*arrowhead*) (see Fig. 13-6). **B:** Color Doppler demonstrates highly eccentric and severe aortic regurgitation based on a large vena contracta and proximal isovelocity surface area (*arrow*). Note that the eccentric regurgitant jet is directed toward the anterior mitral leaflet. This regurgitant jet led to the formation of the pseudoaneurysm. Finally, note the increased soft tissue thickening of the anterior aortic annulus and proximal aorta consistent with aortitis or early abscess formation. All of these finding were confirmed at surgery. LA, left atrium; LV, left ventricle.

- Up to 50% of leaflet perforations, especially those of the mitral valve, are associated with or preceded by a pseudoaneurysm.

Valvular, Annular, Aortic Root, or Myocardial Abscesses

- Abscesses occur in 20% to 40% of cases of IE and are twice as common with prosthetic valves.
- Abscesses are predominant in the aortic posterior annulus, periannular area, aortic-mitral intervalvular fibrosa, posterior aortic root, and interventricular septum (Fig. 13-5) (12,13).
- In prosthetic valves, abscesses are characteristically seen around the sewing ring.
- Rarely, isolated myocardial abscess or infarction can occur due to coronary embolism.
- An abscess appearance is of an amorphous, soft tissue echoreflectant mass (if solid) or of an echolucent and variable-sized mass (if cystic) (12).
- Cystic abscesses as a difference of pseudoaneurysms do not expand and collapse during the cardiac cycle and do not show flow by color Doppler.

Valve Pseudoaneurysm

- Pseudoaneurysms result from direct extension and erosive effect of the infection and shearing forces of flow into a leaflet, intervalvular fibrosa, aortic root or annulus, or from a metastatic infection from aortic regurgitation jet lesion on the ventricular side of the anterior mitral leaflet (Figs. 13-3 and 13-6) (14).
- Pseudoaneurysms are more commonly associated with aortic prosthetic valve IE.
- Pseudoaneurysms are predominant (50–75%) in the aortic-mitral intervalvular fibrosa, then

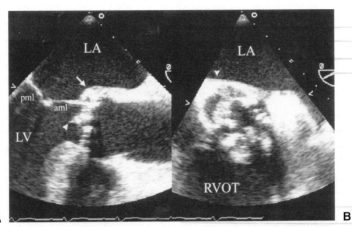

FIG. 13-5. Aortic valve cusp perforation and aortic root abscess. **A:** Transesophageal echocardiographic (TEE) long-axis view of the aortic valve and root demonstrates a perforated noncoronary cusp with a flail portion prolapsing into the left ventricular outflow tract (*arrowhead*). Also note in this view the heterogeneously echoreflectant severe thickening of the posterior aortic annulus and aortic root wall suggestive of aortitis or abscess formation (*arrow*). **B:** This TEE short-axis view demonstrates a severely distorted and sclerosed aortic valve. Also, on the posteromedial aortic root (*arrowhead*), a walled, semilunar shape and partially soft tissue echoreflectant structure is seen. No flow within this structure was demonstrated by color Doppler. These findings are characteristic of an aortic root abscess. aml, anterior mitral leaflet; LA, left atrium; LV, left ventricle; pml, posterior mitral leaflet; RVOT, right ventricular outflow tract.

on the aortic posterior annulus, and rarely, on the base or mid-portions of the aortic cusps or anterior mitral leaflet.

■ Pseudoaneurysms appear as a narrow discontinuity (neck) communicating with a sac or pouchlike structure.

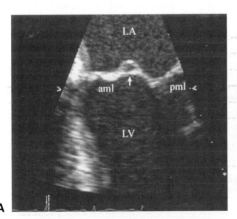
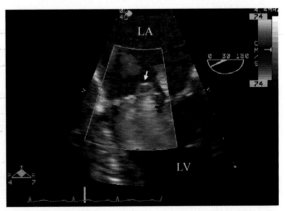

FIG. 13-6. Mitral valve pseudoaneurysm. **A:** This transesophageal echocardiographic four-chamber close-up view of the mitral valve demonstrates in the mid-portion of the anterior mitral leaflet (aml) a small and walled echolucent structure that bulges anteriorly during systole, suggestive of a pseudoaneurysm (*arrow*). **B:** Flow during systole is seen within this structure, confirming a pseudoaneurysm (*arrow*). This patient had severe aortic valve endocarditis with a severe eccentric aortic regurgitant jet directed mainly toward the ventricular side of the mid-portion of the anterior mitral leaflet. By the time the patient went to surgery, a small leaflet perforation in this area was noted. LA, left atrium; LV, left ventricle; pml, posterior mitral leaflet.

- The neck of a pseudoaneurysm opens to the left ventricular outflow tract, and the saccular portion bulges or expands during systole and collapses during diastole.
- The pseudoaneurysm cavity area ranges from <1 cm to 12 cm.

Fistulas

- Extension of the valvular or annular infectious process to the periannular area, aortic-mitral intervalvular fibrosa, or aortic root results in erosion, possible formation of a pseudoaneurysm (approximately 50%), and, ultimately, rupture and communication of the aorta with the left atrium (LA), right atrium, or right ventricle (15,16).
- Rarely, extension of the infection to the interventricular septum can lead to the formation of a fistula that communicates the left ventricle with the right ventricle or right atrium. Color Doppler echo has the most important diagnostic value in the recognition of this complication.

Ring Dehiscence

- Most commonly, prosthetic valve abscesses lead to ring dehiscence.
- Ring dehiscence appears as a discontinuity between the outer border of the sewing ring and the respective annulus.
- The demonstration of a color Doppler jet in this area of discontinuity (during diastole for aortic and systole for mitral valve) is a necessary complementary diagnostic parameter.
- From the transgastric and basal short-axis and mid-esophageal four-chamber, two-chamber, and longitudinal TEE views of the mitral or aortic valve, an estimate of the extent of the ring dehiscence can be made by identifying the circumferential extent of the color Doppler jet around the sewing ring.

Valvular Regurgitation

- In uncomplicated IE, the degree of valvular regurgitation is variable, but generally less than moderate.
- In complicated IE, associated valvular regurgitation is generally moderate or worse (Figs. 13-2 and 13-4).

- Pulsed, continuous wave, and especially color Doppler are of most value in the assessment of the severity and mechanism of regurgitant lesions.

Pitfalls

- TTE has limited sensitivity for the detection of native and prosthetic valve vegetations and associated complications (abscesses, perforations, fistulas).
- Shadowing and reverberations from prosthetic mechanical valves decrease the detection of prosthetic valve vegetations by TTE or TEE.
- Echo does not exclude IE in a patient with other clinical data diagnostic of IE.
- Echo, including TEE, cannot clearly differentiate an active from a healed vegetation.
- Echo, including TEE, cannot completely differentiate an infective vegetation from valve masses seen in patients with malignancies, inflammatory connective tissue diseases (i.e., systemic lupus erythematosus), rheumatic valvulitis, a noninfective flail portion of a native or torn bioprosthetic mitral, or aortic leaflet.
- Localized or nodular valve thickening or calcification, benign leaflet nodules (nodules of Arantii), valve excrescences, suture material around a sewing ring (especially after mitral valve replacement), valve thrombus, or pannus ingrowth may also mimic vegetations.

Diagnostic Accuracy in Infective Endocarditis

Although TEE is not routinely recommended in patients with suspected IE, in the author's opinion and as suggested but not specifically stated by the American College of Cardiology/American Heart Association guidelines and others, TEE should be the primary diagnostic method in patients with clinically suspected IE (Table 13-4) (1–5,9,17).

Detection and Characterization of Valve Vegetations

- TEE has a significantly higher sensitivity but equally high specificity as TTE for detection

TABLE 13-4. *Indications for Transesophageal Echocardiography in Patients with Suspected or Proven Infective Endocarditis*

Technically limited TTE
High clinical suspicion for IE with a negative TTE
High clinical suspicion for IE in patients with *Staphylococcus* bacteremia
In elderly patients with underlying degenerative valvular heart disease
Clinically suspicious for IE and negative blood cultures
Clinically suspicious and bacteremia, but negative or inadequate TTE
Persistent fever or bacteremia
Suspected prosthetic valve endocarditis
Suspected valve complications (≥moderate regurgitation, abscess, perforation, or fistula)
After valve replacement requiring homografts or coronary reimplantation (intraoperative)

IE, infective endocarditis; TTE, transthoracic echocardiography.

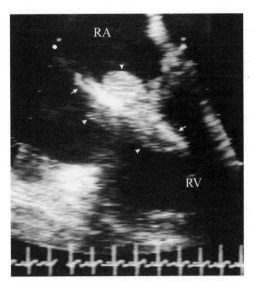

FIG. 13-7. Pacemaker lead vegetation. This transesophageal echocardiographic four-chamber view demonstrates a large mass (*arrowheads*) extending from the right atrium (RA) to the right ventricle (RV) and attached to a pacemaker wire (*arrows*). Mild soft tissue thickening of the tricuspid valve but no valve vegetations were detected. Histopathology of this mass confirmed an infective vegetation.

of native and prosthetic valve vegetations (Table 13-5).

■ TEE is superior to TTE in defining the location, size, shape, mobility, and number of valve vegetations.

■ TEE and TTE probably detect tricuspid valve vegetations with equal frequency, but TEE defines more accurately vegetations' morphology and associated complications.

◆ TEE is also probably more accurate in defining the mechanism of tricuspid regurgitation and the extent of leaflets' and chordal involvement.

■ Pulmonic valve IE and IE associated with pacemakers, automatic implantable cardioverter-defibrillators, or right heart catheters are more often recognized and better characterized by TEE than by TTE.

◆ TEE detects vegetations on these devices in approximately 90% of cases, as compared to ≤30% by TTE (Fig. 13-7) (18).

◆ A lead infection may have a sleevelike appearance rather than a distinct vegetation in 25% of cases.

◆ In these patients, a vegetation size by TEE of < or >10 mm predicts high success and safety rates for percutaneous or surgical lead extraction, respectively.

■ Because TEE is of superior diagnostic value as compared to TTE, most patients with sus-

pected culture-negative IE should undergo TEE.

Detection of Complications

■ The sensitivity of TEE for the detection of abscesses, leaflet perforations, and pseudoaneurysms ranges from 90% to 100%, as compared to 22% to 45% by TTE. The specificity of both techniques is similarly high for leaflet perforations.

■ Similar superiority of TEE as compared to TTE has been reported for detection of bioprosthetic leaflet perforations.

■ Although limited data are available comparing TEE and TTE for the detection of fistulas, in most series, the diagnosis of this abnormality has been made by TEE (15,16).

■ In patients with suspected prosthetic valve IE, TTE provides a complementary assessment of aortic or mitral valve obstruction, aortic

TABLE 13-5. *Detection of Valvular or Paravalvular Complications in Infective Endocarditis (IE)*

Abnormality	TEE		TTE	
	Sensitivity (%)	Specificity (%)	Sensitivity (%)	Specificity (%)
Vegetations[a]	83–100	93–100	17–63	83–98
Abscess	98–100	—	22–28	—
Perforation	95	98	45	98
Pseudoaneurysm	90	—	43	—

[a]Lower TEE sensitivity values apply to prosthetic valves. The reported negative and positive predictive values of TEE for native IE are 98–100% and 95–98%, respectively. Its negative predictive value for prosthetic valve IE is 90%.

regurgitation, and assessment of left atrial and pulmonary artery pressures.

Differential Diagnosis of Infective Endocarditis

- The echo appearance of infective vegetations overlap with that of other noninfective valve masses or similar masses' appearance, such as valve excrescences, ruptured mitral chordae tendinea, torn bioprosthetic leaflets, Libman-Sacks vegetations, rheumatic valvulitis, thrombotic vegetations, and papillary fibroelastoma.
- Some of these echo abnormalities or normal variants may be present in patients with clinically suspected IE (i.e., valve excrescences), may preexist or be caused by IE (ruptured chordae tendinea), or may coexist with infective vegetations (Libman-Sacks vegetations).
- These facts underscore the importance of clinical and microbiologic data in the diagnosis of IE as well as the need for expert echo interpretation.

Valve Excrescences

- Valve excrescences result from the constant bending and buckling of the leaflets, leading to tearing of the subendocardial collagen and elastic fibers with subsequent endothelialization.
- On echo, valve or Lambl's excrescences appear as thin (0.6–2.0 mm in width), elongated (4–16 mm in length), and hypermobile structures seen at the coaptation point of the aortic and mitral valve leaflets and, rarely, on the right-sided valves.
- Excrescences on the aortic valve prolapse into the left ventricular outflow tract during diastole.

- Excrescences on the mitral valve prolapse into the LA during systole.
- Valve excrescences are detected almost exclusively by TEE and are seen in 35% to 40% of apparently healthy subjects, in 45% to 50% of patients undergoing TEE for other reasons than suspected cardioembolism, and in 40% of those undergoing TEE for suspected cardioembolism (see Fig. 1-9A) (19).
- In contrast to valve excrescences, infective vegetations are generally >3 mm in diameter, resolve or change in size or appearance over time, and are usually associated with structural and functional valve abnormalities.
- In a patient with suspected IE, however, it may be difficult to differentiate a valve excrescence from a small or an early-stage infective mass.

Ruptured Chordae Tendinea

- A ruptured chordae is an elongated, hypermobile structure, usually >3 mm in thickness prolapsing into the LA during systole; it is generally associated with prolapse and myxomatous thickening of the respective leaflet and significant and eccentric mitral regurgitation (see Figs. 5-2 through 5-6).
- Therefore, the distinction between a myxomatous ruptured chordae and an infected ruptured chordae can only be made by the integration of clinical and echo data.

Torn Bioprosthetic Leaflet

- The sclerotic degenerative process of a bioprosthetic leaflet can lead to a torn portion of it and can be associated with significant regurgitation.
- A torn aortic leaflet portion prolapses into the left ventricular outflow in diastole, and a

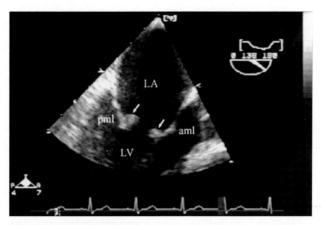

FIG. 13-8. Libman-Sacks vegetations. This transesophageal echocardiographic long-axis view of the mitral valve in a young female with systemic lupus erythematosus demonstrates a small, oval, sessile, and soft tissue echoreflectant mass on the distal portion and atrial side of the anterior (aml) and posterior (pml) mitral leaflets (*arrows*). Mild thickening of the mitral leaflets is noted. Associated symptomatic severe mitral regurgitation led to mitral valve surgery. Histology confirmed masses as Libman-Sacks vegetations. LA, left atrium; LV, left ventricle.

torn leaflet portion of a mitral valve prolapses into the LA in systole (see Chapter 11 and Fig. 11-6).

- A torn leaflet cannot clearly be differentiated from a primary or associated vegetation unless another associated abnormality indicative of valve infection is detected (i.e., vegetation, abscess, or fistula).

Libman-Sacks Endocarditis

- Libman-Sacks vegetations (characteristic of systemic lupus erythematosus) can be mistaken as infective vegetations.
- Libman-Sacks vegetations are located at the leaflet's line of closure, have heterogeneous echoreflectance, are usually sessile but can be elongated, and show mobility dependent on the leaflet motion (Fig. 13-8) (20).
- Infective vegetations can coexist with Libman-Sacks vegetations in the same or different heart valve, however.

Rheumatic Valvulitis

- Acute rheumatic endocarditis is associated with predominantly mild mitral and aortic regurgitation, but moderate to severe lesions uncommonly occur.

- Valve vegetations can be seen in at least 25% of patients with acute rheumatic endocarditis.
- These rheumatic valve masses are located on the body and tip of the leaflets and are predominantly seen on the mitral valve (>80%).
- Therefore, in the appropriate geographic locations, infective versus rheumatic endocarditis may be difficult to differentiate by echo (21).

Nonbacterial Thrombotic Vegetations

- Nonbacterial thrombotic vegetations are seen in patients with malignancies, immunologic, or hypercoagulable states.
- They are associated with underlying mildly thickened or normal leaflets.
- They are located predominantly at the closure margins of the leaflets on the atrial side of the mitral and on the ventricular side of the aortic valve cusps.
- Thus, thrombotic vegetations are indistinguishable from infective vegetations by echo (21).

Papillary Fibroelastoma

- Papillary fibroelastomas are rare benign cardiac tumors seen predominantly on the aortic (aortic side) and mitral valve (atrial side).

■ They are usually small (<2 cm); have heteroge-neous echoreflectance; appear frondlike; are attached to the valve by a stalk, usually away from the coaptation point; and are hypermobile.

■ The underlying leaflet is normal or mini-mally thickened and is usually without valve regurgitation.

■ They are usually incidentally diagnosed or diagnosed when first manifested with sys-temic embolism (22).

Prognostic Value in Infective Endocarditis

■ Patients with large (>10 mm), recently formed and hypermobile vegetations have a higher morbidity and mortality than those with sessile or smaller vegetations (7,23):

◆ Higher rate of failure to therapy.

◆ Higher incidence of embolism [more com-mon with mitral than with aortic or other valve involvement (odds ratio, 2.8)].

◆ Valvular dysfunction or heart failure.

◆ Valve replacement (odds ratio, 2.95).

◆ Higher death rate (odds ratio, 1.55).

◆ Patients with a vegetation size ≤5 mm, 6 to 10 mm, and ≥11 mm have up to a 10%, 20% to 40%, and >50% incidence of complications, respectively.

■ After successful medical therapy, 25% to 30% of native valve vegetations resolve, 15% to 20% decrease in size, 35% to 40% persist unchanged in size, and 10% to 15% increase in size. Persistent vegetations commonly become fibrosed or, rarely, calcified.

■ Patients with significant valve dysfunction (regurgitation, abscesses, perforation, fistula, or pseudoaneurysms) have an operative mor-tality of 15% to 30% and an overall survival at 1 to 2 years of 50% to 70% (12,17,24).

■ Complications other than embolism are more common with aortic valve IE. Therefore, native aortic valve IE carries a worse progno-sis than mitral or right-sided IE.

■ Prosthetic aortic valve IE carries the worst prognosis of all because of the associated high incidence of ring abscesses leading to ring dehiscence, paraprosthetic regurgita-tion, septic embolism, and persistent and recurrent infection after medical or surgical therapy (24).

◆ Patients with uncomplicated and compli-cated prosthetic valve IE have up to 20% and 80% to 100% mortality with medical therapy, respectively.

◆ In these patients, the surgical mortality of uncomplicated and complicated IE is decreased to 10% and 50%, respectively.

◆ Survival may be improved in these patients with early surgery and with the use of homografts or stentless valves.

■ Right-sided IE associated with pacemaker wires and catheters is associated with an in-hospital mortality of 5% to 10% and a 12-month to 24-month mortality of 25% to 30% (18).

■ Finally, despite improvements in medical and surgical therapy, the overall mortality of IE is approximately 20%.

Indicators for Valve Surgery in Infective Endocarditis

■ Echo plays a critical role in identifying most patients with class I recommendations for valve surgery, according to the American Col-lege of Cardiology/American Heart Associa-tion guidelines (Table 13-6) (3,4,12,17,24).

■ Because of the higher diagnostic accuracy of TEE as compared to TTE in detecting com-plications associated with native and pros-thetic valve IE, recommendations for valve surgery are predominantly based on TEE.

Use in Pregnant Patients with Infective Endocarditis

The diagnosis and prognostic value of echo in the pregnant patient with IE is probably similar to that of the nonpregnant patient, but limited data are currently available (25).

Intraoperative Use in Patients with Infective Endocarditis

Intraoperative TEE plays an important role in the immediate postoperative assessment of valve replacement or, infrequently, valve repair in patients with IE.

TABLE 13-6. *Echocardiography Indicators for Valve Surgery in Infective Endocarditis*

Acute aortic or mitral regurgitation with heart failure

Acute aortic regurgitation with tachycardia and early closure of the mitral valve

Valve dysfunction and persistent infection after 7–10 d of appropriate antibiotic therapy

Paravalvular regurgitation (for prosthetic valve), annular or aortic abscess, sinus or aortic true or false aneurysm, fistula formation, or new-onset conduction disturbances

Patients with systemic embolism and persistent valve vegetations despite appropriate antibiotic therapy

Early prosthetic valve endocarditis

Prosthetic valve dysfunction with heart failure

Staphylococcal prosthetic endocarditis not responding to antibiotic therapy

Prosthetic valve infection with gram-negative organisms or organisms with a poor response to antibiotics

Fungal native or prosthetic valve endocarditis

Follow-Up in Patients with Infective Endocarditis

■ No specific guidelines for echo follow-up are available for medically treated uncomplicated IE.

  ◆ Unless earlier clinical indications are present, a repeat echo after completion of antibiotic therapy is appropriate.

■ In cases of complicated IE undergoing valve surgery, a repeat TTE or TEE before discharge and after completion of antibiotic therapy is appropriate.

■ In uncomplicated cases post–valve surgery, echo follow-up guidelines for bioprosthetic and prosthetic valves should be followed (see Chapter 11).

REFERENCES

1. Jassal DS, Lee C, Silversides C, et al. Can structural clinical assessment using modified Duke's criteria improve appropriate use of echocardiography in patients with suspected infective endocarditis? *Can J Cardiol* 2003;19:1017–1022.

2. Greaves K, Mou D, Patel A, et al. Clinical criteria and the appropriate use of transthoracic echocardiography for the exclusion of infective endocarditis. *Heart* 2003;89:273–275.

3. Bonw RO, Carabello B, De Leon AC, et al. ACC/AHA guidelines for the management of patients with valvular heart disease. *J Am Coll Cardiol* 1998;32:1486–1588.

4. Cheitlin MD, Armstrong WF, Aurigemma GP, et al. ACC/AHA/ASE guideline update for the clinical application of echocardiography: summary article. *J Am Coll Cardiol* 2003;42:954–970.

5. Humpl T, McCrindle BW, Smallhorn JF. The relative roles of transthoracic compared with transesophageal echocardiography in children with suspected infective endocarditis. *J Am Coll Cardiol* 2003;41:2068–2071.

6. Michelfelder EC, Ochsner JE, Khoury P, et al. Does assessment of pretest probability of disease improve the utility of echocardiography in suspected endocarditis in children? *J Pediatr* 2003;142:263–267.

7. Vilacosta I, Graupner C, San Roman JA, et al. Risk of embolization after institution of antibiotic therapy for infective endocarditis. *J Am Coll Cardiol* 2002;39:1489–1495.

8. Heidenreich PA, Masoudi FA, Maini B, et al. Echocardiography in patients with suspected endocarditis: a cost-effectiveness analysis. *Am J Med* 1999;107:198–208.

9. Kuruppu JC, Corretti M, Mackowiak P, et al. Overuse of transthoracic echocardiography in the diagnosis of native valve endocarditis. *Arch Intern Med* 2002;162:1715–1720.

10. Spirito P, Rapezzi C, Bellone P, et al. Infective endocarditis in hypertrophic cardiomyopathy: prevalence, incidence, and indications of antibiotic prophylaxis. *Circulation* 1999;99:2132–2137.

11. DeCastro S, Cartoni D, d'Amati G, et al. Diagnostic accuracy of transthoracic and multi-plane transesophageal echocardiography for valvular perforation in acute infective endocarditis: correlation with anatomic findings. *Clin Infect Dis* 2000;30:825–826.

12. Choussat R, Thomas D, Isnard R, et al. Peri-valvular abscesses associated with endocarditis; clinical features and prognostic factors of overall survival in series of 233 cases. Perivalvular Abscesses French Multi-centre Study. *Eur Heart J* 1999;20:232–241.

13. Knosalla C, Weng Y, Yankah AC, et al. Surgical treatment of active infective aortic valve endocarditis with associated peri-annular abscess: 11-year results. *Eur Heart J* 2000;21:490–497.

14. Soejima H, Ogawa H, Hirai N, et al. Infective endocarditis with perivalvular pseudoaneurysm. *Circ J* 2002;66:211–212.

15. Esen AM, Kucukoglu MS, Okcun B, et al. Transesophageal echocardiographic diagnosis of aortico-left atrial fistula in aortic valve endocarditis. *Eur J Echocardiog* 2003;4:221–222.

16. Novak PG, Isserow S, Gudas V, et al. Transesophageal echocardiographic identification of an aortic root to right atrial fistula in a patient with acute streptococcal aortic valve bacterial endocarditis. *J Am Soc Echocardiogr* 2003;16:497–498.

17. Zamorano J, Sanz J, Moreno R, et al. Better prognosis of elderly patients with infectious endocarditis in the era of routine echocardiography and nonrestrictive indications for valve surgery. *J Am Soc Echocardiogr* 2002;15:702–707.

18. Mier-Ewert HK, Gray ME, John RM. Endocardial pacemaker or defibrillator leads with infected vegetations: a single-center experience and consequences of transvenous extraction. *Am Heart J* 2003;146:339–344.

19. Roldan CA, Shively BK, Crawford MH. Valve excrescences: prevalence, evolution and risk for cardioembolism. *J Am Coll Cardiol* 1997;30:1308–1314.

20. Roldan CA, Shively BK, Crawford MH. An echocardiographic study of valvular heart disease associated with systemic lupus erythematosus. *N Engl J Med* 1996;335:1424–1430.

21. Vasan RS, Shrivastava S, Vijayakumar M, et al. Echocardiographic evaluation of patients with acute rheumatic fever and rheumatic carditis. *Circulation* 1996;94:73.

22. Yee HC, Nwosu JE, Lii AD, et al. Echocardiographic features of papillary fibroelastoma and their consequences and management. *Am J Cardiol* 1997;80:811–814.

23. Habib G. Embolic risk in subacute bacterial endocarditis: determinants and role of transesophageal echocardiography. *Curr Cardiol Rep* 2003;5:129–136.

24. Lee R, Moon MR. Homograft valve repair for recurrent prosthetic valve endocarditis. *J Thorac Cardiovasc Surg* 2003;125:725–727.

25. Avila WS, Rossi EG, Ramires JA, et al. Pregnancy in patients with heart disease: experience with 1,000 cases. *Clin Cardiol* 2003;26:135–142.

14

Intracardiac Masses and Systemic Embolism

Gerald A. Charlton

- Acute neurologic ischemic syndromes and suspected peripheral emboli account for a substantial number of referrals to the echocardiography (echo) laboratory.
- Approximately 600,000 patients experience new or recurrent strokes every year, and approximately 14% of patients who survive a first stroke or transient ischemic attack will have a recurrence within 1 year (1).
- It has been estimated that a cardioembolic mechanism is responsible for approximately 20% of ischemic strokes, with another 30% to 40% being labeled as "cryptogenic," many of which may have an underlying cardiac etiology (2,3).
- Echo, both transthoracic (TTE) and transesophageal (TEE), is useful for identifying and characterizing abnormal cardiac masses (tumors, thrombi, and vegetations), as well as potential substrates for thrombus formation or embolization, or both (Table 14-1) (2–4).
- More difficult than finding an abnormality on TTE or TEE that may represent a potential source of embolus is deciding how such findings should alter therapy in an effort to reduce the risk of a recurrent event (5).

ECHOCARDIOGRAPHY

Class I and IIa Indications for Echocardiography in Patients with Neurologic Events or Other Vascular Occlusive Events

- Both TTE and TEE are useful in the evaluation of possible cardiac sources of emboli (Tables 14-2 and 14-3) (2,6).

- TEE is more sensitive for detecting possible cardiac sources of embolism in patients with cerebral ischemia of uncertain etiology.
- The use of TEE in patients with known cardiac disease and underlying indications for chronic anticoagulation (i.e., atrial fibrillation) is questionable, however.
- The most therapeutic benefit of echo appears to be in younger patients without known cardiovascular disease and in older patients with cardiovascular disease, such as hypertension and coronary artery disease, but no concurrent indication for anticoagulation (7).

Characterization of Cardiac Masses and Tumors

- Definitive tissue characterization of cardiac masses cannot be made by echo alone.
- When integrated with the clinical situation, however, information from echo can limit the possible diagnoses and help characterize the mass as a probable tumor, thrombus, or vegetation (Table 14-4).

TABLE 14-1. *Sources of Emboli*

Definite	Probable	Possible
Left ventricular thrombus	Left ventricular aneurysm	Atrial septal aneurysm
Left atrial thrombus	Spontaneous echo contrast	Patent foramen ovale
Vegetations	Cardiomyopathy	
Aortic atheroma		
Cardiac tumors		
Atrial fibrillation		

TABLE 14-2. *Indications for Echocardiography in Patients with Neurologic Events or Other Vascular Occlusive Events*

Clinical scenario	Class
Patients of any age with abrupt occlusion of a major peripheral or visceral artery	I
Younger patients (typically <45 yr) with cerebrovascular events	I
Older patients (typically >45 yr) with neurologic events without evidence of cerebrovascular disease or other obvious cause	I
Patients for whom a clinical therapeutic decision (anticoagulation, etc.) depends on the results of echocardiography	I
Patients with suspicion of embolic disease and with cerebrovascular disease of questionable significance	IIa

From Cheitlin MD, Armstrong WF, Aurigemma GP, et al. ACC/AHA/ASE 2003 guideline update for the application of echocardiography: a report of the American College of Cardiology/American Heart Association Task Force on Practice Guidelines (ACC/AHA/ASE Committee to Update the 1997 Guidelines for the Clinical Application of Echocardiography), 2003, with permission. Available at www.acc.org/clinical/guidelines/echo/index.pdf.

Intraoperative and Periprocedural Echocardiography

- Preoperative echo, especially TEE, is important for planning a surgical approach.
- It is important to define the site of attachment; identify involvement of other structures, such as valve leaflets; and exclude multiple masses.
- TEE is of important diagnostic value for the exclusion of left atrial thrombi before cardioversion in selected patients with atrial fibrillation/flutter and in patients undergoing valvuloplasty for mitral stenosis (8).
- In patients undergoing coronary bypass grafting, intraoperative TEE detection of significant ascending aorta or aortic arch atheromatous disease may alter the site of aortic cannulation and prevent perioperative cerebrovascular events (9).

Follow-Up in Patients with Cardiac Masses and Substrate for or Prior Embolism

- Postoperative echo should document complete excision of cardiac masses.
- Long-term follow-up depends on likelihood of tumor recurrence.

Pitfall

Numerous normal structures may be mistaken for abnormal cardiac masses (Table 14-5).

SPECIFIC EMBOLIC CONDITIONS

Transient Ischemic Attack

Transient ischemic attack is sudden onset of a focal neurologic deficit that resolves spontaneously in ≤24 hours.

Ischemic Stroke

- Ischemic stroke is an acute neurologic injury that persists >24 hours and is caused by local vascular disease or emboli from the heart or a more proximal vessel.

TABLE 14-3. *Recommendations of the Canadian Task Force on Preventive Health Care: Screening for Potential Cardioembolic Sources in Patients with Stroke*

Clinical scenario	Level of evidence	Recommendation
Patients with clinical cardiac disease and no preexisting indications for anticoagulation	Case-control and cross-sectional studies	Fair evidence to recommend echocardiography in this group. Transesophageal echocardiography is preferred initial screening test.
Patients with preexisting indications for anticoagulation or contraindications for anticoagulation	Case-control and cross-sectional studies	Fair evidence to recommend against echocardiography in this patient group.
Patients without clinical cardiac disease	Case-control and cross-sectional studies	Insufficient evidence to recommend for or against echocardiography in this group.

From Kapral MK, Silver FL, with the Canadian Task Force on Preventive Health Care. Preventive health care, 1999 update: 2. Echocardiography for the detection of a cardiac source of embolus in patients with stroke. *CMAJ* 1999;161:989–996, with permission.

TABLE 14-4. *Distinguishing Characteristics of Intracardiac Masses*

Characteristic	Thrombus	Tumor	Vegetation
Location	Left atrial appendage when associated with atrial fibrillation/flutter and mitral stenosis Left atrial body with mitral stenosis and prosthetic mitral valves LV with anterior wall MI and/or left ventricular aneurysm Less frequently with severe global left ventricular systolic dysfunction	LA (myxomas) on fossa ovale area Myocardium Pericardium Valves	Usually on valvular leaflets' coaptation point (atrial side for atrioventricular valves and ventricular side for semilunar valves) Occasionally on ventricular side of anterior mitral leaflet (when aortic valve involvement and AR), ventricular septal wall (in HOCM), chordae tendinea, or Chiari network
Appearance	Usually discrete, oval, multilobar, flat or well-layered, or pedunculated	Variable	Recently formed are soft tissue echoreflectant; are commonly oval, sessile, or pedunculated; and have independent rotatory motion
Associated findings	Underlying etiology usually evident Left ventricular systolic dysfunction or segmental wall motion abnormalities (exception: eosinophilic heart disease)	Intracardiac obstruction, depending on the site of tumor Systemic nonspecific manifestations	Valvular regurgitation usually present Leaflet perforation, leaflet pseudoaneurysm, chordal rupture, aortic root or myocardial abscesses Systemic signs of endocarditis and positive blood cultures Hypercoagulability, malignancy, or connective tissue diseases

AR, aortic regurgitation; HOCM, hypertrophic obstructive cardiomyopathy; LA, left atrium; LV, left ventricle; MI, myocardial infarction.

■ Ischemic stroke excludes hemorrhagic stroke.

Peripheral Embolism

Peripheral embolism is an arterial embolism to a limb or visceral artery originating from a more proximal artery (most commonly the aorta) or the heart.

Paradoxical Embolism

Paradoxical embolism is an arterial embolism that originates in the venous system and gains access to the arterial system via an arteriovenous malformation or intracardiac shunt.

CARDIAC MASSES

Definition

A cardiac mass is an abnormal cardiac structure, such as a tumor, vegetation, or thrombus.

Cardiac Tumors

Cardiac tumors are benign or malignant masses that originate in the heart (primary) or at a distant site and spread to the heart (secondary).

Primary Cardiac Tumors

Myxoma

Definition

Myxoma is the most common cardiac tumor and is benign. It may present with mitral valve obstruction, embolization, or constitutional symptoms.

Diagnostic Methods

■ Myxoma can be identified with TTE, but TEE is indicated to further evaluate location, size, shape, and number of tumors, as well as planning of surgical resection.

TABLE 14-5. *Normal Variants That May Mimic Abnormal Cardiac Masses*[a]

Right ventricle	Moderator band
	Pacemaker leads or catheters
Right atrium	Eustachian valve
	Chiari network
	Pectinate muscles
	Pacemaker leads or catheters
	Lipomatous hypertrophy of the inter-atrial septum
	Fat in tricuspid annulus
	Prominent folds of the superior atrial wall
Left ventricle	Prominent bridging trabeculations
Left atrium	Prominent ridge formed by the junction of the left upper pulmonary vein and lateral wall of atrial appendage
	Pectinate muscles
	Suture line in cardiac transplant patients

[a]See also normal variants in Chapter 1.

- If the tumor obstructs valvular flow, elevated Doppler velocities will be found, mimicking mitral valvular stenosis.

Key Diagnostic Features

- Myxoma occurs mostly in the left atrium (LA) near the fossa ovalis and has a pedunculated, short stalk. It can also arise from the right atrium (RA), left ventricle (LV), or multiple sites.
- It is classically found in the LA during systole, and when large, it prolapses into the mitral orifice in diastole.
- It has heterogeneous echogenicity with occasional calcifications.

Papillary Fibroelastoma

Definition
Papillary fibroelastomas are usually small tumors (≤1 cm) on the mitral or aortic valve, but they may be found on other endocardial surfaces.

Key Diagnostic Features

- Papillary fibroelastomas are usually found on the downstream side of the valve (10).
- They consist of multiple fronds attached to the point of coaptation of the involved valve by a short stalk.

- The underlying valve structure and function is generally normal.
- They are usually diagnosed incidentally or after embolic complications.

Pitfall
Papillary fibroelastoma may be difficult to distinguish from a vegetation.

Other Benign Tumors

Fibromas
Key diagnostic features

- Fibromas are found in the ventricular myocardium.
- They are usually in the septum or anterior free wall.
- Fibromas measure 3 to 10 cm in size, with central calcification.

Pitfall
Fibromas may be confused with rhabdomyomas.

Lipomas
Key diagnostic features
Lipomas occur throughout the heart, in the subepicardium or subendocardium, but mostly in the LV and RA, and are of variable size (1–15 cm).

Prognosis
Fibromas and lipomas are not associated with systemic embolization.

Malignant Cardiac Tumors

- Mesotheliomas, angiosarcomas, fibrosarcomas, and rhabdomyosarcomas are rare, and not associated with embolization.
- Usually begin as intramural tumors, but rapidly extend into the pericardium or cardiac chambers, or both.

Secondary Cardiac Tumors

Definition

- Secondary cardiac tumors are those that originate from another primary site other than the heart.
- They are actually more common than primary cardiac tumors (20–40:1).

Key Diagnostic Features

- Secondary cardiac tumors typically involve the pericardium, leading to pericardial masses and effusion, but they may involve the myocardium or chambers.
- Primary sites include lung, breast, thyroid, esophageal, renal, and melanoma, as well as leukemia and lymphoma.
- They usually appear late in the course of disease.

Intracardiac Thrombi

Definition

Intracardiac thrombi are an abnormal collection of platelets, fibrin, and red blood cells.

Etiology

- Intracardiac thrombi tend to occur where there is low-velocity blood flow or stasis.
- They can be seen in the LV, the LA, on prosthetic heart valves, and in the right heart.

Diagnostic Methods and Accuracy

- TTE has a >90% sensitivity and >85% specificity for detection of left ventricular thrombi and is probably superior to the sensitivity and specificity of TEE, especially for apical thrombi (Fig. 14-1).
- TTE sensitivity is higher with the use of 3.5-MHz and 5.0-MHz transducers, harmonic imaging, and left ventricular cavity-enhancing contrast agents (Fig. 14-1C).
- In some patients, TTE is limited secondary to poor endocardial resolution, chronic lung disease, or obesity. Such patients may require TEE to help identify and define ventricular thrombi.
- Atrial thrombi require TEE for diagnosis, with the appendage best seen at 30 to 40 degrees of rotation from the basilar short-axis view.

Key Diagnostic Features

Left Ventricular Thrombi

- Occur predominantly (>90%) within the first week after an ST-elevation myocardial infarction (MI), with a higher incidence in anterior

than inferior or lateral MI (>20% vs./1%, respectively) (Fig. 14-1) (11).
- Occur most commonly at the apex of the LV in association with an apical aneurysm, apical wall akinesis or dyskinesis, a high (>1.5) wall motion score index, high left ventricular end-systolic and end-diastolic volumes, or an ejection fraction ≤40%.
- Appears as a distinctive left ventricular mass of oval, multilobar, sessile, flat (mimics endocardium), or (usually mobile) pedunculated shape.
- A recent thrombus has similar echoreflectance to that of the myocardium (Fig. 14-1B), in contrast to an old thrombus with heterogeneously increased echoreflectance and, rarely, calcification (Fig. 14-1A).
- With cavity-enhancing contrast, a thrombus appears as a discrete-filling defect in continuity with abnormal (akinetic or dyskinetic) endocardium (Fig. 14-1C), whereas a bridging trabeculation surrounded by contrast appears as a linear-filling defect that separates from a normal or abnormal endocardium during systole (Fig. 14-2).

Left Atrial Thrombi

- Frequently associated with atrial spontaneous echo contrast or "smoke" (Fig. 14-3A,B) (8).
- Usually are found in the appendage in association with atrial fibrillation or flutter, mitral stenosis, or prosthetic mitral valve (Fig. 14-3C).
- Are of soft tissue echoreflectance, irregular shape, and variable size.
- Low atrial velocities (≤40 cm/sec) in those with atrial fibrillation or flutter are predictive of thrombus formation and future embolic events (Fig. 14-3D).

Prognosis

Ventricular or atrial thrombi, especially if pedunculated and mobile, are associated with a high risk of cardioembolism.

Pitfalls

- LV-bridging trabeculations or false tendons are normal variants that can be differentiated

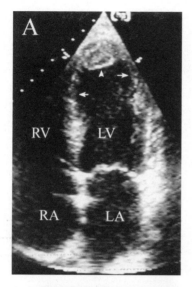

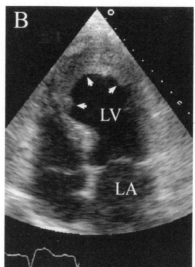

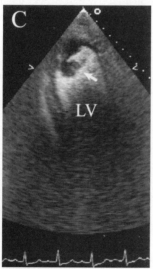

FIG. 14-1. Left ventricular apical thrombi. Oval **(A)** (*arrowhead*) with heterogeneous echoreflectance and underlying thin and akinetic walls (*arrows*), layered **(B)** (*arrows*) with homogeneous soft tissue echoreflectance and associated large left ventricular aneurysm, and bilobar **(C)** (*arrow*) apical thrombus enhanced by a cavity-enhancing contrast agent. All three patients had had anteroapical myocardial infarctions. LA, left atrium; LV, left ventricle; RA, right atrium; RV, right ventricle.

from left ventricular thrombi by the following features (Figs. 14-2 and 1-8A):

◆ Linear or band-like fibromuscular structures traversing the left ventricular cavity in variable directions, more commonly seen in the distal one-third of the LV and apex, single or multiple, more commonly extend from lateral wall to interventricular septum, and are more echoreflectant than the myocardium.

◆ Their separation from the endocardium during systole (forming a systolic slack) and underlying normal inward wall motion and

endocardial thickening also help to differentiate them from thrombi.

■ Pectinate muscles are normal appendage structures that can be differentiated from irregularly shaped masses typical of thrombi by the following features:

◆ Muscle ridges that extend from the lateral to medial wall of the left atrial appendage, appear as nonmobile linear projections of the appendage wall, may or may not traverse the entire appendage cavity, and have similar echoreflectance to that of the appendage wall (see Fig. 1-8B).

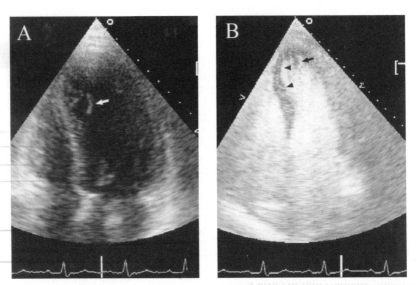

FIG. 14-2. A: Bridging trabeculation (*arrow*) in a patient with an apical myocardial infarction. **B:** Trabeculation is enhanced by an intravenous contrast agent (*arrow*). Also, note apical septal akinesis (*arrowheads*).

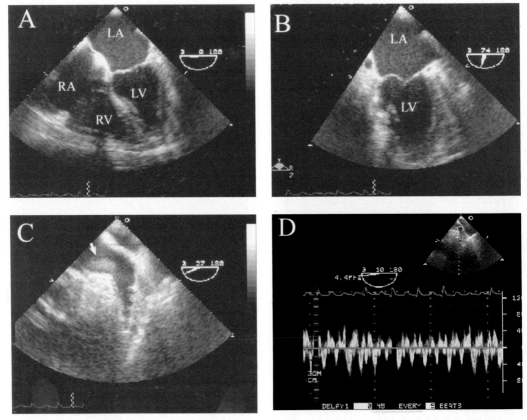

FIG. 14-3. Left atrial thrombi and substrate for thrombus formation. Left atrial spontaneous echocardiography contrast **(A,B)**, left atrial appendage thrombi **(C)**, and low atrial appendage velocities **(D)**. LA, left atrium; LV, left ventricle; RA, right atrium; RV, right ventricle.

Vegetations

Definition

Vegetations are masses composed of microorganisms, platelets, fibrin, and red blood cells, usually attached to valvular structures.

Etiology

- Although vegetations are the *sine qua non* of infective endocarditis, nonbacterial thrombotic vegetations are seen in patients with connective tissue diseases, hypercoagulable states, or malignancy.
- Libman-Sacks vegetations are characteristic of systemic lupus erythematosus.

Diagnostic Methods and Accuracy

- Vegetations can rarely be identified using M-mode echo but are better defined with two-dimensional imaging.
- TEE has high sensitivity and specificity of >95%, whereas TTE has a similar specificity but lower sensitivity of only 45% to 60%.

Key Diagnostic Features

- Vegetations are usually located at the leaflets' coaptation point on the atrial side of atrioventricular valves and on the ventricular side of semilunar valves (Fig. 14-4) (12).
- They are of variable size but generally are >3 mm. Large vegetations are >10 mm.
- They are of variable shape, most commonly globular, but they can be polypoid, tubular, frond-like, elongated, pedunculated, and unilobulated or multilobulated.
- Recent vegetations have homogeneous soft tissue echoreflectance similar to that of the myocardium. Less frequently, they are heterogeneous in appearance. Highly echoreflectant, partially or completely calcified vegetations denote chronic and healed lesions.
- Generally, they are pedunculated or prolapsing masses with independent rotatory mobility.

Prognosis

- Large (>10 mm), recently formed, hypermobile, and mitral valve vegetations have a

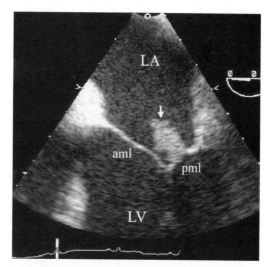

FIG. 14-4. Infective vegetation. Large homogeneously soft tissue echoreflectant vegetation on the posterior mitral valve leaflet (pml) in a patient with multiple embolic events to the central nervous system. aml, anterior mitral leaflet; LA, left atrium; LV, left ventricle.

higher incidence of embolism (odds ratio, 2.8) (13–15).
- Nonbacterial thrombotic or Libman-Sacks vegetations are associated with cardioembolism, independent of their size.

Valve Excrescences

Definition

Valve excrescences are normal structures called *valve* or *Lambl's excrescences* or *fibrin strands*.

Etiology

The constant bending and buckling of the valve leaflets lead to tearing of subendocardial collagen and elastic fibers, which subsequently endothelialize.

Diagnostic Methods

Valve excrescences are detected almost exclusively by TEE in 35% to 40% of apparently healthy subjects, in 45% to 50% of patients undergoing TEE for reasons other than suspected cardioembolism, and in 40% of those undergoing TEE for suspected cardioembolism.

Key Diagnostic Features

- Valve excrescences are thin (up to 2 mm in width), elongated (up to 16 mm in length), and hypermobile (16).
- They are seen mainly at the coaptation point of the aortic or mitral valves' leaflets.
- Those on the aortic valve prolapse to the left ventricular outflow tract during diastole, and those on the mitral valve prolapse into the LA during systole (see Fig. 1-9A).

Prognosis

- Valve excrescences appear to be stable over time.
- They are probably not associated with increased risk of embolization (16).

Pitfall

Large or multiple excrescences may be mistaken for valvular vegetations.

CARDIAC SUBSTRATES FOR THROMBUS FORMATION, EMBOLIZATION, OR BOTH

Definition

A cardiac substrate is not a definitive source of an embolism but is an abnormality that may predispose to thrombus formation or embolization.

Myocardial Infarction

Definition

MI is defined as myocardial necrosis.

Etiology

- MI is usually due to underlying atherosclerosis and abrupt occlusion of a coronary artery.
- Infrequently, it can result from severe coronary vasospasm.
- It is rarely due to *in situ* thrombosis without atherosclerosis or from thromboembolism.

Diagnostic Methods

Diagnostic methods for MI include a combination of clinical history of chest discomfort (angina), diagnostic electrocardiogram changes, and elevated cardiac markers.

Prognosis

Risk of stroke or systemic embolization is higher if MI is associated with atrial fibrillation or a large wall motion abnormality, or both, especially of the anterior wall (Fig. 14-1).

Left Ventricular Aneurysm

Definition

Left ventricular aneurysm is an abnormal, dyskinetic, thin, and scarred region of the LV with an abnormal "bulge" or outpouching during diastole (Fig. 14-1B). Incidence is 8% to 22%.

Etiology

- Left ventricular aneurysm occurs generally within the first week of an MI.
- It is located predominantly (>90%) at the apex after an anterior MI with adverse remodeling of the LV.

Diagnostic Method and Accuracy

Left ventricular aneurysm can be identified by TTE with a sensitivity of >90% (11).

Prognosis

Left ventricular aneurysm is associated with increased risk for thrombus formation and in-hospital and 1-year mortality.

Cardiomyopathy

Definition

Cardiomyopathy is abnormal left ventricular systolic function, usually in the setting of a dilated LV.

Etiology

- Cardiomyopathy is commonly secondary to coronary artery disease, MI, and subsequent aneurysm formation.
- It can be seen as dilated nonischemic cardiomyopathy with severely depressed left ventricular systolic function.

Prognosis

- Anticoagulation for dilated cardiomyopathy without identified thrombus is controversial.
- No randomized clinical trials have been conducted.

Left Atrial/Left Ventricular Pseudocontrast

Definition

- Left atrial/left ventricular pseudocontrast is also called *spontaneous echo contrast.*
- Abnormal "smoke" is seen in cardiac chambers.

Etiology

- Left atrial/left ventricular pseudocontrast is caused by slow blood flow and rouleau formation by the red blood cells.
- It is seen in patients with atrial fibrillation or flutter and low left atrial appendage velocities (Fig. 14-3A,B,D).
- It also can be seen in the LV of patients with severe systolic dysfunction.

Diagnostic Methods

Left atrial/left ventricular pseudocontrast is best identified by TEE (Fig. 14-3A,B), but it can occasionally be seen with TTE (8).

Prognosis

Left atrial/left ventricular pseudocontrast is associated with the presence of thrombi and future embolism.

Aortic Atheroma

Definition

- Aortic atheroma is abnormally increased thickening of the intima of the aorta and is often associated with thrombi, fibrinous material, and cholesterol deposits.
- Aortic atheroma can be flat or sessile and protruding or mobile.
- It is predominantly seen in the aortic arch and descending thoracic aorta.
- Its prevalence in patients with systemic embolism ranges from 20% to 30%, as compared to 5% to 10% in matched controls.

- It may embolize spontaneously or secondary to invasive manipulation, such as during cardiac catheterization.

Diagnostic Methods and Accuracy

- TTE has limited sensitivity and specificity.
- Suprasternal views with harmonic imaging may have diagnostic value.
- TEE has high sensitivity and specificity. Contrast agents may increase diagnostic accuracy of TEE, especially for atheromas in the aortic arch.

Key Diagnostic Features

- Morphologic classifications are as follows (Fig. 14-5):
  - Simple atheroma: smooth; protrudes into the lumen <4 to 5 mm.
  - Complex atheromas: >4 to 5 mm thick, protruding, irregular, ulcerated, or with mobile debris.
  - Grade I: Minimal intimal thickening.
  - Grade II: Extensive intimal thickening.
  - Grade III: Sessile atheroma.
  - Grade IV: Protruding atheroma.
  - Grade V: Mobile atheroma.

Prognosis

- Patients with plaque thickness <1.0 mm, 1.0 to 3.9 mm, or ≥4 mm have odds ratios for emboli of 1.0, 3.9, and 13.8, respectively (4,17).
- Also, patients with plaques ≥4 mm have a >10% recurrence of stroke/year.
- Patients with aortic arch atheroma undergoing heart surgery requiring cardiopulmonary bypass have an approximately 12% incidence or a sixfold increased risk of stroke, as compared to those without atheroma.
  - If mobile plaques are seen in the descending aorta by TEE, up to 40% of patients may have intraoperative stroke or transient ischemic attack.

Patent Foramen Ovale

Definition

Patent foramen ovale (PFO) is an abnormal, small (<5 mm) communication between the LA and RA.

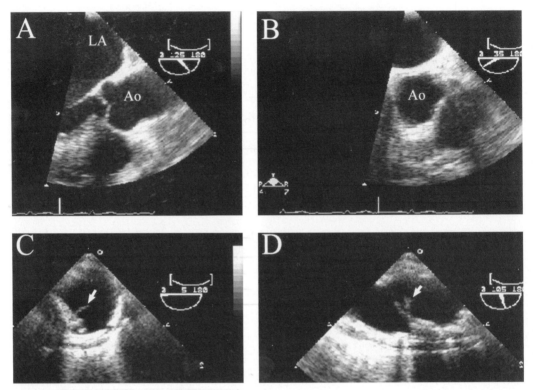

FIG. 14-5. Aortic atheroma. Note the contrasting normal appearance of the ascending aorta (Ao) **(A,B)** as compared with a complex, protruding atheroma with a hypermobile component in the proximal descending aorta (*arrows*) **(C,D)** in a patient with a retinal embolus. LA, left atrium.

Etiology

Failure of the septum secundum and septum primum to fuse causes PFO.

Prevalence

PFO is identified in 10% of the normal population by TTE and up to 30% by TEE; in patients with cryptogenic stroke, it is identified in up to 50%.

Diagnostic Methods and Accuracy

- PFO is diagnosed with TTE or TEE using color flow Doppler (at low Nyquist limit) or (more commonly) agitated saline contrast, or both, with TEE being more sensitive.
- PFO usually requires saline contrast for definitive diagnosis, which demonstrates presence of contrast bubbles in LA within three cardiac cycles of complete opacification of the right heart (Fig. 14-6).

Prognosis

- PFO can lead to abnormal right to left shunting if right atrial pressure exceeds left atrial pressure, either transiently or chronically (18,19).
- PFO is a potential source of paradoxical emboli.
- Four-year risk of recurrent stroke is approximately 2.3%, which is not significantly different from patients without this finding.

Atrial Septal Aneurysm

Definition

- Atrial septal aneurysm is characterized by hypermobile, redundant tissue in the interatrial septum in the region of the fossa ovalis.
- The base of the aneurysm is >15 mm, with a total excursion into the RA and LA exceeding 11 mm. The entire interatrial septum may be aneurysmal (Figs. 14-7 and 14-8).

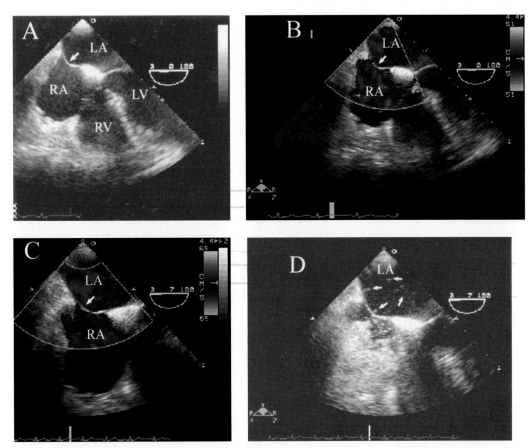

FIG. 14-6. Atrial septal aneurysm with patent foramen ovale. **A:** Transesophageal echocardiographic four-chamber view of an atrial septal aneurysm (*arrow*). **B,C:** No evidence of interatrial communication or patent foramen ovale was found by color Doppler with a Nyquist limit at 50–60 cm/sec at the atrial septal aneurysm (*arrows*). **D:** By saline contrast study, trivial amount of bubbles was seen crossing into the left atrium (LA) (*arrows*). LV, left ventricle; RA, right atrium; RV, right ventricle.

- Frequently (>70%) associated with a PFO.
- May serve as potential source of emboli, independent of association with PFO.

Prevalence

Atrial septal aneurysm occurs in 1% to 5% of the healthy population and up to 22% of patients with cryptogenic stroke.

Diagnostic Methods

- Atrial septal aneurysm is best identified on TTE using the subcostal or apical four-chamber view and on TEE using the four-chamber view from the mid-esophageal transverse plane.

- Agitated saline contrast injection is indicated to evaluate for PFO, which worsens the prognosis (Fig. 14-6).
- Saline contrast study in combination with transcranial Doppler is currently used for detection of characteristic Doppler velocity patterns suggestive of microemboli (from bubbles traversing into the LA and systemic circulation) (20).

Prognosis

- Four-year risk of recurrent stroke in patients with isolated atrial septal aneurysm is low for patients taking aspirin, and it is not significantly different when compared to subjects without these findings (18,19,21).

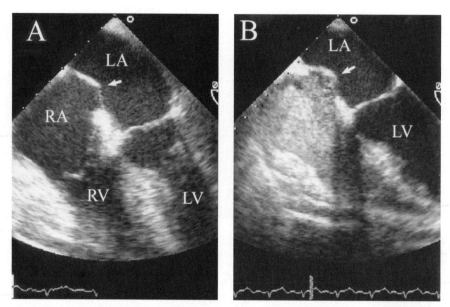

FIG. 14-7. Atrial septal aneurysm. **A:** Transesophageal echocardiographic four-chamber view of an atrial septal aneurysm (*arrows*) with no evidence of patent foramen ovale by saline contrast study **(B)**. LA, left atrium; LV, left ventricle; RA, right atrium; RV, right ventricle.

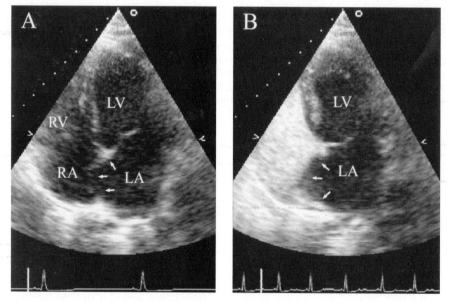

FIG. 14-8. Atrial septal aneurysm. **A,B:** Atrial septal aneurysm of the entire septum (*arrows*). **B:** No evidence of interatrial communication by saline contrast study. LA, left atrium; LV, left ventricle; RA, right atrium; RV, right ventricle.

■ Four-year risk of recurrent stroke in patients with atrial septal aneurysm and PFO is high (15.2%), with a hazard ratio of 4.17 when compared to subjects without these findings, even when patients are given aspirin.

■ There is low risk of cerebrovascular events or embolic stroke when atrial septal aneurysm is found incidentally.

REFERENCES

1. American Heart Association. 2000 Heart and Stroke Statistical Update. Dallas: American Heart Association, 1999.
2. Kapral MK, Silver FL, with the Canadian Task Force on Preventive Health Care. Preventive health care, 1999 update: 2. Echocardiography for the detection of a cardiac source of embolus in patients with stroke. *CMAJ* 1999;161:989–996.
3. O'Brien PJ, Thiemann DR, McNamara RL, et al. Usefulness of transesophageal echocardiography in predicting mortality and morbidity in stroke patients without clinically known cardiac sources of embolus. *Am J Cardiol* 1998;81:1144–1151.
4. Tunick PA, Nayar AC, Goodkin GM, et al. Effect of treatment on the incidence of stroke and other emboli in 519 patients with severe thoracic aortic plaque. *Am J Cardiol* 2002;90:1320–1325.
5. Wolf PA, Clagett P, Easton D, et al. Preventing ischemic stroke in patients with prior stroke and transient ischemic attack: a statement for healthcare professionals from the Stroke Council of the American Heart Association. *Stroke* 1999;30:1991–1994.
6. Cheitlin MD, Armstrong WF, Aurigemma GP, et al. ACC/AHA/ASE 2003 guideline update for the application of echocardiography: a report of the American College of Cardiology/American Heart Association Task Force on Practice Guidelines (ACC/AHA/ASE Committee to Update the 1997 Guidelines for the Clinical Application of Echocardiography), 2003. Available at www.acc.org/clinical/guidelines/echo/index.pdf.
7. Labovitz AJ for the STEPS Investigators. Transesophageal echocardiography and unexplained cerebral ischemia: a multicenter follow-up study. *Am Heart J* 1999;137:1082–1087.
8. Seidl K, Rameken M, Rogemuller A, et al. Embolic events in patients with atrial fibrillation and effective anticoagulation: value of transesophageal echocardiography to guide direct-current cardioversion: final results of the Ludwigshafen Observation Cardioversion Study. *J Am Coll Cardiol* 2002;29:1436–1442.
9. Schwammenthal E, Schwammenthal Y, Tanne D, et al. Transcutaneous detection of aortic arch atheromas by suprasternal harmonic imaging. *J Am Coll Cardiol* 2002;39:1127–1132.
10. Yee HC, Nwosu JE, Lii AD, et al. Echocardiographic features of papillary fibroelastoma and their consequences and management. *Am J Cardiol* 1997;80:811–814.
11. Neskovic AN, Marinkovic J, Bojic M, et al. Predictors of left ventricular thrombus formation and disappearance after anterior wall myocardial infarction. *Eur Heart J* 1998;19:908–916.
12. Heidenreich PA, Masoudi FA, Maini B, et al. Echocardiography in patients with suspected endocarditis: a cost-effectiveness analysis. *Am J Med* 1999;107:198–208.
13. Vilacosta I, Graupner C, San Roman JA, et al. Risk of embolization after institution of antibiotic therapy for infective endocarditis. *J Am Coll Cardiol* 2002;39:1489–1495.
14. Zamorano J, Sanz J, Moreno R, et al. Better prognosis of elderly patients with infectious endocarditis in the era of routine echocardiography and nonrestrictive indications for valve surgery. *J Am Soc Echocardiogr* 2002;15:702–707.
15. Habib G. Embolic risk in subacute bacterial endocarditis: determinants and role of transesophageal echocardiography. *Curr Cardiol Rep* 2003;5:129–136.
16. Roldan CA, Shively BK, Crawford MH. Valve excrescences: prevalence, evolution and risk for cardioembolism. *J Am Coll Cardiol* 1997;30:1308–1314.
17. Donnan GA, Davis SM, Jones EF, et al. Aortic source of brain embolism. *Curr Treat Options Cardiovasc Med* 2003;5:211–219.
18. Mas J-L, Arquizan C, Lamy C, et al. Recurrent cerebrovascular events associated with patent foramen ovale, atrial septal aneurysm, or both. *N Engl J Med* 2001;345:1740–1746.
19. Rodriguez CJ, Homma S, Sacco RL, et al. Race-ethnic differences in patent foramen ovale, atrial septal aneurysm, and right atrial anatomy among ischemic stroke patients. *Stroke* 2003;34:2097–2102.
20. Zanchetta M, Rigatelli G, Onorato E. Intracardiac echocardiography and transcranial Doppler ultrasound to guide closure of patent foramen ovale. *J Invasive Cardiol* 2003;15:93–96.
21. Burger AJ, Sherman HB, Charlamb MJ. Low incidence of embolic strokes with atrial septal aneurysms: a prospective, long-term study. *Am Heart J* 2000;139:149–152.

15

Diseases of the Aorta

Robert J. Siegel and Takashi Miyamoto

- Most chronic disorders of the aorta are without symptoms. Approximately 40% of patients with ascending aortic aneurysm are asymptomatic, as are most patients with Marfan syndrome, pseudoaneurysm, and sinus of Valsalva aneurysms.
- Aortic atheromatosis is also asymptomatic until acutely manifested with a transient ischemic attack, stroke, or peripheral embolism.
- Acute aortic disorders (aortic dissection and rupture, intramural hematoma, and penetrating aortic ulcer) generally present with severe chest pain that usually radiates to the back, retrosternal or interscapular pain, dyspnea, dysphagia, or extremity pain.
  - ◆ Aortic dissection, rupture of aortic sinus of Valsalva, or trauma with flail aortic cusps may result in severe acute aortic regurgitation (AR) and acute severe heart failure.
- The physical examination in chronic or acute disorders of the aorta is nonspecific, nonsensitive, and therefore of limited diagnostic value.

CLASS I INDICATIONS FOR ECHOCARDIOGRAPHY IN AORTIC DISEASES

Transthoracic echocardiography (TTE) and particularly transesophageal echocardiography (TEE) are of important diagnostic value in patients with aortic diseases (Table 15-1) (1–5).

M-MODE AND TWO-DIMENSIONAL ECHOCARDIOGRAPHY

Imaging of the Aorta

Ascending Aorta: Best Imaging Planes

The ascending aorta begins at the aortic valve and extends 5 to 6 cm to the junction with the aortic arch.

Transthoracic Echocardiography

- M-mode parasternal long-axis and short-axis view by two-dimensional guidance.
- Two-dimensional left parasternal long-axis and short-axis view and suprasternal view.
- Apical five-chamber view with anterior angulation of the transducer.
- Right parasternal long-axis view.
- Sometimes subcostal imaging.
- Enhance imaging of superior portion of ascending aorta by moving transducer to higher interspaces [origin of aorta beneath third left intercostal space (ICS) and courses toward second right ICS].
- Enhance image quality with steeper left lateral decubitus position (brings aorta closer to chest wall).
- Apical five-chamber view allows assessment of flow by pulse Doppler.
- Suprasternal view allows high-quality pulse Doppler antegrade flow.

Transesophageal Echocardiography

- Multiplane probe at angle of 120 to 135 degrees generally allows assessment of long axis of

TABLE 15-1. *Class I Indications for Echocardiography in Thoracic Aortic Diseases*

Aortic dissection, diagnosis, location, and extent.[a]

Aortic aneurysm.

Aortic intramural hematoma.[a]

Aortic rupture.[a]

Aortic root dilatation in Marfan syndrome or other connective tissue syndromes.

Degenerative or traumatic aortic disease with clinical atheroembolism.[a]

Follow-up of aortic dissection, especially when complication or progression is suspected.[a]

First-degree relative of a patient with Marfan syndrome or other connective tissue disorder.

The hemodynamically unstable multiple-injury patient without obvious chest trauma but with a mechanism of injury suggesting potential cardiac or aortic injury (deceleration or crush).[a]

Widening of the mediastinum and postinjury-suspected aortic injury.[a]

Follow-up study on victims of serious blunt or penetrating trauma.

Surgical repair of aortic dissection with possible aortic valve involvement and valve replacement requiring homografts or coronary reimplantation (intraoperative).

[a]Transesophageal echocardiography is the sonographic technique of choice for these conditions.

aorta from aortic valve to just below innominate artery (may image up to 10 cm of aorta).

- Short-axis views at 0 to 30 degrees. The aortic segments just beneath the arch cannot be visualized due to the trachea being interposed between the ascending aorta and the esophagus.
- A deep transgastric approach can visualize the ascending aorta. Multiplane imaging at 0, 90, and 120 degrees allows images of the proximal 3 to 5 cm of ascending aorta.

Epiaortic Imaging (Intraoperative)

- Imaging of ascending aorta by direct application of transducer on aorta in sterile sheath.
- Primarily used to reduce intraoperative stroke risk by identifying sites of significant atherosclerosis or atheroma and to choose sites for aortic cannulation or cross-clamping.
- Epiaortic guidance of aortic cannulation and cross-clamping to reduce intraoperative stroke risk.
- More accurate than TEE for detection and assessment of ascending aortic atherosclerosis.
- Sensitivity and specificity for ascending atherosclerosis are 100%, compared to TEE sen-

sitivity and specificity of 100% and 60%, respectively.

- **Pitfalls**
  - Needs to be done intraoperatively and under sterile conditions.
  - Potential for contamination of surgical field.
  - Logistics are more complex than intraoperative TEE.
  - Need to use stand-off for epiaortic probe to visualize the aortic wall (e.g., sterile, saline-filled bag or glove).

Aortic Arch: Best Imaging Planes

The aortic arch begins beneath the upper edge of the second right ICS and joins the descending thoracic aorta posterior to the fourth ICS.

Transthoracic Echocardiography

- TEE imaging is best from the suprasternal notch. By scanning with transducer inferoposterolateral (left), imaging plane aligns with long axis of aortic arch (left carotid to the right, innominate artery to the left). The right pulmonary artery is beneath the aortic arch.
- Nearness of suprasternal notch to aortic arch makes imaging routinely feasible, and left carotid and subclavian arteries are detected in 90% and innominate in 60% of cases (5), with both longitudinal and transverse planes.
- Right parasternal view may be useful.
- Right or left supraclavicular imaging of arch, or both, are also sometimes feasible.
- Doppler flow toward descending thoracic aorta.
- Normal systolic flow away from transducer is followed by early diastolic reversal (Fig. 15-1), mid-diastolic antegrade flow, and again reversal of flow at end-diastole.
- Low wall filters may be needed to detect normal Doppler flow pattern due to low-velocity diastolic flow.

Transesophageal Echocardiography

- Esophagus posterior to aorta at level of arch (Fig. 15-1).
- High esophageal imaging at 0 and 130 degrees with posterior and medial flexion yields longitudinal views of arch.
- Other multiplane views yield cross-sectional views at multiple levels.

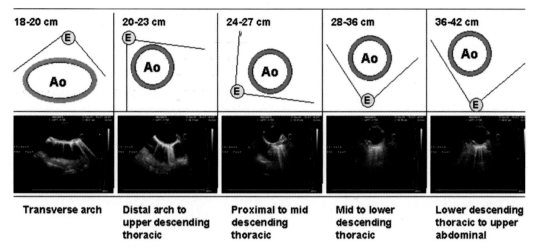

18-20 cm	20-23 cm	24-27 cm	28-36 cm	36-42 cm

Transverse arch	Distal arch to upper descending thoracic	Proximal to mid descending thoracic	Mid to lower descending thoracic	Lower descending thoracic to upper abdominal

FIG. 15-1. Aortic imaging. Transesophageal echocardiographic (TEE) images of aorta (Ao) and schematic showing relationship of esophagus to aorta at varying levels of the TEE probe from insertion site at the bite-block. TEE shows transverse scan plane at distance (in centimeters) from bite-block.

Epiaortic Imaging (Intraoperative)

Intraoperative epiaortic imaging is as described in Ascending Aorta.

Descending Thoracic Aorta: Best Imaging Planes

The descending thoracic aorta begins at the lower edge of fourth left ICS.

Transthoracic Echocardiography

- Parasternal long axis allows short-axis view of descending thoracic aorta seen beneath heart at the site of atrioventricular groove.
- Longitudinal view of aorta is obtained by lateral angulation and rightward rotation of transducer (feasible in >65% of cases).
- Apical two-chamber view with medial tilt of transducer.
- Subcostal view allows imaging of distal descending aorta and proximal abdominal aorta.
- In presence of left pleural effusion, imaging thoracic aorta from right lateral decubitus position is feasible.
- Doppler is best done from suprasternal notch due to parallel flow.

Transesophageal Echocardiography

- Aorta is posterolateral to esophagus (Fig. 15-1).

- Short-axis plane seen at 0 degrees and long-axis plane at 90 degrees.
- Comprehensive imaging from abdominal aorta to aortic arch is often best accomplished during "pull-back" of probe from the transgastric position, with probe inserted to 45 to 50 cm from bite-block to approximately 15 to 20 cm from bite-block.
- During pull-back, rotation is required to keep short-axis aortic images in the center of the screen due to aorta becoming more anterior and rightward as the probe is pulled in a cephalad direction.
- Flow is perpendicular to ultrasound. Thus, it is not possible to obtain accurate maximal Doppler flow velocities of aorta.
- In descending aorta in transverse view (0 degrees), color flow Doppler reflects counterclockwise swishing direction of blood flow. In a longitudinal view (90 degrees), color flow Doppler reveals red pattern toward head and blue toward diaphragm.

Intravascular Ultrasound

- Intravascular ultrasound (IVUS) uses catheters with high-frequency (20–40 MHz) miniature transducers to image within blood vessels (3).
- IVUS is used more commonly to image the descending thoracic aorta.
- IVUS yields high-resolution images.

- IVUS has documented utility in assessment of aortic dissection, trauma, aneurysm, and coarctation.
- IVUS is used for assessment and deployment of endovascular grafts for aneurysm, as well as dissection.
- **Pitfalls**
  - ◆ IVUS has no Doppler capability, no steerability, and limited penetration due to high frequency.
  - ◆ It requires fluoroscopy in the catheterization laboratory or a specialized operating room.
  - ◆ TTE should be the first choice in clinically stable situations to assess the ascending aorta.

Aortic Aneurysm

Definition

Aortic aneurysm is the dilatation of an aortic segment ≥1.5 times the normal diameter. The intimal, media, and adventitia all are present.

Normal Diameters

- Aortic annulus: 2.6 ± 0.3 cm in males and 2.3 ± 0.2 cm in females.
- Sinus of Valsalva: 3.4 ± 0.3 cm in males and 3.0 ± 0.3 cm in females.
- Ascending aorta: <3.7 cm, 1.4–2.1 cm/m^2, 2.9 ± 0.3 cm in males, and 2.6 ± 0.3 cm in females.
- Descending aorta: 1.0–1.6 cm/m.

Types

- Fusiform: Uniform dilatation of entire aortic circumference (75% of aneurysms).
- Saccular: Localized expansion resulting in a balloon-type (eccentric) dilatation of a segment of the wall with a narrow neck. Often contains clot within aortic lumen.

Etiology

Ascending Aorta

Etiology of an aortic aneurysm in the ascending aorta includes atherosclerosis (most common), hypertension, Marfan syndrome, bicuspid aortic valve, aortic coarctation, infection (syphilis, tuberculosis, salmonella), nonspecific aortitis, Turner's and Noonan's syndrome, familial aortic root dilatation, and annuloaortic ectasia.

Arch and Descending Aorta

The etiology of an aortic aneurysm in the arch and descending aorta includes atherosclerosis and Marfan syndrome.

Key Diagnostic Features

- TTE is adequate to detect and characterize ascending aortic aneurysms located at the sinuses and sinotubular positions (2,4,5).
- TEE is more accurate than TTE in detecting distal ascending aortic aneurysm and aneurysm of the arch and descending aorta.
  - ◆ Accurate for assessment of size and defining underlying aortic wall pathology (sclerosis, calcification, atherosclerosis, dissection).
  - ◆ Dilatation of aorta (>3.7 cm).
  - ◆ Systolic expansion of aorta.
  - ◆ Left atrial compression.
  - ◆ Aortic valve mid-systolic closure.
  - ◆ AR may be present.
- TEE transverse (0 degrees) and longitudinal planes (90 degrees) generally are best to define aneurysm shape, size, morphology, extent, and plaque size, as well as presence of thrombus.

Prognosis

- Five-year survival is related to diameter of ascending aorta: ≤6 cm is 61%, and >6 cm is 38%. The 5-year survival for descending thoracic aortic aneurysm with diameter >6 cm is 39%.
- In atherosclerotic aneurysm, the need for surgery has to be individualized due to comorbid diseases.
- The operative mortality rate ranges from 2% to 21%, and there is a high risk of rupture with aneurysm >6 cm.

Pitfalls

Transthoracic Echocardiography

TTE has limited sensitivity and specificity for aortic dimension due to tangential imaging and for aortic wall pathology due to distance from

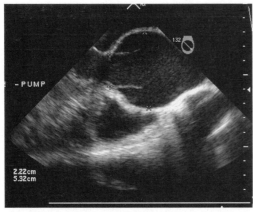
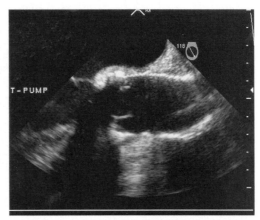

A   B

FIG. 15-2. Marfan syndrome. Transesophageal echocardiographic image of ascending aorta (long-axis, multiplane view) in a Marfan patient with marked dilatation of the aorta at the sinus of Valsalva **(A)**. **B:** After the post-Bentall procedure (composite conduit and valve prosthesis). The aortic conduit is visualized.

transducer, calcification in aorta, and limited windows (6).

Transesophageal Echocardiography

TEE does not usually allow visualization of aorta adjacent to the trachea or the innominate artery and much of the abdominal aorta.

Marfan Syndrome

Definition

Marfan syndrome includes abnormalities of the skeleton, eye, cardiovascular system, pulmonary system, skin, central nervous system, and family history.

Etiology

■ Marfan syndrome is an autosomal-dominant connective tissue disorder.
■ Approximately 25% of cases have no family history.

Key Diagnostic Features

Major Criteria

■ Dilatation of the ascending aorta with or without AR and involving at least the sinuses of Valsalva (Fig. 15-2).

♦ Initially affects most proximal aorta.
♦ In children and adults ≤45 years of age, aorta rarely dilates distal to root.
♦ AR secondary to dilatation of aortic sinotubular ridge.
♦ AR is rare when ascending aorta ≤4.0 cm.
♦ AR is almost always present if ascending aorta >6.0 cm.
■ Dissection of the ascending aorta.
♦ Dissection begins in root and often progresses to iliacs.
♦ Retrograde dissection can involve coronaries and can rupture into pericardium.

Minor Criteria

■ Mitral valve prolapse with or without mitral valve regurgitation.
■ Dilatation of main pulmonary artery in the absence of valvular or peripheral pulmonic stenosis or any other obvious cause in patients younger than 40 years of age.
■ Calcification of the mitral annulus in patients younger than the age of 40 years *or*
■ Dilatation or dissection of the descending thoracic or abdominal aorta in patients younger than the age of 50 years.
■ For the cardiovascular system to be involved, a major criterion or only one of the minor criteria must be present.

TABLE 15-2. *Aortic Root Dimension in Marfan Syndrome and Risk*

Low risk (<4 cm)	Moderate risk (≥4.0 cm)	High risk[a] (>5.0 cm)
Pregnancy not contraindicated.	Pregnancy contraindicated due to risk of aortic dissection or rupture.	Prophylactic surgery generally recommended when aorta ≥5.0–5.5 cm. Some centers recommend surgery at 4.8 cm or if rate of increase in aortic root ≥5 mm in 6 mo. If patient has family history of sudden cardiovascular death, consider surgery before 5.0 cm.

[a]Six-centimeter aorta has >10% chance of rupture in 1 yr.

Pregnancy

Pregnancy is contraindicated if aorta >4 cm due to increased risk of aortic dissection (Table 15-2).

Prognosis

- Life expectancy is primarily determined by cardiovascular involvement, especially the aorta.
- Beta-blockade reduces the progression of aortic root dilatation in some patients.
- Prophylactic aortic root replacement improves prognosis.
- Low risk if aorta <4 cm.
- High risk if aorta >5 cm.

Indicator for Prophylactic Aortic Surgery

- Ascending aorta replacement if diameter >5.0 to 5.5 cm.
  - ◆ Some centers advocate 4.8 cm.
  - ◆ Progression of dilatation >5 mm in 6 months.
  - ◆ Symptomatic AR.
  - ◆ Descending thoracic aorta replacement if diameter >6.0 cm.
- Additional risk factors are associated with increased risk of aortic dissection, including aortic dilatation extending beyond the sinus of Valsalva, a rapid rate of dilatation >2 mm/year or 5%/year, and family history of aortic dissection.

Follow-Up

- Annual TTE to assess aortic root, AR, and mitral regurgitation.
- Perform serial TTE more frequently if the aortic root is dilated, the aorta is enlarging between examinations, or during pregnancy.

Aortic Dissection

Definition

- Aortic dissection is a tear in the aortic intima that results in blood entering the media and dissecting the aortic wall.
- The blood-filled space becomes the false lumen.

Etiology

- Genetic diseases causing cystic medial necrosis, such as Marfan syndrome and Ehlers–Danlos syndrome (type IV).
- Bicuspid aortic valve.
- Systemic hypertension (seen in 80% of cases with dissection).
- Pregnancy, aortic coarctation, aging, direct aortic trauma (e.g., status post–cardiac surgery with cannula insertion into aorta, at sites of aortic transection for valve or root replacement, aortic anastomotic sites for coronary artery bypass grafts), and cocaine use.
- Aortic dissection is a medical emergency; thus, time to treatment is essential.
- Although TTE is useful, TEE is much more sensitive and specific and, therefore, it is the primary imaging modality (Table 15-3) (1–3,7–9).
- TEE, therefore, should not be delayed by TTE by more than a few minutes, if at all.

Classification

DeBakey

- Type I: Involves ascending, arch and descending thoracic aorta (70% of cases).
- Type II: Involves ascending aorta alone (up to arch; 5% of cases).

TABLE 15-3. *Diagnostic Accuracy of Echocardiography for Aortic Dissection[a,b]*

Imaging test	Sensitivity	Specificity
Transthoracic echo-cardiography	59% (37/62)	98% (43/44)
Transesophageal echocardiography	83% (39/48)	98% (25/26)

[a]Standard of reference: surgery (62), autopsy (7), angiography (64).
[b]Highest sensitivity and specificity with experienced operator and multiplane probe.

- Type III: Involves descending thoracic aorta ± abdominal aorta (25% of cases).

Stanford

- A: All dissections involving ascending aorta.
- B: All dissections not involving ascending aorta.

Key Diagnostic Features

Transthoracic Echocardiography

- TTE M-mode and two-dimensional echocardiography (echo) are of diagnostic value in dissection of ascending aorta, but TEE should still be immediately performed (Table 15-4).
- Dilatation of aortic root (>42 mm).
- Aortic valve cusp prolapse and mid-systolic closure of aortic valve.
- Diastolic fluttering of mitral valve and left ventricular volume overload due to AR.
- Demonstration of aortic intimal flap in multiple views as a thin, mobile, linear structure.

- Demonstration of true (perfusing) lumen with systolic expansion and false (nonperfusing) lumen with systolic compression.
- Compression of left atrium by aorta.
- Pericardial effusion with or without tamponade finding.
- Left pleural effusion.
- Left ventricular wall motion abnormalities if it extends to coronary aorta.

Transesophageal Echocardiography

- Dilated aorta.
- Linear, mobile, intimal flap with erratic motion separating the true and false lumen of the aorta (Fig. 15-3).
- Intimal flap is more mobile in systole and diastole if true and false lumen are communicating.
- Expansion of true lumen and compression of false lumen with systole.
- Stasis or thrombus in nonperfusing false lumen is due to reduced flow.
- Intimal tears are predominantly (70%) seen in the ascending aorta; 20% to 25% are seen in the descending aorta.
- Identification of coronary artery involvement (most commonly right coronary artery).
- Identification of AR, aortic valve prolapse, pleural effusion, pericardial effusion or tamponade.
  - ◆ Pericardial effusion found in 33% of type I, 45% of type II, and 6% of type III dissections.
  - ◆ Pericardial effusion is associated with a worse prognosis.
- Detection of site of penetrating aortic ulcer.
- AR is present in 52% of type I, 64% of type II, and 8% of type III dissections.

TABLE 15-4. *Differentiating Perfusing (True) from Nonperfusing (False) Lumen of Aortic Dissection*

Perfusing lumen	Nonperfusing lumen
Smaller	Larger
Systolic expansion	Systolic compression
On inner (anterior) curvature	Diastolic expansion
Spontaneous contrast or thrombus, or both, unusual	On outer (posterior) curvature
Echocardiographic contrast enters this lumen first	Spontaneous contrast or thrombus, or both, frequent
Continuous flow Doppler and pulse Doppler signals easy to obtain	Delayed entrances or no opacification with echocardiographic contrast (depends on communication)
Doppler forward flow during systole	Continuous flow Doppler and pulse Doppler signals often weak or not present
At site of communication, flow from perfusing into nonperfusing lumen detected by continuous flow or pulse Doppler	Doppler flow delayed, absent, or even retrograde

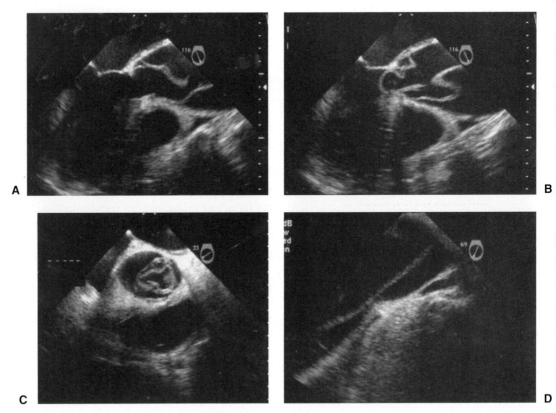

FIG. 15-3. Aortic dissection. Multiplane transesophageal echocardiographic image of ascending aortic dissection in long-axis views **(A,B)** and short-axis view **(C)**. The intimal flaps are mobile and compliant. The dissection extends throughout the entire aortic arch **(D)**.

- Detection of flow in perfusing and nonperfusing lumens.
- Detection by color flow and pulse Doppler of site(s) of communication between true and false lumen (multiple sites in 28% of cases).
  - ◆ Flow is generally bidirectional (75%) at site of communication.
- Detection of dissection entry site.

Pitfalls

Transthoracic Echocardiography

TTE allows limited imaging resolution of aorta.

Transesophageal Echocardiography

- TEE may result in false-positive diagnosis of Stanford type A (DeBakey type II) due to reverberation artifacts in ascending aorta.
  - ◆ Generally, it is due to right pulmonary artery or posterior aortic wall motion.

- ◆ Use M-mode echo to overcome reverberation artifacts usually seen in the ascending aorta.
- ◆ Use of color flow Doppler and echo contrast may eliminate artifact.
- False-negative diagnosis is due to small dissections involving upper ascending aorta or proximal arch due to "TEE blind spot" secondary to air in trachea.
- Normal innominate or azygos vein may be misinterpreted as false lumen or dissection flap. Use saline contrast in arm vein to opacify innominate or azygos vein to differentiate it from a false lumen.
- False-negative may occur in the presence of thrombosed false lumen or immobile intimal flaps. Echo contrast may improve detection of intimal flap, especially when flap is small or nonmobile.
- TEE is limited in assessment of arch vessels (e.g., brachiocephalic, carotid, and subclavian

arteries); however, for acute operation, branch vessel detection generally is not critical.

■ There is a blind spot between the esophagus and left main stem bronchus and the distal ascending aorta.

■ The test is dependent on TEE operator experience, skill, and judgment.

■ Echo contrast is helpful in identifying true and false aortic lumen.

Prognosis

Stanford Type A Dissection (DeBakey Type I and II)

■ If untreated, type A dissection has a 10% to 15% mortality rate in the first 6 hours, 30% to 35% within the first 24 hours, 60% at 72 hours, and 75% to 80% at 3 weeks.

■ Death is due to aortic dissection and rupture (>70% hemopericardium).

■ Presence of pericardial effusion and AR is associated with worse prognosis.

■ Type A dissection (DeBakey types I and II) requires emergency surgery.

Stanford Type B Dissection (DeBakey Type III)

■ If asymptomatic and medically treated, type B has a 15% to 20% mortality over 24 to 36 months.

■ Surgical management is recommended if patient is symptomatic; aorta is >6.0 cm; or if complications of leak are present, such as mediastinal periaortic fluid or hematoma, or pericardial or pleural effusion.

Aortic Intramural Hematoma

Definition

Aortic intramural hematoma is a localized separation of layers of the aortic wall by blood in the absence of an intimal tear or a penetrating ulcer, due to rupture of vasa vasorum of media.

Etiology

■ Etiology of aortic intramural hematoma includes systemic hypertension and blunt trauma.

■ It constitutes 8% to 15% of patients with an acute aortic syndrome.

Key Diagnostic Features

■ Aortic intramural hematoma is most common in the descending thoracic aorta (Fig. 15-4) (1,2,7,10,11).

■ Aortic intramural hematoma is characterized by a ≥7 mm circular/crescentic enlargement of the aortic wall, measuring 1 to 20 cm in length.

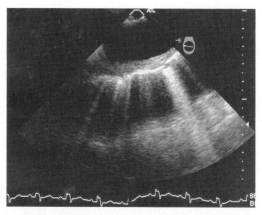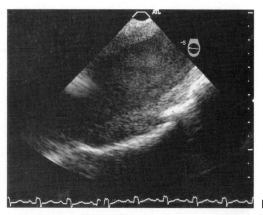

A   B

FIG. 15-4. Aortic intramural hematoma. Transesophageal echocardiographic view of an aortic arch intramural hematoma. **A:** The aortic wall is thickened, and the echodensity is indicative of thrombus. No intimal flap is present, and echocardiographic contrast **(B)** does not show evidence of delayed flow or a false channel.

TABLE 15-5. *Multiplane Transesophageal Echocardiography Sensitivity and Specificity in Acute Aortic Syndromes[a]*

Abnormality	Sensitivity (%)	Specificity (%)
Dissection	98–100	98
Intramural hematoma	90–100	91–99
Traumatic rupture	93–100	98–100

[a]Insufficient data available on penetrating ulcers.

- There is no evidence of an intimal flap or flow by Doppler in the aortic wall.
- Echolucency within the thickened aortic wall suggests thrombus.
- Intimal calcifications are centrally displaced.
- Echocontrast agents do not enter the zone of aortic wall thickening and facilitate identification of aortic internal surface.
- The aorta is dilated, and there are no false lumen.

Diagnostic Accuracy

- TEE has a sensitivity of 90% to 100% and a specificity of 91% to 99% (Tables 15-5 and 15-6). Sensitivity is generally lower than for dissection.
- Serial studies are often helpful in identifying progression to dissection or healing.

Prognosis

- Approximately one-third of patients go on to develop typical dissection.
- Twenty-five percent to 30% of patients progress to aortic rupture.
- Involvement of ascending aorta (as with dissection) has a worse prognosis.
- Emergency surgery, therefore, is recommended for ascending aorta involvement. If there is involvement of the descending thoracic aorta, pursue medical management of blood pressure and beta-blockade and reserve surgery only if ischemic or hemorrhagic complications are present.

Pitfalls

- Aortic wall thickening may be nonspecific and can be seen with atherosclerosis.

TABLE 15-6. *Diagnostic Accuracy of Multiplane Transesophageal Echocardiography (TEE) and Helical Chest Computed Tomography (CT) for the Identification of Traumatic Arterial Injuries in Consecutive Patients Sustaining Severe Blunt Chest Trauma[a]*

Diagnostic accuracy	Multiplane TEE (%)	Helical Chest CT (%)
Sensitivity	93	73
Specificity	100	100
Negative predictive value	99	95
Positive predictive value	100	100

[a]It is important to note that helical chest CT identified all traumatic subadventitial injuries necessitating surgical repair and provided no false-positive result.

- Intramural hematoma and atherosclerosis can have concentric, diffuse thickening.
- Intramural hematoma often coexists with atherosclerotic disease.
- The echo-free zone diagnostic of intramural hematoma is not always readily identified.
- It may be difficult to distinguish aortic intramural hematoma from dissection.

Penetrating Aortic Ulcer

Definition

- Ulcerated atherosclerotic plaque erodes through the intima into the media, creating a localized dissection and hematoma.
- The aortic ulcer communicatoes with the aortic lumen, and the localized dissection is limited by severe calcifications and arteriosclerosis.

Etiology

- There is a high prevalence of systemic hypertension in penetrating aortic ulcer.
- It constitutes 6% to 9% of acute aortic syndrome.

Key Diagnostic Features

- Penetrating aortic ulcer most often involves the descending thoracic aorta (Fig. 15-5) (1,2,7,12,13).
- Ulcer crater, no intimal flap, no false lumen.

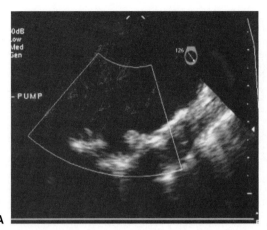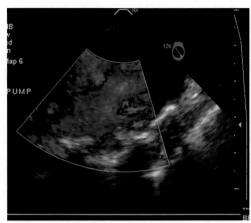

FIG. 15-5. Penetrating atherosclerotic ulcer. **A:** Transesophageal echocardiography demonstrates a penetrating aortic ulcer in the aortic arch. **B:** Color flow mapping reveals flow into the ulcer crater.

- Extensive atherosclerosis and dilated aorta.
- Continuous wave and pulse wave Doppler demonstrate flow into ulcer crater.
- Echo contrast opacifies aortic lumen and ulcer crater.

Pitfalls

- Penetrating aortic ulcer is seen most frequently in the descending aorta, but one needs to meticulously scan the arch, preferably with a TEE multiplane probe, as it is easy to miss an ulcer in the arch.
- Acoustic shadowing from calcium in aortic wall can obscure its detection.

Aortic Rupture

Definition

- Aortic rupture is aortic perforation with partial or complete transection.
- Trauma results in shear injury due to high-speed deceleration, leading to separation of intima and media and entrance of blood through small intimal tear.
- Located in ascending aorta (5%) proximal to origin of subclavian artery.
- Located in descending aorta (95%) just distal to left subclavian artery.
- TEE is the primary diagnostic modality for detection of aortic trauma or rupture (1–3,7,14).

Etiology

- Aortic rupture results from progression of aortic dissection, intramural hematoma, or penetrating ulcer.
- It is also caused by trauma due to motor vehicle accidents or falls (e.g., from a ladder, building, and so forth).
- It is seen in 4.8% of patients presenting to the operating room with blunt thoracic trauma.

Key Diagnostic Features

Aortic Rupture

- Aortic dissection.
- Acute AR.
- Pleural effusion, pericardial effusion ± tamponade.
- Periaortic fluid or hematoma (Fig. 15-6).
- Perforation at site of penetrating atherosclerotic ulcer.
- Color flow Doppler through perforation site.
- Echo contrast enters pleural, pericardial space, or periaortic space.

Aortic Trauma

- Echogenic flap or intraluminal mass distal to the isthmus.
- Flap traversing the lumen within limited region in the aorta.

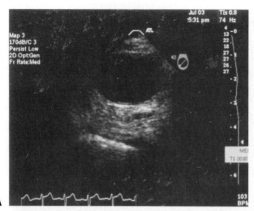 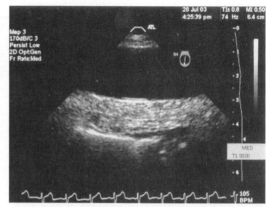

FIG. 15-6. Periaortic hematoma. Transesophageal echocardiography (TEE) shows a large periaortic hematoma in **(A)** short-axis and **(B)** long-axis views of the descending thoracic aorta. TEE was performed in the emergency room to evaluate this severely hypotensive patient who had been in a motor vehicle accident.

- Echogenic mass resembling a thrombus in the aortic arch or near the isthmus.
- Intraluminal or mural echogenic masses, or both (presumably thrombi, often mobile).
- Mediastinal hematoma.
- Increased distance between aorta and transducer.

Diagnostic Accuracy

Sensitivity is 100%, and specificity is 98% for TEE and aortic rupture (Tables 15-5 and 15-6).

Pitfalls

- Large intimal tears in aorta are easy to identify, but small tears can be missed.
- Insensitive to tear or rupture of branch vessels.

Pseudoaneurysm of the Aorta

Native Aorta Pseudoaneurysm

Definition

- Native aorta pseudoaneurysm is a ruptured aorta contained by the adventitia.
- At autopsy, native aorta pseudoaneurysms represent 1% to 8% of all aortic aneurysms.

Etiology

- Native aorta pseudoaneurysms occur post–aortic valve replacement or surgery of ascending aorta.
- Native aorta pseudoaneurysm also results from trauma, infection (tuberculosis), or aortitis (Takayasu).
- Etiology also includes penetrating atherosclerotic ulcers.

Key Diagnostic Features

- Native aorta pseudoaneurysm involves one segment of the wall, resulting in ballooning or outgrounding (Fig. 15-7) (1,2,15).
- Clot is generally detected within "pseudoaneurysm."
- Flow is present in lumen of aorta and within "pseudoaneurysm" with pulse and color Doppler.
- It may mimic abscess, annuloaortic dehiscence (due to endocarditis), and ligamentum arteriosum aneurysm.

Aortic Graft Pseudoaneurysm

Definition

- Aortic graft pseudoaneurysm is a false lumen or cavity due to leaking of blood at the aortic anastomosis site of a vascular graft and the native aorta.
- It is located proximal or distal to vascular graft anastomosis to aorta.
- It occurs at coronary reimplantation sites with Bentall or Ross procedures, or at the implan-

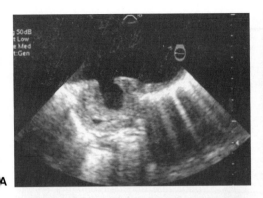
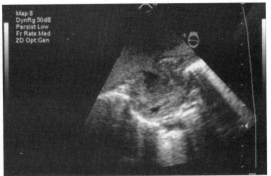
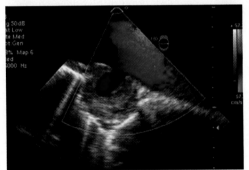
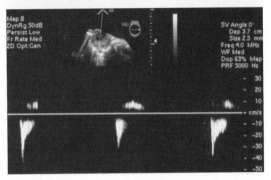

FIG. 15-7. Aortic pseudoaneurysm. Transesophageal echocardiography identifies a narrow-necked pseudoaneurysm proximal to the ligamentum arteriosus. **A:** The pseudoaneurysm contains clot. Echocontrast demonstrates flow into the cavity **(B)** as does color flow **(C)** and pulse wave Doppler **(D)**.

tation site in aorta for saphenous vein or arterial coronary bypass grafts.

Key Diagnostic Features

- Aortic enlargement.
- Echolucent area adjacent to aorta or to aortic graft.
- Flow in pseudoaneurysm by pulse and color flow Doppler.
- Echo contrast agents are useful, as they may opacify false lumen, cavity, or channel.

Pitfalls

- The location of pseudoaneurysm is often difficult to image by TTE.
- TEE imaging is limited to assessing a pseudoaneurysm at the distal ascending aorta.

Aortic Atheromatosis

Definition

- Aortic atheromatosis is a flat or senile, protruding or mobile atheroma in the thoracic aorta.

- It has a prevalence of 20% to 30% in patients with embolic events, compared to 5% to 10% in apparently healthy persons.
- It has a prevalence of 42% to 50% in patients with unexplained stroke.

Etiology

The etiology of aortic atheromatosis is atherosclerosis.

Key Diagnostic Features

Transthoracic Echocardiography

- Parasternal long-axis view, suprasternal view of the aortic arch, and apical two-chamber view of the descending thoracic aorta may demonstrate increased echodensity, brightness, and acoustic shadowing of aortic wall indicative of fibrocalcific plaques (Fig. 15-8) (2,16–18).
- Suprasternal views with harmonic imaging has been reported to be useful in detecting protruding atheromas (18).

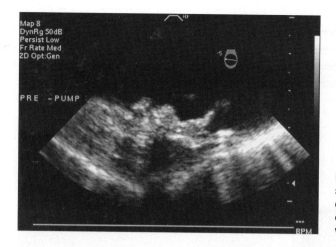

FIG. 15-8. Aortic atheroma. Transesophageal echocardiography reveals complex, protruding aortic arch atheroma more than 6 mm in thickness with a very irregular, jagged surface.

- Increased echodensity and brightness on parasternal long-axis view of aorta at site of sinotubular junction are often associated with severe aortic atherosclerosis.

Transesophageal Echocardiography

- TEE shows increased echodensity and thickening of the intima of the aorta, often associated with irregularity or disruption of the intimal surface.
- Plaque may be sessile, protruding, or mobile.

Morphologic Classification

- Grade I: Minimal intimal thickening.
- Grade II: Extensive intimal thickening.
- Grade III: Sessile atheroma.
- Grade IV: Protruding atheroma (Fig. 15-8).
- Grade V: Mobile atheroma.

Diagnostic Accuracy

- TTE has limited sensitivity and specificity.
- TEE has high sensitivity and specificity.

Prognosis

- Severe aortic atherosclerosis carries a high mortality and morbidity.
- Plaque thickness and morphology are the most important factors for determining embolic risk.
- Plaques <1.0 mm have an odds ratio of 1.0 for emboli.
- Plaques 1.0 to 3.9 mm have an odds ratio of 3.9.
- Plaques ≥4 mm have an odds ratio of 13.8.

- Protruding, pedunculated, mobile, or ulcerated plaque.
- Patients with plaques ≥4 mm have a 12% recurrence of stroke within 1 year.
- Aortic atheromatosis is an important cause of stroke during heart surgery requiring cardiopulmonary bypass, with an approximately 12% incidence of stroke when aortic arch atheromas are seen (six times higher than when not seen).
- If mobile plaques are seen in descending aorta by TEE, up to 40% of patients may have intraoperative cerebrovascular accident.
- Descending thoracic aortic disease is predictive of ascending aortic disease; therefore, if intraoperatively significant plaquing in arch or descending aorta, or both, is seen, epiaortic imaging is suggested to better assess ascending aorta for cross-clamp and cannulation sites.

Sinus of Valsalva Aneurysm

Definition

- Sinus of Valsalva aneurysm is a dilatation of the aortic sinus of Valsalva.
- It may be acquired or congenital and present with or without rupture.

Etiology

- Sinus of Valsalva aneurysm is most commonly congenital; other causes include Marfan syndrome, infective endocarditis, and surgical repair of ventricular septal defect.

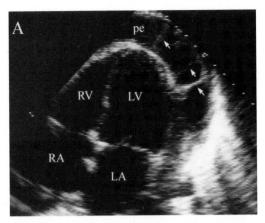 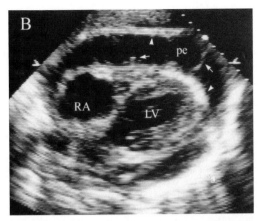

FIG. 16-1. Infectious pericarditis. Transthoracic echocardiographic apical **(A)** and subcostal **(B)** four-chamber views in a patient with infectious pericarditis demonstrate a large pericardial effusion (pe), significant parietal and visceral pericardial thickening (*arrowheads*), and partial and complete fibrous bands extending from the visceral to the parietal pericardium (*arrows*). LA, left atrium; LV, left ventricle; RA, right atrium; RV, right ventricle.

sion is not seen in ≥30% of patients with clinical pericarditis.

- Also, pericardial effusion does not establish the diagnosis of pericarditis. Patients with uremia, nephrosis, malnutrition, and heart failure have small pericardial effusions without pericarditis.
- Loculated pericardial effusions are uncommon in patients with clinical pericarditis.

Pericardial Effusion

- Pericardial effusion is a separation of the visceral and parietal pericardium by fluid (>30 mL) and is associated with a decrease motion of the parietal pericardium.
- *Small pericardial effusion* (<100 mL) is seen only posterior to the left ventricle (LV), distal to the atrioventricular groove, and with <1 cm separation of the pericardial layers.
- *Moderate pericardial effusion* (100–500 mL) is seen when fluid accumulation is circumferential, extends posterior to the left atrium, and the separation of pericardial layers is still <1 cm.
- *Large pericardial effusion* (>500 mL) is seen when there is circumferential fluid accumulation, >1 cm separation of pericardial layers, and anteroposterior or mediolateral heart swinging within the pericardial sac.

- *Loculated effusion* is focal, usually single, of variable size and location, and fluid is surrounded by thickened pericardium. These effusions are common post–cardiac surgery (especially after valve surgery).
- *Intrapericardial strands or fibrous bands* are aggregates of fibrin, thrombus, or rarely tumor and are indicative of inflammation. They extend from the visceral to parietal pericardium as partial or complete band-like structures with linear, undulated, or hypermobile appearance (Fig. 16-1).

Differential Diagnosis of Pericardial Effusion

- *Epicardial fat* has a speckled or granular echoreflectance; is seen anterior, anteroapical, and posterolateral to the right ventricle, rarely posterior to the LV; and is more prevalent in the elderly, obese, diabetic, and women (<1% in those <30 years old, and up to 15% in those >80 years old). Thus, an anterior echo-free space is usually epicardial fat rather than a loculated pericardial effusion.
- *A left pleural effusion* extends behind the descending aorta, in contrast to a posterior pericardial effusion that extends anterior to the descending aorta and posterior to the left atrium.

Pitfalls

- Low sensitivity for detecting pericardial thickening (40–60%) or nodules or masses (<40%) (5).
- Low sensitivity for detection of loculated pericardial effusions in patients after cardiac surgery.
- Unable to accurately differentiate type of pericardial fluid (blood, pus, exudate, or transudate).

CARDIAC TAMPONADE

Definition

- Cardiac tamponade is pericardial effusion leading to an increased intrapericardial pressure (>3 mm Hg);
- Compression and decreased filling of right and left heart chambers;
- Increased and equalization of intrapericardial, right heart, pulmonary artery diastolic, and pulmonary capillary wedge pressures; and
- Decreased cardiac output and blood pressure and increased heart rate and systemic vascular resistance.

Common Etiologies

Etiologies of cardiac tamponade include cancer (breast, lung, melanoma, or lymphoma; 30–60% of cases), uremia (10–15% of cases), acute or chronic idiopathic pericarditis (5–15% of cases), infection (5–10%) of cases, anticoagulation (5–10% of cases), connective tissue diseases (2–6% of cases), and Dressler's or postpericardiotomy syndromes (1–2% of cases) (6).

Pathophysiology

- Normally, with inspiration there is an increase in negative intrathoracic and intrapleural pressures leading to a decrease in intrapericardial (>5 mm Hg) and right heart pressures, resulting in an increased venous return. A simultaneously decreased pressure in the pulmonary veins results in a decreased left heart filling.
- In tamponade and during inspiration, a mild decrease in intrapericardial and right heart pressures results in increased right ventricular filling, leftward septal displacement that limits left ventricular filling, and decreased pressure in the pulmonary veins that further decreases left ventricular filling.
- The end-result is a low cardiac output, low blood pressure, and low pulse volume during inspiration (*pulsus paradoxus*).

Echocardiography

- The onset and severity of echo manifestations in cardiac tamponade vary according to the following:
  - ◆ Rate and severity of fluid accumulation (global or localized).
  - ◆ Patient's intravascular volume status (i.e., low-pressure tamponade in volume depletion).
  - ◆ Associated myocardial disease (i.e., absent chamber compression and pulsus paradoxus if high right ventricular or left ventricular end-diastolic pressure).
  - ◆ Underlying pericardial disease (effusive-constriction if pericardial thickening or fibrosis present).
- Clinically evident cardiac tamponade is highly predictive of echo findings of tamponade. In contrast, in patients without overt clinical cardiac tamponade, echo identifies those with no to mild hemodynamic compromise.
- Patients with loculated pericardial effusions or hematomas have atypical clinical, echo, or hemodynamic findings of tamponade. In these patients, echo has the highest diagnostic value.
- Thus, cardiac tamponade is a clinical syndrome with a spectrum of severity rather than an all or none phenomenon, and an accurate diagnosis requires integration of clinical, echo, and hemodynamic data.

M-Mode and Two-Dimensional Echocardiography

Best Imaging Planes

- M-mode TTE parasternal long-axis or short-axis and subcostal views.
- Two-dimensional (2D) TTE parasternal long-axis and short-axis views, apical and subcostal four-chamber views.

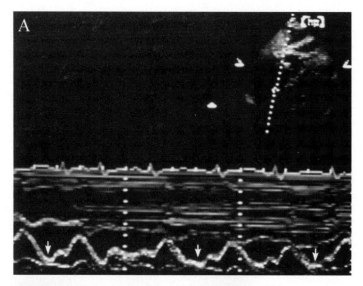

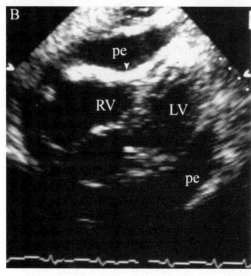

FIG. 16-2. Cardiac tamponade. **A:** M-mode echocardiography of the posterolateral right ventricular wall in a patient with cardiac tamponade demonstrates significant right ventricular diastolic collapse (*arrow*). **B:** The two-dimensional subcostal four-chamber view demonstrates a large pericardial effusion (pe) and significant right ventricular diastolic collapse (*arrowhead*). LV, left ventricle; RV, right ventricle.

- Transesophageal echo (TEE) transgastric short-axis and long-axis and mid-esophageal four-chamber views.

Key Diagnostic Features

- M-mode defines better than 2D echo the presence, timing, and severity of right ventricular diastolic collapse, which occurs during early diastole and resolves in late diastole (Fig. 16-2).
- By M-mode, decreased stroke volume during inspiration results in a decreased mitral valve opening and E-F slope.

- M-mode may also identify pericardial thickening.
- 2D echo defines more accurately than M-mode the size of a pericardial effusion, the diastolic collapse of right and left heart chambers, and the presence and degree of pericardial thickening and adhesions (Table 16-3).
- By 2D echo, a pericardial effusion with filamentous structures or fibrinous strands or bands suggests an inflammatory etiology (infectious, malignant, or hemorrhagic) (Fig. 16-1).
- In patients with blunt or penetrating chest trauma, a pericardial effusion with or without

TABLE 16-3. *Characteristics of Right Heart Diastolic Compression in Cardiac Tamponade*

Right atrium	Right ventricle
Occurs when IPP is ≥4 mm Hg	Occurs when IPP ≥6–8 mm Hg
Most common and earliest finding	Occurs after right atrial compression
High sensitivity but low specificity and positive predictive value	Lower sensitivity than right atrial compression, but higher specificity and positive and negative predictive values
Occurs during late diastole/early systole and is worse during expiration or apnea	Occurs during early diastole; may be transient or last throughout early and mid-diastole and disappear after atrial contraction
Duration of one-third or more of cardiac cycle is a better predictor of tamponade	Degree and duration of right ventricular collapse do not correlate with severity of cardiac tamponade
Best noted on mid-portion of right atrial lateral wall	Best noted on right ventricular anterior and postero-lateral wall and infundibulum
Best seen from apical and subcostal views	Best seen from parasternal long-axis and short-axis views and subcostal view

IPP, intrapericardial pressure.

findings of tamponade is highly predictive of cardiac perforation, coronary artery laceration, or aortic rupture, and it indicates the need for immediate open thoracotomy.

■ In a critically ill patient requiring emergent pericardiocentesis, a small amount of saline contrast injected into the pericardial space is useful to assess the location of the pericardiocentesis needle and to ensure the safety of the procedure (Fig. 16-3).

Pitfalls

■ No single M-mode or 2D echo parameter is pathognomonic of cardiac tamponade.
■ M-mode and 2D echo are less accurate in the diagnosis of atypical forms of tamponade.
■ M-mode and 2D echo have limited sensitivity and specificity in the detection of pericardial thickening.

Pulsed Doppler Echocardiography

Best Imaging Planes

■ TTE apical four-chamber view for assessment of mitral and pulmonary veins inflows.

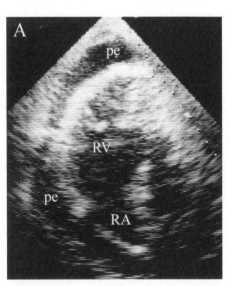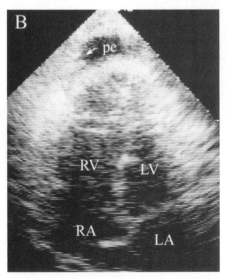

FIG. 16-3. Cardiac tamponade. **A:** Transthoracic echocardiographic apical four-chamber view in a patient with cardiac tamponade and acute decompensation demonstrates a large pericardial effusion (pe) requiring an emergent successful echocardiography-guided pericardiocentesis. **B:** To confirm the intrapericardial location of the puncture needle, a small amount of saline contrast was injected. Note the pericardial space almost completely filled with saline contrast (*arrow*). LA, left atrium; LV, left ventricle; RA, right atrium; RV, right ventricle.

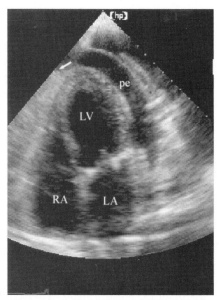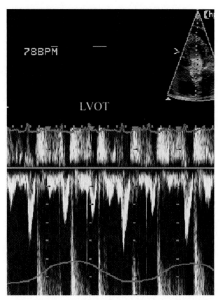

FIG. 16-4. Cardiac tamponade. **A:** Two-dimensional apical four-chamber view demonstrates a large pericardial effusion (pe) with significant fibrinous material (*arrow*) obliterating the pericardial space next to the lateral wall of the right ventricle (RV). **B:** Pulsed Doppler velocities in the left ventricular outflow tract (LVOT) demonstrate significant (>40%) respiratory variability. LA, left atrium; LV, left ventricle; RA, right atrium.

■ TTE apical five-chamber or three-chamber view to assess left ventricular outflow tract flow velocities.

■ TTE subcostal view for assessment of flow in the hepatic veins.

Key Diagnostic Features

Tricuspid and Mitral Inflow Patterns

■ During inspiration, there is an exaggerated increase in the tricuspid early (E) and late (A) inflow velocities from >35% to 80% and >25% to 50%, respectively (normal variability, 10–25%).

■ During inspiration, there is an exaggerated decrease of mitral inflow velocities of 30% to 50% (approximately one-half of the effect on right-sided velocities).

◆ Similar changes occur in the pulmonic and aortic valves (Fig. 16-4).

◆ A decrease in left atrial preload during inspiration leads to a decrease in left atrial to left ventricular pressure gradient and to a prolongation of left ventricular isovolu-

mic relaxation time (time from aortic valve closure to mitral valve opening) of >70% or usually >150 msec (normal ≤110 msec).

◆ Reverse changes occur with expiration.

Hepatic Veins' Flow Patterns

■ Normally and during inspiration, systolic flow velocities are higher than diastolic velocities, and the systolic and diastolic reversal velocities are minimal.

■ In cardiac tamponade, there is a marked predominance of systolic as compared to diastolic velocities and a reduction in the normal increase of flow during inspiration.

■ During expiration and the first cardiac cycle, there is a marked decrease or even reversal of the diastolic flow.

Pitfalls

■ Doppler flow patterns are less accurate in patients with high right ventricular or left ventricular diastolic pressures caused by preexistent pulmonary hypertension, cor pulmonale, or other myocardial or valvular heart disease.

■ Flow patterns in the hepatic veins cannot be assessed in one-third of patients with suspected cardiac tamponade and are less reliable in patients with atrial fibrillation, severe tricuspid regurgitation, and in those on positive-pressure ventilation.

Atypical Cardiac Tamponade

Cardiac Tamponade without Pulsus Paradoxus

■ Cardiac tamponade without right ventricular collapse and pulsus paradoxus occurs in patients with high right ventricular or left ventricular end-diastolic pressure. In these patients, right ventricular to left ventricular interdependence (septal deviation) and variability of stroke volume during inspiration is less accentuated or is absent.

■ Included in this group are patients with positive-pressure ventilation, atrial septal defect, pulmonary hypertension with cor pulmonale, right ventricular myocardial infarction, hypervolemia, left ventricular systolic or diastolic dysfunction, and moderate or severe aortic regurgitation.

Low-Pressure Cardiac Tamponade

Low intravascular volume leading to low end-diastolic pressures can be associated with right atrial, right ventricular, or, rarely, left ventricular diastolic collapse without clinical evidence of tamponade (7).

Acute and Subacute Localized Cardiac Tamponade

■ With acute bleeding into the pericardium (after heart surgery or coronary artery perforation post–percutaneous coronary intervention; right heart perforation after pacemaker, automated implantable cardioverter-defibrillator, or central venous pressure lines; aortic dissection; and blunt or penetrating chest trauma), cardiac tamponade occurs with small or loculated pericardial effusions (8–11).

◆ Post–cardiac surgery, loculated effusions are generally small to moderate in size, appear as an echolucent fluid or a highly reflective and irregular mass (hematoma), and occur commonly anterior and lateral to the right atrium and right ventricular free wall, causing isolated right atrial or right ventricular compression (Fig. 16-5).

◆ Compression of the left atrium or LV are also common in these patients.

■ Risk factors for tamponade in patients post–cardiac surgery include the following:

◆ Anticoagulation (>85% of patients).

◆ Valve replacement (≥40% of patients).

◆ Loculated effusions (≥30% of patients).

◆ Post–cardiotomy syndrome (≥30% of patients).

■ Tamponade occurs more commonly 3 days to 3 months after surgery, but it can occur earlier.

■ Equalization of pressures occur in ≤50% of these patients. Thus, sinus tachycardia, elevated jugular venous pressure, hypotension, and pulsus paradoxus are present in only 50%, 40%, 30%, and 20%, respectively.

Pleural Effusion and Cardiac Tamponade

Rarely, a large pleural effusion (infectious or hemorrhagic) can produce right ventricular or left ventricular diastolic compression and echo and clinical manifestations of tamponade.

Summary

No echo finding is pathognomonic of cardiac tamponade; therefore, its diagnosis requires integration of clinical, echo, and hemodynamic data (Table 16-4).

CONSTRICTIVE PERICARDITIS

Definition

■ Constrictive pericarditis is cardiac compression caused by a thickened, fused, fibrosed, or calcified pericardium, with or without pericardial effusion, resulting in high filling pressures and decreased ventricular filling.

■ Restrained ventricular filling after the first one-third of diastole leads to a rapid and

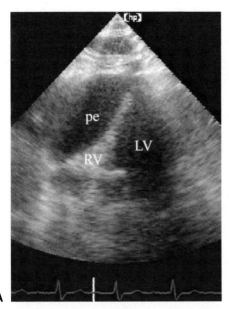
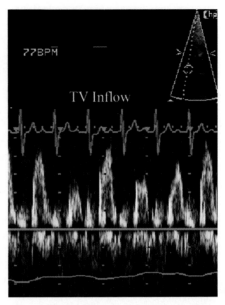

FIG. 16-5. Atypical cardiac tamponade. **A:** A technically difficult subcostal four-chamber two-dimensional echocardiogram in a patient post–cardiac surgery demonstrates a large loculated pericardial effusion (pe) completely obliterating the right ventricle (RV) during diastole. **B:** Note the significant (>50%) respiratory variability of the tricuspid inflow pulsed Doppler velocities (TV Inflow). The patient underwent successful surgical drainage of the effusion. LV, left ventricle.

marked elevation and equalization of ventricular end-diastolic and mean atrial pressures ("square root sign").

■ With the exception of lesser degree of inspiratory increase of flow to the right heart (no decrease in intrapericardial pressure due to fused and fibrosed pericardium), the patho-physiology of constrictive or effusive-constrictive pericarditis is similar to that of cardiac tamponade.

Common Etiologies

■ Constrictive pericarditis is caused by any type of acute pericarditis resulting in pericardial thickening, fibrosis, and calcification (12).
  ◆ In a general population, idiopathic or viral infection are common.
  ◆ In tertiary care centers, malignancy, autoimmunity, and post–cardiotomy syndrome are more common (13).
■ Tuberculosis causes constriction in immuno-compromised patients and in developing countries.
■ Constriction is generally progressive, but it exists in acute, subacute, and chronic forms.
■ Transient constriction (lasting a few days) commonly follows acute pericarditis with or without pericardial effusion.
■ Manifestations of constriction post–cardiac surgery can occur 1 to 5 years later (13).

TABLE 16-4. *Echocardiography Findings in Cardiac Tamponade*

Finding	Frequency (%)
Moderate to large pericardial effusion	≥95
Right atrial diastolic compression	≥90
Right ventricular diastolic compression	≥60
Variable transmitral and tricuspid inflow with respiration	≥75
Plethoric inferior vena cava	≥60
Abnormal hepatic veins' flow pattern	≥60
Abnormal pulmonary veins' flow pattern	≥50
Rarely, left atrial or left ventricular diastolic compression	≤30

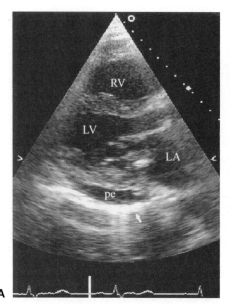 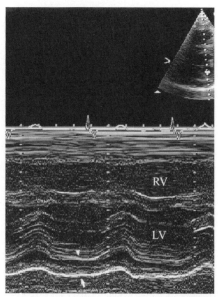

FIG. 16-6. Constrictive pericarditis. **A:** Two-dimensional parasternal long-axis view demonstrates a posterior loculated pericardial effusion (pe) with predominant parietal pericardial thickening (*arrow*). The corresponding M-mode **(B)** demonstrates pericardial thickening (*arrow*), parallel motion of the posterior parietal and visceral pericardium due to adhesions, characteristic posterior wall diastolic flattening (*arrowhead*), abnormal septal motion, and restrained inward motion of the anterior wall of the right ventricle (RV) due to adhesions to the sternum. LA, left atrium; LV, left ventricle.

Echocardiography

M-Mode and Two-Dimensional Echocardiography

Key Diagnostic Features

- Normal pericardial thickness as determined by TEE M-mode is 1.2 ± 0.8 mm (14).
- Pericardial thickening >3 mm or calcification is highly predictive of constrictive pericarditis, but up to 18% of patients with proven constriction have histologically abnormal pericardium with normal thickness (Fig. 16-6) (15).
- Pericardial thickening is more easily seen anterior to the right ventricular free wall and posterior to the LV.
- M-mode detects pericardial thickening and calcification in 50% to 75% of those with surgically proven constriction. TEE is superior to TTE for detection of pericardial thickening.
- Pericardial thickening or calcification can be patchy or diffuse, and its detection is improved in the presence of pericardial fluid.

- Pericardial calcification denotes chronicity and is an independent predictor of perioperative mortality.
- Pericardial adhesions are evident by a decreased or absent sliding motion of the parietal and visceral pericardium, most noticeable in the right ventricular anterior wall. They are best seen anterior and posterolateral to the right ventricular wall from TTE long parasternal and subcostal views, respectively.
- Abrupt flattening of the left ventricular posterior wall at mid-diastole and late diastole due to the sudden interruption of left ventricular filling (Fig. 16-6) and a steep mitral valve E to F slope are characteristic findings.
- Early mitral valve closure due to decreased left ventricular filling and a high left ventricular end-diastolic pressure and premature opening of the pulmonic valve due to a high right ventricular end-diastolic pressure are also common findings.
- Exaggerated septal anterior motion (toward the right ventricle) or early septal diastolic bounce due to higher left ventricular diastolic pressure

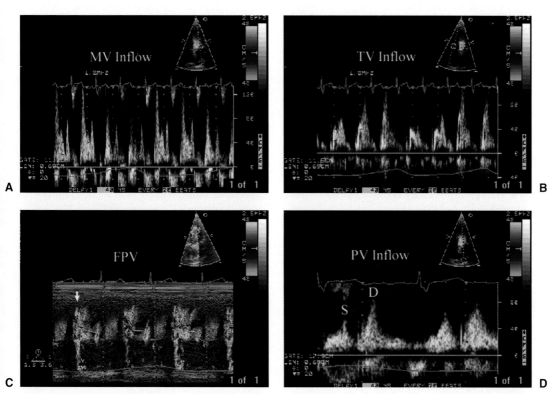

FIG. 16-7. Constrictive pericarditis. Doppler echocardiography in the patient from Figure 16-6 demonstrates hemodynamics consistent with constrictive pericarditis. **A:** Mitral valve inflow (MV Inflow) demonstrates a constrictive pattern, with an early diastolic transmitral velocity (E wave)/atrial filling transmitral velocity (A wave) ratio >1.5, short E acceleration and deceleration times, and significant respiratory variability of E velocities. **B:** Similarly, the tricuspid valve inflow (TV Inflow) demonstrates significant respiratory variability. **C:** Color M-mode flow propagation velocity (FPV) of left ventricular filling demonstrates a velocity of >100 cm/sec (*arrow*). **D:** The pulmonary vein inflow (PV Inflow) demonstrates decreased systolic (S) as compared with diastolic (D) velocities consistent with left atrial hypertension.

during early filling, and atrial systolic notch (transient posterior or toward the LV septal displacement after atrial activation) immediately followed by an early diastolic notch (displacement toward the right ventricle) are also characteristic common findings.

■ Inferior vena cava and hepatic veins' dilatation are additional features.

Pitfalls

■ M-mode or 2D echo manifestations of constriction are multiple but less sensitive and specific than those of cardiac tamponade.

■ 2D echo detects abnormal septal motion associated with constriction with less precision than M-mode echo.

■ The correlation of pericardial thickening with hemodynamic or autopsy evidence of constriction is <40% due to frequent irregular, localized, or patchy pericardial thickening.

■ Thus, no single M-mode or 2D echo finding is pathognomonic of constrictive pericarditis.

Pulsed Doppler Echocardiography: Key Diagnostic Features

■ The *mitral inflow* shows a *constrictive pattern* seen in >90% of patients (Fig. 16-7) (16–19).

◆ During expiration, the E peak velocity is predominant and usually <90 cm/sec, and the E deceleration time is short (<160 msec).

- ◆ The atrial filling transmitral velocity (A wave) peak velocity is one-third to one-half of the early diastolic transmitral velocity (E wave) velocity (<50 cm/sec).
- ◆ The E/A ratio is ≥1.5.
- ◆ The isovolumic relaxation time is short and is usually <80 msec.
- A small proportion of patients (≤10%) show a *restrictive filling pattern*.
  - ◆ E peak velocity is more predominant, and the E deceleration is even shorter (<120 msec).
  - ◆ The A wave velocity is lower (<25% of the E velocity), and the E/A ratio is >2.
  - ◆ Patients with marked left atrial hypertension may have blunted or absent respiratory variation in Doppler mitral E velocity. Head-up tilt or sitting position decreases left ventricular preload and may unmask the characteristic respiratory variation of the mitral E velocity (20).
- The *pulmonary veins' Doppler flow pattern* during expiration is also characteristic (Fig. 16-7).
  - ◆ Low peak systolic velocity (usually <50 cm/sec).
  - ◆ Predominant peak diastolic velocity (<70 cm/sec).
  - ◆ A systolic to diastolic peak velocity ratio of <1.
  - ◆ Low peak atrial reversal velocity of <20 cm/sec.
- Finally, the *hepatic veins' flow* shows a characteristic W pattern.
  - ◆ Decreased systolic and diastolic flow.
  - ◆ Increased corresponding late systolic and diastolic flow reversals.
- Tissue Doppler.
  - ◆ Myocardial velocities at the basal lateral mitral annulus with a sampling gate of 10 mm and a Nyquist limit of 15 to 20 cm/sec; early diastolic (Em) velocities are generally ≥8 cm, and Em acceleration and deceleration rates are ≥1 m/sec^2 (21).
  - ◆ The ratio of mitral inflow (E) over mitral annulus Em is generally >10 and <15 (22).
- Flow propagation velocity.
  - ◆ From the four-chamber or two-chamber TTE or TEE, color M-mode flow propagation of the left ventricular filling with the cursor

aligned within the main direction of the mitral inflow demonstrates velocities generally >80 cm/sec, but velocities ≥100 cm/sec are highly diagnostic (Fig. 16-7) (21).

Effusive-Constrictive Pericarditis: Key Diagnostic Features

- The diagnosis of effusive-constrictive pericarditis is confirmed when, after pericardiocentesis, a decrease in the intrapericardial pressure is associated with a persistently elevated intracardiac pressure (23).
- This is an uncommon clinical syndrome, can be subacute or chronic, and is characterized by the presence of a moderate to large pericardial effusion, pericardial thickening and adhesion, and Doppler echo features suggestive of cardiac tamponade and constriction.
- Causes of this condition are similar to those of cardiac tamponade and constrictive pericarditis.

Pitfalls

- No Doppler echo finding is pathognomonic of constrictive pericarditis.
- In patients with constrictive pericarditis and marked left atrial hypertension, mitral and pulmonary veins' Doppler inflow patterns are less diagnostic.
- Flow patterns of the hepatic veins can be masked by a systolic reversal in patients with significant tricuspid regurgitation or by a limited diastolic flow during sinus tachycardia.
- Echo is less accurate than computed tomography (CT) and magnetic resonance imaging for defining the presence and severity of pericardial thickening.

Summary

No single echo finding is pathognomonic of constrictive pericarditis; therefore, the diagnosis of constrictive pericarditis is based on the integration of all echo abnormalities and complemented by clinical, CT or magnetic resonance imaging, and hemodynamic findings (Table 16-5).

TABLE 16-5. *Echocardiography Findings in Constrictive Pericarditis*

Finding	Frequency (%)
Pericardial thickening	30–40
Pericardial calcification	<10
Pericardial effusion[a]	25–30
Normal or mildly enlarged atria	≥75
Abnormal septal diastolic motion	≥70
Constrictive Doppler pattern of the mitral or tricuspid valve inflow	≥90
Restrictive mitral inflow Doppler pattern	<10
Left atrial hypertension	≥95
Abnormal pulmonary veins' flow Doppler pattern	≥95
Plethoric inferior vena cava	≥70
Abnormal hepatic veins' flow Doppler pattern exacerbated by expiration	≥75

[a]These patients commonly have effusive-constrictive pericarditis.

DIFFERENTIATION OF CONSTRICTIVE PERICARDITIS FROM RESTRICTIVE CARDIOMYOPATHY

■ The clinical and hemodynamic differentiation of constrictive pericarditis from restrictive cardiomyopathy is difficult.

■ Doppler echo plays an important role in their differentiation, but not a single finding is specific enough of each condition.

■ Differentiation of these two conditions requires integration of clinical, hemodynamic, Doppler echo, and CT or magnetic resonance imaging data. In some patients, the diagnosis of constriction is made only after surgery (Table 16-6).

DIAGNOSTIC ACCURACY FOR THE DETECTION OF PERICARDIAL DISEASES

Cardiac Tamponade

■ In patients with clinical cardiac tamponade, right atrial or right ventricular diastolic collapse is seen in ≥90% of patients. In these patients, right atrial collapse is as common as right ventricular diastolic collapse (Table 16-7).

■ In patients without clinical cardiac tamponade, right atrial diastolic collapse is seen in approximately 30% of patients, and right ventricular collapse is seen in 10% of patients.

■ Right atrial diastolic compression has high sensitivity (up to 90%), but low specificity (60–80%) and positive predictive value (50–60%) for cardiac tamponade.

■ Right ventricular diastolic compression has low sensitivity (≥60%), but high specificity (≥90%) and positive and negative predictive value (≅ 80% for both) for cardiac tamponade.

■ In patients with localized tamponade, the sensitivity of right ventricular diastolic compression is low (48–77%).

■ The diagnostic accuracy of 2D echo is higher in patients with large and circumferential pericardial effusions.

■ In patients with clinical cardiac tamponade, the sensitivity and specificity of hepatic veins' flow pattern is 75% and 91%, respectively, but they are lower in those without clinical tamponade.

■ The combination of hepatic veins' flow patterns with right heart chamber compression improves the specificity and positive predictive value of echo for detection of cardiac tamponade.

■ In patients post–cardiac surgery and hemodynamically unstable, echo, especially TEE, is probably more accurate than hemodynamics in defining the presence of global or localized cardiac tamponade.

Constrictive Pericarditis

■ Using a cut-off value of 3 mm pericardial thickness, the sensitivity and specificity of pericardial thickening for detection of constrictive pericarditis are 95% and 86%, respectively.

■ Assessment of pericardial thickening by TEE correlates with CT.

■ From expiration to inspiration, a >30% fall in mitral E velocity, a 20% to 30% fall in systolic and predominantly diastolic peak velocity of the pulmonary veins' flow, a reciprocal >40% increase in the tricuspid E velocity, and a 50% increase of the isovolumic relaxation time have a sensitivity of >85% and a specificity of >90% for constrictive pericarditis.

TABLE 16-6. *Differentiation of Constrictive Pericarditis from Restrictive Cardiomyopathy*

Diagnostic method	Constrictive pericarditis	Restrictive cardiomyopathy
M-mode or 2D	Pericardial thickening >3 mm	Normal pericardium (<2 mm)
	Posterior wall diastolic flattening	Abnormal appearance and increased myocardial thickness
	Normal myocardium	
	Normal left ventricular cavity	Small left ventricular cavity
Doppler	Constrictive mitral inflow pattern (>90%)	Restrictive mitral inflow pattern (>90%)
	>15–30% ↓ mitral E peak and pulmonary vein systolic and diastolic velocities from expiration to inspiration	<15% ↓ mitral E peak and pulmonary vein systolic and diastolic velocities from expiration to inspiration
	Pulmonary veins' systolic/diastolic ratio ≥0.65	Pulmonary veins' systolic/diastolic ratio ≤0.40
	Mitral annulus tissue Doppler velocity ≥8 cm/sec	Mitral annulus tissue Doppler velocity <8 cm/sec
	Em acceleration/deceleration rates >1 m/sec^2	Em acceleration/deceleration rates <1 m/sec^2
	Flow propagation velocity >100 cm/sec	Flow propagation velocity <100 cm/sec
	During expiration, >50% ↑ in hepatic veins' diastolic reversal and ↓ systolic and diastolic forward flow velocities by >25% and >50%, respectively	Predominant forward diastolic hepatic vein flow, ↑ systolic and diastolic reversals during inspiration
	>50% ↑ IVRT from expiration to inspiration	
Hemodynamics	LVEDP-RVEDP ≤5 mm Hg[a]	LVEDP–RVEDP >5 mm Hg
	PASP <55 mm Hg	PASP >55 mm Hg
	RVEDP/RVSP >1/3[b]	RVEDP/RVSP <1/3
	Left ventricular or right ventricular dip and plateau filling	

2D, two-dimensional; IVRT, isovolumic relaxation time; LVEDP, left ventricular end-diastolic pressure; PASP, pulmonary artery systolic pressure; RVEDP, right ventricular end-diastolic pressure; RVSP, right ventricular systolic pressure.

[a]This parameter has a 60% sensitivity and 71% specificity for constrictive pericarditis.
[b]This parameter has a 93% sensitivity and 57% specificity for constrictive pericarditis.

- Other series report that a respiratory variability of the mitral E velocity of >10% and a pulmonary venous peak diastolic velocity of >18% predict constrictive pericarditis with sensitivities of 84% and 79% and specificities of 91% and 91%, respectively (21).
- Lateral mitral annulus velocity >8 cm/sec predicts constriction with a sensitivity of 89% and a specificity of 100% (21).

TABLE 16-7. *Sensitivity, Specificity, and Predictive Value of Right Heart Diastolic Compression for the Detection of Cardiac Tamponade*

Abnormality	Sensitivity (%)	Specificity (%)	PPV (%)	NPV (%)
Right atrial collapse	68	66	52	80
Right ventricular collapse	60	90	77	81
Right atrial and right ventricular collapse	45	92	74	76
Any collapse	90	65	58	92
Abnormal pulmonary veins' flow	75	91	82	88
Abnormal hepatic vein flow and one right-heart chamber collapse	67	91	80	84
Abnormal hepatic vein flow and two right-heart chambers collapse	37	98	90	75

NPV, negative predictive value; PPV, positive predictive value.

- A mitral inflow color M-mode flow propagation velocity of >100 cm/sec predicts constriction with a sensitivity of 74% and a sensitivity of 91% (21).
- During expiration, a decrease in the hepatic veins' diastolic reversal increase of >50% and a decrease in the systolic and diastolic forward flow velocities of >25% and >50%, respectively, have a sensitivity of 68% and a specificity of 100% for constrictive pericarditis.

USE IN THE PREGNANT PATIENT WITH PERICARDIAL DISEASES

- The causes, morbidity, and mortality of pericardial diseases during pregnancy are probably similar to those of a general population.
- The value of echo for detection and management of pericardial diseases in the pregnant patient are also similar to those of a general population.
- Currently available data on the diagnostic and therapeutic role of echo in pregnant patients with pericardial diseases are based on isolated or small series of case reports.
- To prevent radiation exposure to the fetus, echo-guided pericardiocentesis using the apical approach should be the primary choice in the management of pregnant patients with cardiac tamponade.

USE IN THE TREATMENT AND FOLLOW-UP OF PATIENTS WITH PERICARDIAL DISEASES

Pericarditis

- In a patient with clinical pericarditis, the absence of pericardial effusion or thickening may indicate a good prognosis on medical therapy and does not warrant repeat echo after completion of treatment.
- Patients with a pericardial effusion of any size may have a worse clinical course than those without effusion, and this warrants repeat echo after completion of antiinflammatory therapy to assess for resolution or increase of effusion.

Cardiac Tamponade and Echocardiography-Guided Percutaneous Pericardiocentesis

- An echo-guided pericardiocentesis is highly successful (96–99%), safe (0–1.2% of major complications), and spares most patients (>80%) of other interventions (24–26).
- Echo defines accurately the distance the pericardiocentesis needle should traverse the subcutaneous tissue to the parietal pericardium, identifies interposing organs (stomach or liver from the subxiphoid view or lung from the apical approach), defines the desired needle angulation from the puncture site, and localizes the needle's shaft-draining catheter position.
- If the needle or catheter position is uncertain and blood is aspirated, a small amount (2–5 mL) of saline or other contrast agent can be injected through the puncture needle to opacify the pericardial space and accurately identify the position of puncture needle or draining catheter (Fig. 16-3) (27).
- Finally, 2D echo determines if a pericardial effusion was partial or completely drained, if fluid reaccumulates before pulling out a drainage, and defines the need of a pericardial window.
- Patients with echo findings suggestive of tamponade but who are asymptomatic and without physical findings of tamponade can be managed conservatively and have repeat echo at least weekly.
- In patients who have undergone surgical drainage of a pericardial effusion or a pericardiectomy, follow-up Doppler echo defines the success of these procedures.

Constrictive Pericarditis

- No specific echo follow-up guidelines are available for these patients.
- Patients treated medically should have a follow-up study after maximally tolerated therapy to reassess hemodynamics.
- Follow-up echo 4 to 6 weeks after surgery may provide an assessment of the success of pericardiectomy.

REFERENCES

1. Foster E. Pericardial effusion: a continuing drain on our diagnostic acumen. *Am J Med* 2000;109:169–170.
2. Cheitlin MD, Armstrong WF, Aurigemma GP, et al. ACC/AHA/ASE guideline update for the clinical application of echocardiography: summary article. *J Am Coll Cardiol* 2003;42:954–970.
3. Sagrista-Sauleda J, Merce J, Permanyer-Miralda G, et al. Clinical clues to the causes of pericardial effusions. *Am J Med* 2000;109:95–101.
4. Sagrista-Sauleda J, Angel J, Permanyer-Miralda G, et al. Long-term follow-up of idiopathic chronic pericardial effusion. *N Engl J Med* 1999;341:2054–2059.
5. Auer J, Berent R, Eber B. Pitfalls in the diagnosis of pericardial effusion by echocardiography. *Heart* 1999;82:613.
6. Merce J, Sagrista-Sauleda J, Permanyer-Miralda G, et al. Correlation between clinical and Doppler echocardiographic findings in patients with moderate and large pericardial effusion: implications for the diagnosis of cardiac tamponade. *Am Heart J* 1999;138:759–764.
7. Dwivedi SK, Saran R, Narain VS. Left ventricular diastolic collapse in low-pressure cardiac tamponade. *Clin Cardiol* 1998;21:224–226.
8. Steiner MA, Marshall JJ. Coronary sinus compression as a sign of cardiac tamponade. *Cathet Cardiovasc Diagn* 2000;49:455–458.
9. Dardas PS, Tsikaderis DD, Makrigiannakis K, et al. Complete left atrial obliteration due to localized tamponade after coronary artery perforation during PTCA. *Cathet Cardiovasc Diagn* 1998;45:61–63.
10. Chan D. Echocardiography in thoracic trauma. *Emerg Med Clin North Am* 1998;16:191–207.
11. Tsang TS, Freeman WK, Barnes ME, et al. Rescue echocardiographically guided pericardiocentesis for cardiac perforation complicating catheter-based procedures. The Mayo Clinic experience. *J Am Coll Cardiol* 1998;32:1345–1350.
12. Mehta A, Mehta M, Jain A. Constrictive pericarditis. *Clin Cardiol* 1999;22:334–344.
13. Dardas P, Tsikaderis D, Ioannides E, et al. Constrictive pericarditis after coronary artery bypass surgery as a cause of unexplained dyspnea: a report of five cases. *Clin Cardiol* 1998;21:691–694.
14. Ling LH, Oh JK, Tei C, et al. Pericardial thickness measured with transesophageal echocardiography: feasibility and potential clinical usefulness. *J Am Coll Cardiol* 1997;29:1317–1323.
15. Talreja DR, Edwards WD, Danielson GK, et al. Constrictive pericarditis in 26 patients with histologically normal pericardial thickness. *Circulation* 2003;108:1852–1857.
16. McCully RB, Higano ST, Oh JK. Diagnosis of constrictive pericarditis. *Circulation* 1999;99:2476.
17. Henein MY, Rakhit RD, Sheppard MN, et al. Restrictive pericarditis. *Heart* 1999;82:389–392.
18. Mayers RB, Spodick DH. Constrictive pericarditis: clinical and pathophysiologic characteristics. *Am Heart J* 1999;138:219–232.
19. Cheng TO. Doppler features of constrictive pericarditis. *Circulation* 1997;96:3799–3800.
20. Oh JK, Tajik AJ, Appleton CP, et al. Preload reduction to unmask the characteristic Doppler features of constrictive pericarditis. A new observation [see comments]. *Circulation* 1997;95:796–799.
21. Rajagopalan N, Garcia MJ, Rodriguez L, et al. Comparison of new Doppler echocardiographic methods to differentiate constrictive pericardial heart disease and restrictive cardiomyopathy. *Am J Cardiol* 2001;87:86–94.
22. Ha JW, Oh JK, Ling LH, et al. Annulus paradoxus. Transmitral flow velocity to mitral annular velocity is inversely proportional to pulmonary capillary wedge pressure in patients with constrictive pericarditis. *Circulation* 2001;104:976–978.
23. Sagrista-Sauleda J, Angel J, Sanchez A, et al. Effusive-constrictive pericarditis. *N Engl J Med* 2004;350:469–475.
24. Tsang T, Barnes M, Hayes S, et al. Clinical and echocardiographic characteristics of significant pericardial effusions following cardiothoracic surgery and outcomes of echo-guided pericardiocentesis for management. *Chest* 1999;116:322–331.
25. Salem K, Mulji A, Lonn E. Echocardiographically guided pericardiocentesis—the gold standard for the management of pericardial effusion and cardiac tamponade. *Can J Cardiol* 1999;15:1251–1255.
26. Tsang TSM, Freeman WK, Sinak LJ, et al. Echocardiographically guided pericardiocentesis: evolution and state-of-the-art technique. *Mayo Clin Proc* 1998;73:647–652.
27. Muhler EG, Engelhardt W, Von Bernuth G. Pericardial effusions in infants and children: injection of echo contrast medium enhances the safety of echocardiographically-guided pericardiocentesis. *Cardiol Young* 1998;8:506–508.

Subject Index

Page numbers followed by *f* indicate figures; those followed by *t* indicate tables.

A

A wave, 5t, 10
  age-related changes in, 5t, 10
  in cardiac tamponade, 227
  in constrictive pericarditis, 231f, 232
  in diastolic dysfunction, ventricular, 59, 60, 61,
    61f–64f
  in mitral regurgitation, 91, 91f
  ratio to E wave. *See* E/A ratio
  in tissue Doppler, 8, 64, 66
    in dilated cardiomyopathy, 64f, 66f
    in hypertrophic cardiomyopathy, 65f
    normal values for, 8f–9f, 10t, 67t
Abscess in infective endocarditis, 180, 181f
  detection of, 183, 184t
  prognosis in, 186
Acute coronary syndromes, 25–36
  contrast echocardiography in, 27, 28f
  diagnostic and prognostic features in, 27–28
    after treatment, 33–36
  history and physical examination in, 25
  indications for echocardiography in, 26, 26t
  myocardial ischemia and infarction in. *See* Myo-
    cardial ischemia and infarction
Adenosine in stress echocardiography, 36–37, 37t
Age-related changes, 5t
  in mitral inflow patterns, 5t, 8f–9f, 10, 60f
Amyloidosis, 58
Aneurysm
  of aorta, 208–209
    in Valsalva sinus, 218–219, 219f
  and aortic valve perforation in endocarditis, 179f
  of interatrial septum, 22, 200–203, 201f, 202f
  left ventricular, 195f, 198
    post–myocardial infarction, 30, 30f, 198
Angina
  chronic stable, 36–37
  post–myocardial infarction, 28
  unstable, 27, 28f
    diagnostic and prognostic features in, 36, 36t
    indications for echocardiography in, 26
Annulus
  of aortic valve, 4t, 14
  of mitral valve, 4t, 13
    calcification of, 89–90, 101
    systolic descent of, 6, 44
  of pulmonic valve, 5t, 18
  of tricuspid valve, 5t, 17
Antihypertensive drug therapy, 53

Aorta, 14–15, 204–219
  aneurysm of, 208–209
    in Valsalva sinus, 218–219, 219f
  arch of, 4t, 15, 206–207
    aneurysm of, 208, 209
    in ductus arteriosus patency, 169
    intraoperative echocardiography of, 207
  ascending, 14–15, 205–206
    aneurysm of, 208, 209
    intraoperative echocardiography of, 206
  atheroma of. *See* Atheroma, aortic
  coarctation of, 170–172
  color Doppler of. *See* Color Doppler, of aorta
  descending, 4t, 15, 207–208
    aneurysm of, 208, 209
  disorders of, 204–219
    indications for echocardiography in, 205, 206t
    symptoms in, 205
  dissection of, 210–213, 212f
    definition of, 210
    diagnostic accuracy of echocardiography in,
      211, 211t
    differential diagnosis in, 211t
    in Marfan syndrome, 209
  hematoma of, 216, 216f
    intramural, 213f, 213–214, 214t
  M-mode and two-dimensional echocardiography
    of, 14, 205–208
    in coarctation, 170–171, 171f
    in dissection, 211, 212
  in Marfan syndrome, 208, 209f, 209–210
  pseudoaneurysm of, 216–217, 217f
  root of, 4t
    abscess in endocarditis, 180, 181f
    diastolic diameter of, 14
    motion of, 6, 6f, 12f, 15, 42
    sclerosis of, 113
    wall thickness of, 12f, 14, 113
  rupture of, 214t, 215–216
  sinuses of, 4t, 14
    aneurysm in, 218–219, 219f
  trauma of, 213, 214t, 215–216
  tubular, 4t, 15
    in aortic regurgitation, 113
  ulcer of, penetrating, 214–215, 215f
Aortic valve, 4t, 12f, 13–14
  annulus of, 4t, 14
  Aranti nodes on, 20
  bicuspid, 113